FREE Study Skills DVD Offer

Dear Customer,

Thank you for your purchase from Mometrix! We consider it an honor and a privilege that you have purchased our product and we want to ensure your satisfaction.

As a way of showing our appreciation and to help us better serve you, we have developed a Study Skills DVD that we would like to give you for <u>FREE</u>. This DVD covers our *best practices* for getting ready for your exam, from how to use our study materials to how to best prepare for the day of the test.

All that we ask is that you email us with feedback that would describe your experience so far with our product. Good, bad, or indifferent, we want to know what you think!

To get your FREE Study Skills DVD, email <u>freedvd@mometrix.com</u> with *FREE STUDY SKILLS DVD* in the subject line and the following information in the body of the email:

- The name of the product you purchased.
- Your product rating on a scale of 1-5, with 5 being the highest rating.
- Your feedback. It can be long, short, or anything in between. We just want to know your impressions and experience so far with our product. (Good feedback might include how our study material met your needs and ways we might be able to make it even better. You could highlight features that you found helpful or features that you think we should add.)
- Your full name and shipping address where you would like us to send your free DVD.

If you have any questions or concerns, please don't hesitate to contact me directly.

Thanks again!

Sincerely,

Jay Willis
Vice President
<u>jay.willis@mometrix.com</u>
1-800-673-8175

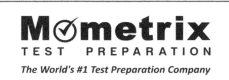

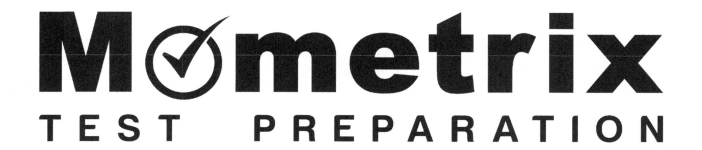

Adult CCRN
Study Guide
2021 and 2022

Adult Critical Care Registered
Nurse Exam Secrets Review Book

Full-Length Practice Test

Detailed Answer
Explanations

4th Edition
Prep

Written and edited by Mometrix Test Prep

Printed in the United States of America

This paper meets the requirements of ANSI/NISO Z39.48-1992 (Permanence of Paper).

Mometrix offers volume discount pricing to institutions. For more information or a price quote, please contact our sales department at sales@mometrix.com or 888-248-1219.

Mometrix Media LLC is not affiliated with or endorsed by any official testing organization. All organizational and test names are trademarks of their respective owners.

Paperback
ISBN 13: 978-1-5167-1816-0
ISBN 10: 1-5167-1816-X

DEAR FUTURE EXAM SUCCESS STORY

First of all, **THANK YOU** for purchasing Mometrix study materials!

Second, congratulations! You are one of the few determined test-takers who are committed to doing whatever it takes to excel on your exam. **You have come to the right place.** We developed these study materials with one goal in mind: to deliver you the information you need in a format that's concise and easy to use.

In addition to optimizing your guide for the content of the test, we've outlined our recommended steps for breaking down the preparation process into small, attainable goals so you can make sure you stay on track.

We've also analyzed the entire test-taking process, identifying the most common pitfalls and showing how you can overcome them and be ready for any curveball the test throws you.

Standardized testing is one of the biggest obstacles on your road to success, which only increases the importance of doing well in the high-pressure, high-stakes environment of test day. Your results on this test could have a significant impact on your future, and this guide provides the information and practical advice to help you achieve your full potential on test day.

Your success is our success

We would love to hear from you! If you would like to share the story of your exam success or if you have any questions or comments in regard to our products, please contact us at **800-673-8175** or **support@mometrix.com**.

Thanks again for your business and we wish you continued success!

Sincerely,
The Mometrix Test Preparation Team

Need more help? Check out our flashcards at:
http://mometrixflashcards.com/CCRN

TABLE OF CONTENTS

Introduction

Thank you for purchasing this resource! You have made the choice to prepare yourself for a test that could have a huge impact on your future, and this guide is designed to help you be fully ready for test day. Obviously, it's important to have a solid understanding of the test material, but you also need to be prepared for the unique environment and stressors of the test, so that you can perform to the best of your abilities.

For this purpose, the first section that appears in this guide is the **Secret Keys**. We've devoted countless hours to meticulously researching what works and what doesn't, and we've boiled down our findings to the five most impactful steps you can take to improve your performance on the test. We start at the beginning with study planning and move through the preparation process, all the way to the testing strategies that will help you get the most out of what you know when you're finally sitting in front of the test.

We recommend that you start preparing for your test as far in advance as possible. However, if you've bought this guide as a last-minute study resource and only have a few days before your test, we recommend that you skip over the first two Secret Keys since they address a long-term study plan.

If you struggle with **test anxiety**, we strongly encourage you to check out our recommendations for how you can overcome it. Test anxiety is a formidable foe, but it can be beaten, and we want to make sure you have the tools you need to defeat it.

Secret Key #1 – Plan Big, Study Small

There's a lot riding on your performance. If you want to ace this test, you're going to need to keep your skills sharp and the material fresh in your mind. You need a plan that lets you review everything you need to know while still fitting in your schedule. We'll break this strategy down into three categories.

Information Organization

Start with the information you already have: the official test outline. From this, you can make a complete list of all the concepts you need to cover before the test. Organize these concepts into groups that can be studied together, and create a list of any related vocabulary you need to learn so you can brush up on any difficult terms. You'll want to keep this vocabulary list handy once you actually start studying since you may need to add to it along the way.

Time Management

Once you have your set of study concepts, decide how to spread them out over the time you have left before the test. Break your study plan into small, clear goals so you have a manageable task for each day and know exactly what you're doing. Then just focus on one small step at a time. When you manage your time this way, you don't need to spend hours at a time studying. Studying a small block of content for a short period each day helps you retain information better and avoid stressing over how much you have left to do. You can relax knowing that you have a plan to cover everything in time. In order for this strategy to be effective though, you have to start studying early and stick to your schedule. Avoid the exhaustion and futility that comes from last-minute cramming!

Study Environment

The environment you study in has a big impact on your learning. Studying in a coffee shop, while probably more enjoyable, is not likely to be as fruitful as studying in a quiet room. It's important to keep distractions to a minimum. You're only planning to study for a short block of time, so make the most of it. Don't pause to check your phone or get up to find a snack. It's also important to **avoid multitasking**. Research has consistently shown that multitasking will make your studying dramatically less effective. Your study area should also be comfortable and well-lit so you don't have the distraction of straining your eyes or sitting on an uncomfortable chair.

The time of day you study is also important. You want to be rested and alert. Don't wait until just before bedtime. Study when you'll be most likely to comprehend and remember. Even better, if you know what time of day your test will be, set that time aside for study. That way your brain will be used to working on that subject at that specific time and you'll have a better chance of recalling information.

Finally, it can be helpful to team up with others who are studying for the same test. Your actual studying should be done in as isolated an environment as possible, but the work of organizing the information and setting up the study plan can be divided up. In between study sessions, you can discuss with your teammates the concepts that you're all studying and quiz each other on the details. Just be sure that your teammates are as serious about the test as you are. If you find that your study time is being replaced with social time, you might need to find a new team.

Secret Key #2 – Make Your Studying Count

You're devoting a lot of time and effort to preparing for this test, so you want to be absolutely certain it will pay off. This means doing more than just reading the content and hoping you can remember it on test day. It's important to make every minute of study count. There are two main areas you can focus on to make your studying count:

Retention

It doesn't matter how much time you study if you can't remember the material. You need to make sure you are retaining the concepts. To check your retention of the information you're learning, try recalling it at later times with minimal prompting. Try carrying around flashcards and glance at one or two from time to time or ask a friend who's also studying for the test to quiz you.

To enhance your retention, look for ways to put the information into practice so that you can apply it rather than simply recalling it. If you're using the information in practical ways, it will be much easier to remember. Similarly, it helps to solidify a concept in your mind if you're not only reading it to yourself but also explaining it to someone else. Ask a friend to let you teach them about a concept you're a little shaky on (or speak aloud to an imaginary audience if necessary). As you try to summarize, define, give examples, and answer your friend's questions, you'll understand the concepts better and they will stay with you longer. Finally, step back for a big picture view and ask yourself how each piece of information fits with the whole subject. When you link the different concepts together and see them working together as a whole, it's easier to remember the individual components.

Finally, practice showing your work on any multi-step problems, even if you're just studying. Writing out each step you take to solve a problem will help solidify the process in your mind, and you'll be more likely to remember it during the test.

Modality

Modality simply refers to the means or method by which you study. Choosing a study modality that fits your own individual learning style is crucial. No two people learn best in exactly the same way, so it's important to know your strengths and use them to your advantage.

For example, if you learn best by visualization, focus on visualizing a concept in your mind and draw an image or a diagram. Try color-coding your notes, illustrating them, or creating symbols that will trigger your mind to recall a learned concept. If you learn best by hearing or discussing information, find a study partner who learns the same way or read aloud to yourself. Think about how to put the information in your own words. Imagine that you are giving a lecture on the topic and record yourself so you can listen to it later.

For any learning style, flashcards can be helpful. Organize the information so you can take advantage of spare moments to review. Underline key words or phrases. Use different colors for different categories. Mnemonic devices (such as creating a short list in which every item starts with the same letter) can also help with retention. Find what works best for you and use it to store the information in your mind most effectively and easily.

Secret Key #3 – Practice the Right Way

Your success on test day depends not only on how many hours you put into preparing, but also on whether you prepared the right way. It's good to check along the way to see if your studying is paying off. One of the most effective ways to do this is by taking practice tests to evaluate your progress. Practice tests are useful because they show exactly where you need to improve. Every time you take a practice test, pay special attention to these three groups of questions:

- The questions you got wrong
- The questions you had to guess on, even if you guessed right
- The questions you found difficult or slow to work through

This will show you exactly what your weak areas are, and where you need to devote more study time. Ask yourself why each of these questions gave you trouble. Was it because you didn't understand the material? Was it because you didn't remember the vocabulary? Do you need more repetitions on this type of question to build speed and confidence? Dig into those questions and figure out how you can strengthen your weak areas as you go back to review the material.

Additionally, many practice tests have a section explaining the answer choices. It can be tempting to read the explanation and think that you now have a good understanding of the concept. However, an explanation likely only covers part of the question's broader context. Even if the explanation makes sense, **go back and investigate** every concept related to the question until you're positive you have a thorough understanding.

As you go along, keep in mind that the practice test is just that: practice. Memorizing these questions and answers will not be very helpful on the actual test because it is unlikely to have any of the same exact questions. If you only know the right answers to the sample questions, you won't be prepared for the real thing. **Study the concepts** until you understand them fully, and then you'll be able to answer any question that shows up on the test.

It's important to wait on the practice tests until you're ready. If you take a test on your first day of study, you may be overwhelmed by the amount of material covered and how much you need to learn. Work up to it gradually.

On test day, you'll need to be prepared for answering questions, managing your time, and using the test-taking strategies you've learned. It's a lot to balance, like a mental marathon that will have a big impact on your future. Like training for a marathon, you'll need to start slowly and work your way up. When test day arrives, you'll be ready.

Start with the strategies you've read in the first two Secret Keys—plan your course and study in the way that works best for you. If you have time, consider using multiple study resources to get different approaches to the same concepts. It can be helpful to see difficult concepts from more than one angle. Then find a good source for practice tests. Many times, the test website will suggest potential study resources or provide sample tests.

Practice Test Strategy

When you're ready to start taking practice tests, follow this strategy:

UNTIMED AND OPEN-BOOK PRACTICE

Take the first test with no time constraints and with your notes and study guide handy. Take your time and focus on applying the strategies you've learned.

TIMED AND OPEN-BOOK PRACTICE

Take the second practice test open-book as well, but set a timer and practice pacing yourself to finish in time.

TIMED AND CLOSED-BOOK PRACTICE

Take any other practice tests as if it were test day. Set a timer and put away your study materials. Sit at a table or desk in a quiet room, imagine yourself at the testing center, and answer questions as quickly and accurately as possible.

Keep repeating timed and closed-book tests on a regular basis until you run out of practice tests or it's time for the actual test. Your mind will be ready for the schedule and stress of test day, and you'll be able to focus on recalling the material you've learned.

Secret Key #4 – Pace Yourself

Once you're fully prepared for the material on the test, your biggest challenge on test day will be managing your time. Just knowing that the clock is ticking can make you panic even if you have plenty of time left. Work on pacing yourself so you can build confidence against the time constraints of the exam. Pacing is a difficult skill to master, especially in a high-pressure environment, so **practice is vital**.

Set time expectations for your pace based on how much time is available. For example, if a section has 60 questions and the time limit is 30 minutes, you know you have to average 30 seconds or less per question in order to answer them all. Although 30 seconds is the hard limit, set 25 seconds per question as your goal, so you reserve extra time to spend on harder questions. When you budget extra time for the harder questions, you no longer have any reason to stress when those questions take longer to answer.

Don't let this time expectation distract you from working through the test at a calm, steady pace, but keep it in mind so you don't spend too much time on any one question. Recognize that taking extra time on one question you don't understand may keep you from answering two that you do understand later in the test. If your time limit for a question is up and you're still not sure of the answer, mark it and move on, and come back to it later if the time and the test format allow. If the testing format doesn't allow you to return to earlier questions, just make an educated guess; then put it out of your mind and move on.

On the easier questions, be careful not to rush. It may seem wise to hurry through them so you have more time for the challenging ones, but it's not worth missing one if you know the concept and just didn't take the time to read the question fully. Work efficiently but make sure you understand the question and have looked at all of the answer choices, since more than one may seem right at first.

Even if you're paying attention to the time, you may find yourself a little behind at some point. You should speed up to get back on track, but do so wisely. Don't panic; just take a few seconds less on each question until you're caught up. Don't guess without thinking, but do look through the answer choices and eliminate any you know are wrong. If you can get down to two choices, it is often worthwhile to guess from those. Once you've chosen an answer, move on and don't dwell on any that you skipped or had to hurry through. If a question was taking too long, chances are it was one of the harder ones, so you weren't as likely to get it right anyway.

On the other hand, if you find yourself getting ahead of schedule, it may be beneficial to slow down a little. The more quickly you work, the more likely you are to make a careless mistake that will affect your score. You've budgeted time for each question, so don't be afraid to spend that time. Practice an efficient but careful pace to get the most out of the time you have.

6

Secret Key #5 – Have a Plan for Guessing

When you're taking the test, you may find yourself stuck on a question. Some of the answer choices seem better than others, but you don't see the one answer choice that is obviously correct. What do you do?

The scenario described above is very common, yet most test takers have not effectively prepared for it. Developing and practicing a plan for guessing may be one of the single most effective uses of your time as you get ready for the exam.

In developing your plan for guessing, there are three questions to address:

- When should you start the guessing process?
- How should you narrow down the choices?
- Which answer should you choose?

When to Start the Guessing Process

Unless your plan for guessing is to select C every time (which, despite its merits, is not what we recommend), you need to leave yourself enough time to apply your answer elimination strategies. Since you have a limited amount of time for each question, that means that if you're going to give yourself the best shot at guessing correctly, you have to decide quickly whether or not you will guess.

Of course, the best-case scenario is that you don't have to guess at all, so first, see if you can answer the question based on your knowledge of the subject and basic reasoning skills. Focus on the key words in the question and try to jog your memory of related topics. Give yourself a chance to bring the knowledge to mind, but once you realize that you don't have (or you can't access) the knowledge you need to answer the question, it's time to start the guessing process.

It's almost always better to start the guessing process too early than too late. It only takes a few seconds to remember something and answer the question from knowledge. Carefully eliminating wrong answer choices takes longer. Plus, going through the process of eliminating answer choices can actually help jog your memory.

Summary: Start the guessing process as soon as you decide that you can't answer the question based on your knowledge.

How to Narrow Down the Choices

The next chapter in this book (**Test-Taking Strategies**) includes a wide range of strategies for how to approach questions and how to look for answer choices to eliminate. You will definitely want to read those carefully, practice them, and figure out which ones work best for you. Here though, we're going to address a mindset rather than a particular strategy.

Your chances of guessing an answer correctly depend on how many options you are choosing from.

How many choices you have	How likely you are to guess correctly
5	20%
4	25%
3	33%
2	50%
1	100%

You can see from this chart just how valuable it is to be able to eliminate incorrect answers and make an educated guess, but there are two things that many test takers do that cause them to miss out on the benefits of guessing:

- Accidentally eliminating the correct answer
- Selecting an answer based on an impression

We'll look at the first one here, and the second one in the next section.

To avoid accidentally eliminating the correct answer, we recommend a thought exercise called **the $5 challenge**. In this challenge, you only eliminate an answer choice from contention if you are willing to bet $5 on it being wrong. Why $5? Five dollars is a small but not insignificant amount of money. It's an amount you could afford to lose but wouldn't want to throw away. And while losing $5 once might not hurt too much, doing it twenty times will set you back $100. In the same way, each small decision you make—eliminating a choice here, guessing on a question there—won't by itself impact your score very much, but when you put them all together, they can make a big difference. By holding each answer choice elimination decision to a higher standard, you can reduce the risk of accidentally eliminating the correct answer.

The $5 challenge can also be applied in a positive sense: If you are willing to bet $5 that an answer choice *is* correct, go ahead and mark it as correct.

Summary: Only eliminate an answer choice if you are willing to bet $5 that it is wrong.

Which Answer to Choose

You're taking the test. You've run into a hard question and decided you'll have to guess. You've eliminated all the answer choices you're willing to bet $5 on. Now you have to pick an answer. Why do we even need to talk about this? Why can't you just pick whichever one you feel like when the time comes?

The answer to these questions is that if you don't come into the test with a plan, you'll rely on your impression to select an answer choice, and if you do that, you risk falling into a trap. The test writers know that everyone who takes their test will be guessing on some of the questions, so they intentionally write wrong answer choices to seem plausible. You still have to pick an answer though, and if the wrong answer choices are designed to look right, how can you ever be sure that you're not falling for their trap? The best solution we've found to this dilemma is to take the decision out of your hands entirely. Here is the process we recommend:

Once you've eliminated any choices that you are confident (willing to bet $5) are wrong, select the first remaining choice as your answer.

Whether you choose to select the first remaining choice, the second, or the last, the important thing is that you use some preselected standard. Using this approach guarantees that you will not be enticed into selecting an answer choice that looks right, because you are not basing your decision on how the answer choices look.

This is not meant to make you question your knowledge. Instead, it is to help you recognize the difference between your knowledge and your impressions. There's a huge difference between thinking an answer is right because of what you know, and thinking an answer is right because it looks or sounds like it should be right.

Summary: To ensure that your selection is appropriately random, make a predetermined selection from among all answer choices you have not eliminated.

Test-Taking Strategies

This section contains a list of test-taking strategies that you may find helpful as you work through the test. By taking what you know and applying logical thought, you can maximize your chances of answering any question correctly!

It is very important to realize that every question is different and every person is different: no single strategy will work on every question, and no single strategy will work for every person. That's why we've included all of them here, so you can try them out and determine which ones work best for different types of questions and which ones work best for you.

Question Strategies

READ CAREFULLY

Read the question and answer choices carefully. Don't miss the question because you misread the terms. You have plenty of time to read each question thoroughly and make sure you understand what is being asked. Yet a happy medium must be attained, so don't waste too much time. You must read carefully, but efficiently.

CONTEXTUAL CLUES

Look for contextual clues. If the question includes a word you are not familiar with, look at the immediate context for some indication of what the word might mean. Contextual clues can often give you all the information you need to decipher the meaning of an unfamiliar word. Even if you can't determine the meaning, you may be able to narrow down the possibilities enough to make a solid guess at the answer to the question.

PREFIXES

If you're having trouble with a word in the question or answer choices, try dissecting it. Take advantage of every clue that the word might include. Prefixes and suffixes can be a huge help. Usually they allow you to determine a basic meaning. Pre- means before, post- means after, pro - is positive, de- is negative. From prefixes and suffixes, you can get an idea of the general meaning of the word and try to put it into context.

HEDGE WORDS

Watch out for critical hedge words, such as *likely, may, can, sometimes, often, almost, mostly, usually, generally, rarely,* and *sometimes*. Question writers insert these hedge phrases to cover every possibility. Often an answer choice will be wrong simply because it leaves no room for exception. Be on guard for answer choices that have definitive words such as *exactly* and *always*.

SWITCHBACK WORDS

Stay alert for *switchbacks*. These are the words and phrases frequently used to alert you to shifts in thought. The most common switchback words are *but, although,* and *however*. Others include *nevertheless, on the other hand, even though, while, in spite of, despite, regardless of*. Switchback words are important to catch because they can change the direction of the question or an answer choice.

10

FACE VALUE

When in doubt, use common sense. Accept the situation in the problem at face value. Don't read too much into it. These problems will not require you to make wild assumptions. If you have to go beyond creativity and warp time or space in order to have an answer choice fit the question, then you should move on and consider the other answer choices. These are normal problems rooted in reality. The applicable relationship or explanation may not be readily apparent, but it is there for you to figure out. Use your common sense to interpret anything that isn't clear.

Answer Choice Strategies

ANSWER SELECTION

The most thorough way to pick an answer choice is to identify and eliminate wrong answers until only one is left, then confirm it is the correct answer. Sometimes an answer choice may immediately seem right, but be careful. The test writers will usually put more than one reasonable answer choice on each question, so take a second to read all of them and make sure that the other choices are not equally obvious. As long as you have time left, it is better to read every answer choice than to pick the first one that looks right without checking the others.

ANSWER CHOICE FAMILIES

An answer choice family consists of two (in rare cases, three) answer choices that are very similar in construction and cannot all be true at the same time. If you see two answer choices that are direct opposites or parallels, one of them is usually the correct answer. For instance, if one answer choice says that quantity x increases and another either says that quantity x decreases (opposite) or says that quantity y increases (parallel), then those answer choices would fall into the same family. An answer choice that doesn't match the construction of the answer choice family is more likely to be incorrect. Most questions will not have answer choice families, but when they do appear, you should be prepared to recognize them.

ELIMINATE ANSWERS

Eliminate answer choices as soon as you realize they are wrong, but make sure you consider all possibilities. If you are eliminating answer choices and realize that the last one you are left with is also wrong, don't panic. Start over and consider each choice again. There may be something you missed the first time that you will realize on the second pass.

AVOID FACT TRAPS

Don't be distracted by an answer choice that is factually true but doesn't answer the question. You are looking for the choice that answers the question. Stay focused on what the question is asking for so you don't accidentally pick an answer that is true but incorrect. Always go back to the question and make sure the answer choice you've selected actually answers the question and is not merely a true statement.

EXTREME STATEMENTS

In general, you should avoid answers that put forth extreme actions as standard practice or proclaim controversial ideas as established fact. An answer choice that states the "process should be used in certain situations, if..." is much more likely to be correct than one that states the "process should be discontinued completely." The first is a calm rational statement and doesn't even make a definitive, uncompromising stance, using a hedge word *if* to provide wiggle room, whereas the second choice is a radical idea and far more extreme.

BENCHMARK

As you read through the answer choices and you come across one that seems to answer the question well, mentally select that answer choice. This is not your final answer, but it's the one that will help you evaluate the other answer choices. The one that you selected is your benchmark or standard for judging each of the other answer choices. Every other answer choice must be compared to your benchmark. That choice is correct until proven otherwise by another answer choice beating it. If you find a better answer, then that one becomes your new benchmark. Once you've decided that no other choice answers the question as well as your benchmark, you have your final answer.

PREDICT THE ANSWER

Before you even start looking at the answer choices, it is often best to try to predict the answer. When you come up with the answer on your own, it is easier to avoid distractions and traps because you will know exactly what to look for. The right answer choice is unlikely to be word-for-word what you came up with, but it should be a close match. Even if you are confident that you have the right answer, you should still take the time to read each option before moving on.

General Strategies

TOUGH QUESTIONS

If you are stumped on a problem or it appears too hard or too difficult, don't waste time. Move on! Remember though, if you can quickly check for obviously incorrect answer choices, your chances of guessing correctly are greatly improved. Before you completely give up, at least try to knock out a couple of possible answers. Eliminate what you can and then guess at the remaining answer choices before moving on.

CHECK YOUR WORK

Since you will probably not know every term listed and the answer to every question, it is important that you get credit for the ones that you do know. Don't miss any questions through careless mistakes. If at all possible, try to take a second to look back over your answer selection and make sure you've selected the correct answer choice and haven't made a costly careless mistake (such as marking an answer choice that you didn't mean to mark). This quick double check should more than pay for itself in caught mistakes for the time it costs.

PACE YOURSELF

It's easy to be overwhelmed when you're looking at a page full of questions; your mind is confused and full of random thoughts, and the clock is ticking down faster than you would like. Calm down and maintain the pace that you have set for yourself. Especially as you get down to the last few minutes of the test, don't let the small numbers on the clock make you panic. As long as you are on track by monitoring your pace, you are guaranteed to have time for each question.

DON'T RUSH

It is very easy to make errors when you are in a hurry. Maintaining a fast pace in answering questions is pointless if it makes you miss questions that you would have gotten right otherwise. Test writers like to include distracting information and wrong answers that seem right. Taking a little extra time to avoid careless mistakes can make all the difference in your test score. Find a pace that allows you to be confident in the answers that you select.

KEEP MOVING

Panicking will not help you pass the test, so do your best to stay calm and keep moving. Taking deep breaths and going through the answer elimination steps you practiced can help to break through a stress barrier and keep your pace.

Final Notes

The combination of a solid foundation of content knowledge and the confidence that comes from practicing your plan for applying that knowledge is the key to maximizing your performance on test day. As your foundation of content knowledge is built up and strengthened, you'll find that the strategies included in this chapter become more and more effective in helping you quickly sift through the distractions and traps of the test to isolate the correct answer.

Now it's time to move on to the test content chapters of this book, but be sure to keep your goal in mind. As you read, think about how you will be able to apply this information on the test. If you've already seen sample questions for the test and you have an idea of the question format and style, try to come up with questions of your own that you can answer based on what you're reading. This will give you valuable practice applying your knowledge in the same ways you can expect to on test day.

Good luck and good studying!

Cardiovascular

Acute Coronary Syndromes

Acute coronary syndrome (ACS) is the impairment of blood flow through the coronary arteries, leading to ischemia of the cardiac muscle. Angina frequently occurs in ACS, manifesting as crushing pain substernally, radiating down the left arm or both arms. However, in females, elderly, and diabetics, symptoms may appear less acute and include nausea, shortness of breath, fatigue, pain/weakness/numbness in arms, or no pain at all (*silent ischemia*). There are multiple classifications of angina:

- **Stable angina:** Exercise-induced, short lived, relieved by rest or nitroglycerin. Other precipitating events include decrease in environmental temperature, heavy eating, strong emotions (such as fright or anger), or exertion, including coitus.
- **Unstable angina** (preinfarction or crescendo angina): A change in the pattern of stable angina, characterized by an increase in pain, not responding to a single nitroglycerin or rest, and persisting for >5 minutes. May cause a change in EKG, or indicate rupture of an atherosclerotic plaque/beginning of thrombus formation. Treat as a medical emergency, indicates impending MI.
- **Variant angina** (Prinzmetal's angina): Results from spasms of the coronary arteries. Associated with or without atherosclerotic plaques, and is often related to smoking, alcohol, or illicit stimulants, but can occur cyclically and at rest. Elevation of ST segments usually occurs with variant angina. Treatment is nitroglycerin or calcium channel blockers.

NSTEMI AND STEMI

Non–ST-segment elevation MI (NSTEMI): ST elevation on the electrocardiogram (ECG) occurs in response to myocardial damage resulting from infarction or severe ischemia. The absence of ST elevation may be diagnosed as unstable angina or NSTEMI, but cardiac enzyme levels increase with NSTEMI, indicating partial blockage of coronary arteries with some damage. Symptoms are consistent with unstable angina, with chest pain or tightness, pain radiating to the neck or arm, dyspnea, anxiety, weakness, dizziness, nausea, vomiting, and "heartburn." Initial treatment may include nitroglycerin, β-blockers, antiplatelet agents, or antithrombotic agents. Ongoing treatment may include β-blockers, aspirin, statins, angiotensin-converting enzyme inhibitors, angiotensin-receptor blockers, and clopidogrel. Percutaneous coronary intervention is not recommended.

ST-segment elevation MI (STEMI): This more severe type of MI involves complete blockage of one or more coronary arteries with myocardial damage, resulting in ST elevation. Symptoms are those of acute MI. As necrosis occurs, Q waves often develop, indicating irreversible myocardial damage, which may result in death, so treatment involves immediate reperfusion before necrosis can occur.

15

Q-WAVE AND NON-Q-WAVE MYOCARDIAL INFARCTIONS

Formerly classified as transmural or non-transmural, myocardial infarctions are now classified as Q-wave or non-Q-wave:

- **Q-Wave:**
  - o Characterized by series of abnormal Q waves (wider and deeper) on ECG, especially in the early AM (related to adrenergic activity).
  - o Infarction is usually prolonged and results in necrosis.
  - o Coronary occlusion is complete in 80-90% of cases.
  - o Q-wave MI is often, but not always, transmural.
  - o Peak CK levels occur in about 27 hours.
- **Non-Q-Wave**
  - o Characterized by changes in ST-T wave with ST depression (usually reversible within a few days).
  - o Usually reperfusion occurs spontaneously, so infarct size is smaller. Contraction necrosis related to reperfusion is common.
  - o Non-Q-wave MI is usually non-transmural.
  - o Coronary occlusion is complete in only 20-30%.
  - o Peak CK levels occur in 12-13 hours.
  - o Reinfarction is common.

MYOCARDIAL INFARCTIONS

LOCATIONS AND TYPES

Myocardial infarctions are classified according to their location and the extent of injury. Transmural myocardial infarction involves the full thickness of the heart muscle, often producing a series of Q waves on ECG. While an MI most frequently damages the left ventricle and the septum, the right ventricle may be damaged as well, depending upon the area of the occlusion:

- **Anterior** (V_2 to V_4): occlusion in the proximal left anterior descending (LAD) or left coronary artery. Reciprocal changes found in leads II, III, aV_F.
- **Lateral** (I, aV_L, V_5, V_6): occlusion of the circumflex coronary artery or branch of left coronary artery. Often causes damage to anterior wall as well; Reciprocal changes found in leads II, III, aV_F.
- **Inferior/diaphragmatic** (II, III, aV_F): occlusion of the right coronary artery and causes conduction malfunctions. Reciprocal changes found in leads I and aV_L.
- **Right ventricular** (V_{4R}, V_{5R}, V_{6R}) occlusion of the proximal section of the right coronary artery and damages the right ventricle and the inferior wall. No reciprocal changes should be noted on an ECG.
- **Posterior** (V_8, V_9): occlusion in the right coronary artery or circumflex artery and may be difficult to diagnose. Reciprocal changes found in V_1-V_4.

CLINICAL MANIFESTATIONS AND DIAGNOSIS

A myocardial infarction (commonly known as a "heart attack") occurs when either an embolus or vasospasm blocks blood flow through the coronary arteries, causing tissue ischemia and eventual necrosis. **Clinical manifestations of myocardial infarction** may vary considerably. More than half of all patients present with acute MIs with no prior history of cardiovascular disease.

Signs/symptoms: Angina with pain in chest that may radiate to neck or arms, palpitations, hypertension or hypotension, dyspnea, pulmonary edema, dependent edema, nausea/vomiting, pallor, skin cold and clammy, diaphoresis, decreased urinary output, neurological/psychological disturbances: anxiety, light-headed, headache, visual abnormalities, slurred speech, and fear.

Diagnosis is based on the following:

- ECG obtained immediately to monitor heart changes over time. Typical changes include T-wave inversion, elevation of ST segment, abnormal Q waves, tachycardia, bradycardia, and dysrhythmias.
- Echocardiogram: decreased ventricular function possible, especially transmural MI.
- Labs:
  - Troponin: Increases within 3-6 hours, peaks 14-20; elevated for up to 1-2 weeks.
  - Creatinine kinase (CK-MB): Increases 4-8 hours and peaks at about 24 hours (earlier with thrombolytic therapy or PTCA).
  - Ischemia Modified albumin (IMA): Increase within minutes, peak 6 hours and return to baseline; verify with other labs.
  - Myoglobin: Increases in 30 minutes-4 hours, peaks 6-7 hours. While an increase is not specific to an MI, a failure to increase can be used to rule out an MI.

Acute Peripheral Vascular Insufficiency

CAROTID ARTERY STENOSIS

The common carotid artery branches from the subclavian artery and then bifurcates into the external carotid and internal carotid arteries. This point of bifurcation is a common site for development of plaques, causing **carotid artery stenosis** that interferes with cranial blood flow. When stenosis develops slowly, collateral vessels may form to aid circulation, but sudden occlusion can cause permanent brain damage and death. Most stenosis is caused by atherosclerosis, with increasing incidence with age. Most ischemia relates to an embolism or thrombus formation.

Symptoms of occlusion are often asymptomatic; however, they include severe pain, anxiety, and those symptoms common to brain attacks (hemiparesis, confusion, aphasia, and diplopia).

Diagnosis: Duplex ultrasound (combining conventional ultrasound with Doppler, determines blood flow and obstruction), CT scan, MRA or angiogram (will indicate degree of blockage).

Treatment may include:

- Medications: anticoagulants and thrombolytics.
- Carotid endarterectomy (recommended if stenosis >60%): poses the danger of a post-procedure stroke due to plaque dislodgement or increased blood flow to narrowed vessels, so the benefits must be carefully weighed.
- Carotid stents/angioplasty (newer non-invasive approaches).

CAROTID ENDARTERECTOMY

A **carotid endarterectomy** involves clamping the carotids and then opening and removing the plaque that is occluding the artery. A shunt may be inserted during the procedure to ensure blood supply to the brain. Postoperative complications may include:

- **Hematoma:** May obstruct respiration; watch closely for increased respiratory effort, swelling near airway.
- **Hypertension:** Especially in the first 48 postoperative hours, may increase risk of neurologic impairment and hematoma.
- **Hypotension:** Usually resolves in 24-48 hours, but may indicate myocardial infarction.
- **Hyperperfusion syndrome:** Caused by inadequate vasoconstriction of vessels dilated from long-term diminished blood flow can cause hemorrhage and edema, *usually identified by severe unilateral headache relieved by raising head.*
- **Hemorrhage:** May be fatal or cause severe impairment.
- **Stroke:** Risk of dislodged plaque forming embolus; frequent neurological checks are crucial.

PERIPHERAL ARTERIAL AND VENOUS INSUFFICIENCY

Characteristics of peripheral arterial and venous insufficiency are listed below:

- **Arterial Insufficiency:**
  - **Pain:** Ranging from intermittent claudication to severe and constant shooting pain.
  - **Pulses:** Weak or absent.
  - **Skin:** Rubor on dependency, but pallor of foot on elevation; pale, shiny, and cool skin with loss of hair on toes and foot. Nails are thick and ridged.
  - **Ulcers:** Painful, deep, circular, often necrotic ulcers on toe tips, toe webs, heels, or other pressure areas.
  - **Edema:** Minimal.
- **Venous Insufficiency:**
  - **Pain:** Aching/cramping.
  - **Pulses:** Strong/present.
  - **Skin:** Brownish discoloration around ankles and anterior tibial area.
  - **Ulcers:** Varying degrees of pain in superficial, irregular ulcers on medial or lateral malleolus and sometimes the anterior tibial area.
  - **Edema:** Moderate to severe.

ACUTE PERIPHERAL VASCULAR INSUFFICIENCY

Acute peripheral arterial insufficiency can occur when sudden occlusion of a blood vessel causes tissue ischemia, ultimately leading to cellular death and necrosis. This can occur as a result of traumatic injury or non-traumatic events such as arterial thrombus or embolism, vasospasm, or severe swelling (compartment syndrome). Risk factors for acute peripheral arterial insufficiency include age, tobacco use, diabetes mellitus, hyperlipidemia and hypertension.

- **Signs and symptoms**: Classic 6 P's: Pain (extreme, unrelieved by narcotics), pallor, pulselessness, poikilothermia (the inability to regulate body temperature; extremity is room temperature), paresthesias, and paralysis (late).
- **Diagnosis**: Ultrasound, angiography, and physical exam. Labs: coagulation studies, CBC, BMP, creatinine phosphokinase.
- **Treatment**: Re-establishment of blood flow to the affected area.

- Arterial thrombus or embolism: mechanical thrombolysis may be performed to remove the clot occluding the vessel.
  - *Trauma*: Surgical repair of the severed/injured vessels. Fasciotomy may be performed in the event of compartment syndrome to relieve pressure.
  - *Other treatment options:* Hyperbaric oxygen therapy, anti-platelet therapy for the prevention of arterial thrombosis and anti-coagulant therapy for the prevention of venous thrombosis.

ACUTE VENOUS THROMBOEMBOLISM

Acute venous thromboembolism (VTE) is a condition that includes both deep vein thrombosis (DVT) and pulmonary emboli (PE). VTE may be precipitated by invasive procedures, lack of mobility, and inflammation, so it is a common complication in critical care units. *Virchow's triad* comprises common risk factors: blood stasis, injury to endothelium, and hypercoagulability. Some patients may be initially asymptomatic, but **symptoms** may include:

- Aching or throbbing pain.
- Positive Homan's sign (pain in calf when foot is dorsiflexed).
- Unilateral erythema and edema.
- Dilation of vessels.
- Cyanosis.

Diagnosis: ultrasound and/or D-dimer test, which test the serum for cross-linked fibrin derivatives. CT scan, pulmonary angiogram, and ventilation-perfusion lung scan may be used to diagnose pulmonary emboli.

Treatment includes:

- Medications: IV heparin, tPA, or other anticoagulation; analgesia for pain.
- Surgical: May have to surgically remove clot if large.
- Bed rest, elevation of affected limb; stockings on ambulation.

Prevention: Use of sequential compression devices (SCDs) or foot pumps, routine anticoagulant use for those at highest risk (Heparin SQ), early and frequent ambulation.

VASCULAR INTERVENTIONS

Vascular interventions are required when a patient has a condition that is decreasing blood flow to the limbs, causing ischemia-related damage. Conditions that require a vascular intervention include acute occlusion (embolus), severe unresponsive vascular disease, ruptured/dissecting aneurysm, damaged vessels, or congenital defect.

- **Bypass grafts:** The MD uses a harvested vein from another part of the body (saphenous usually) or synthetic graft to bypass the occlusion. Because veins have valves, they must be reversed or stripped of valves prior to attachment; however, synthetic grafts have a higher failure rate. A common peripheral bypass is the femoro-popliteal (Fem-pop) bypass, extending from the femoral artery around the blockage to the popliteal artery.
- **Embolectomy:** A catheter is inserted into the blocked artery and threaded through the thrombus. Then a balloon on the tip is inflated, and the physician removes the catheter, removing the clot with it.

- **Aortic Aneurysm Repair:** Intense procedure, requiring an open incision and the patient to be placed on cardiopulmonary bypass. The affected area is resected and replaced with a vascular or Dacron graft.

Nursing considerations: Monitor and control blood pressure carefully to protect patency and integrity of the grafts. Neurologic and renal function should also be carefully monitored, as emboli could block renal or cerebral artery. Frequent neuro, urine output, vascular and dressing checks.

Possible Complications: Pulmonary infection, graft-site infection, renal dysfunction, occlusion, hemorrhage, embolus/thrombus.

PERIPHERAL STENTS

Peripheral vascular stenting may be utilized as an intervention in the treatment of peripheral vascular insufficiency. Often performed in interventional radiology, the interventionalist uses balloon angioplasty to unblock the vessel under fluoroscopic guidance. A small balloon attached to a catheter is inserted into the occluded vessel and inflated to expand the arterial wall and compress the blockage. A small metal tube (stent) is then placed to support the vessel and maintain its patency. Stents are primarily made of stainless steel or a metal alloy. This intervention helps to restore circulation to the affected area and prevent restenosis of the vessel. There are different types of stents available based on the type of vessel affected and the type of lesion. Stenting may be used in both peripheral and coronary arteries.

- **Indications:** Stenting may be the initial choice of intervention in patients with iliac, renal, subclavian or carotid stenosis. Stenting may be indicated in patients with severe claudication, non-healing ulcers of the extremities, ischemic pain with rest and in patients who have a high operative risk. Peripheral stenting often results in shorter hospital stays and shorter recovery times in comparison with surgical intervention.
- **Complications:** Complications that may occur in patients undergoing peripheral stenting include: bleeding, infection, arterial spasm or rupture, dissection of the vessel, restenosis or thrombus formation within the vessel and intravascular fracture of the stent.

FEM-POP BYPASS

Femoropopliteal (Fem-Pop) bypass is used for femoral artery disease in order to bypass an occluded femoral artery above or below the knee. Either a man-made or a vein graft (such as the saphenous vein) is used and is sewn above the blocked area to the femoral artery and below to the popliteal artery, allowing the blood to bypass the occluded area. In addition to the incisions in the affected leg, if a vein graft is obtained from the other leg, the patient may also have a long incision where the vein was removed. Edema in the surgical sites is common and may persist for up to 3 months. Femoral popliteal bypass surgery is indicated for peripheral vascular insufficiency that does not respond to medical treatment, causes severe intermittent claudication and/or ischemic resting pain, and results in gangrene or other non-healing wounds, especially if the limb is at risk for amputation because of impaired oxygenation. The limb(s) must be monitored carefully in the postoperative period for color, sensation, warmth, and ability to move.

Pulmonary Edema, Aortic Aneurysm, and Aortic Rupture

ACUTE CARDIAC-RELATED PULMONARY EDEMA

Acute cardiac-related pulmonary edema occurs when heart failure results in fluid overload, leading to third-spacing of fluid into the interstitial spaces of the lungs. Pulmonary edema may result from MI, chronic HF, volume overload, ischemia, or mitral stenosis.

Symptoms include severe dyspnea, cough with blood-tinged frothy sputum, wheezing/rales/crackles on auscultation, cyanosis, and diaphoresis.

Diagnosis: Auscultation, chest x-ray, and echocardiogram.

Treatment includes:

- Sitting position with 100% oxygen by mask to achieve PO_2 >60%.
- Non-invasive pressure support ventilation (BiPAP) or endotracheal intubation and mechanical ventilation.
- Morphine sulfate 2-8 mg (IV for severe cases), repeated every 2-4 hours as needed – decreases pre-load and anxiety.
- IV diuretics (furosemide ≥40 mg or bumetanide ≥1 mg) to provide venous dilation and diuresis.
- Nitrates as a bolus with an infusion – decrease pre-load.
- Inhaled β-adrenergic agonists or aminophylline for bronchospasm.
- Digoxin IV for tachycardia.
- ACE inhibitors, nitroprusside to reduce afterload.

DISSECTING AORTIC ANEURYSM

A **dissecting aortic aneurysm** occurs when the wall of the aorta is torn and blood flows between the layers of the wall, dilating and weakening it until it risks rupture (which has a 90% mortality). Aortic aneurysms are more than twice as common in males as females, but females have a higher mortality rate, possibly due to increased age at diagnosis.

Abdominal aortic aneurysms (AAA) are usually related to atherosclerosis, but may also result from Marfan syndrome, Ehlers-Danlos disease, and connective tissue disorders. Rupture usually does not allow time for emergent repair, so identifying and correcting before rupture is essential. Different classification systems are used to describe the type and degree of dissection. Common classification:

- **DeBakey classification** uses anatomic location as the focal point:
  - *Type I* begins in the ascending aorta but may spread to include the aortic arch and the descending aorta (60%). This is also considered a proximal lesion or Stanford type A.
  - *Type II* is restricted to the ascending aorta (10-15%). This is also considered a proximal lesion or Stanford type A.
  - *Type III* is restricted to the descending aorta (25-30%). This is considered a distal lesion or Stanford type B.
- Types I and II are thoracic and type III is abdominal.

AORTIC ANEURYSMS

Aortic aneurysms are often asymptomatic, but when symptomatic, patients present with substernal pain, back pain, dyspnea and/or stridor (from pressure on trachea), cough, distention of neck veins, palpable and pulsating abdominal mass, edema of neck and arms.

Diagnosis: X-ray, CT, MRI, Cardiac cath, TEE/transthoracic echocardiogram.

Treatment includes:

- **Anti-hypertensives** to reduce systolic BP, such as β-blockers (esmolol) or Alpha-β-blocker combinations (labetalol) to reduce force of blood as it leaves the ventricle to reduce pressure against aortic wall. IV vasodilators (sodium nitroprusside) may also be needed.
- **Intubation and ventilation** may be required if the patient is hemodynamically unstable.
- **Analgesia/sedation** to control anxiety and pain.
- **Surgical repair:** *Type I and II* are usually repaired surgically because of the danger of rupture and cardiac tamponade. *Type III (abdominal)* is often followed medically and surgery only if the aneurysm is >5.5cm or rapidly expanding. There are two types of surgical repair:
  - *Open:* Patient placed on cardiopulmonary bypass, and through an abdominal incision the damaged portion is removed, and a graft is sutured in place.
  - *Endovascular:* A stent graft is fed through the arteries to line the aorta and exclude the aneurysm.

Complications: Myocardial infarction, renal injury, and GI hemorrhage/ischemic bowel, which may occur up to years after surgery. Endo-leaks can occur with a stent graft, increasing risk of rupture.

AORTIC RUPTURE

Aortic rupture is a catastrophic breakage of the aorta, generally as the result of trauma or rupture of an aortic aneurysm. Aortic rupture (spontaneous) most commonly occurs in the abdominal aorta. The patient typically experiences a severe tearing pain and loses consciousness from hypovolemic shock as the blood pours out of the aorta. Tachycardia occurs and the patient may exhibit cyanosis. An ecchymotic area may appear in the flank area because of retroperitoneal pooling of blood. Diagnostic tests include ultrasound or CT. Survival depends on the size of the tear, the amount of blood loss, and the length of time until surgical repair. About 90% of patients die prior to surgery. An aortic occlusion balloon to stem bleeding may be placed temporarily in order to stabilize the patient. Surgical repair may be via an open procedure of endovascular therapy. Risk factors include male gender, older age, smoking, history of MI, family history of abdominal aortic aneurysm, and peripheral arterial disease, and hypertension.

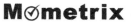

Cardiac Trauma, Cardiogenic Shock, and Cardiac Tamponade

BLUNT CARDIAC TRAUMA AND TRAUMATIC INJURY TO THE GREAT VESSELS

Blunt cardiac trauma most often occurs as the result of motor vehicle accidents, falls, or other blows to the chest. This can result in respiratory distress, rupture of the great vessels, and cardiac tamponade/increasing intrathoracic pressure. The right atrium and right ventricle are the most commonly injured because they are anterior to the rest of the heart. While not definitive, echocardiogram in conjunction with CPK MB levels is useful in predicting complications. Because diagnosis is challenging until complications appear, every patient with suspected blunt chest trauma should receive an ECG upon admission/STAT. If abnormalities are present, continuous monitoring with should be done for 24-48 hours. Decreased cerebral perfusion/anoxia may result in severe agitation with combative behavior.

Traumatic injuries to the great vessels most commonly result from severe decelerating blunt force or penetrating injuries, with aortic trauma the most common. If the aorta is torn, it will result in almost instant death, but in some cases, there is an incomplete laceration to the intimal lining (innermost membrane) of the aorta, causing an aortic hematoma or bulging. This lining, the adventitia, is quite strong and often will contain the rupture long enough to allow surgical repair.

Diagnosis: chest x-ray or CT; transesophageal echocardiogram to verify.

Treatment: STAT surgical repair to avoid eventual rupture, during which other vessels are examined for clotting or internal injuries.

PENETRATING CARDIAC INJURIES

The incidence of **penetrating cardiac injuries** has been on the rise, primarily associated with gunshot injuries and stabbings. The extent of damage caused by a stab wound is often easier to assess than gunshot wounds, which may be multiple and often result in unpredictable and widespread damage not only to the heart but other structures. Mortality rates are very high in the first hour after a penetrating cardiac injury, so it is imperative that the patient be taken immediately to a trauma center rather than attempts made to stabilize the person at the site. NEVER attempt to remove the object in the field/without a physician present. The primary complications:

- **Exsanguination** is frequently related to gunshot wounds, and prognosis is very poor. This may lead to hemothorax and hemorrhagic shock.
- **Cardiac tamponade** is more common with knife wounds, but prognosis is fairly good with surgical repair. Cardiac tamponade often presents with three classic symptoms, known as Beck's triad that should be quickly recognized: muffled heart sounds, low arterial blood pressure, and jugular vein distention.
- **Pneumothorax**: Deviated trachea, increasing SVR, tachypnea and anxiety all may indicate tension pneumothorax, which is a medical emergency. It is treated by emergent insertion of chest tube or needle aspiration of trapped air. Open wounds can be emergently dressed with a three-sided dressing until chest tube can be inserted to create a "flutter valve" effect and allow trapped air to escape.

Nursing Considerations: Management includes controlling bleeding, giving fluids and pressors for blood pressure, preparing patient for surgery, and monitoring for the above-mentioned complications.

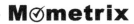

CARDIOGENIC SHOCK

In **cardiogenic shock,** the heart fails to pump enough blood to provide adequate circulation and oxygen to the body. The primary cause of cardiogenic shock is acute myocardial infarction, especially an anterior wall MI. Other causes include papillary muscle/ ventricular septal rupture, pericarditis/myocarditis, prolonged tachyarrhythmia, and hypotensive medications.

Signs/Symptoms: Hypotension, altered mental status secondary to decreased cerebral circulation, oliguria, tachypnea or tachycardia, cool extremities, jugular venous distension and pulmonary edema possible.

Diagnosis: ABGs: metabolic acidosis, hypoxia, hypocapnia; lactic acidosis, BNP, BUN and K ↑; EKG: arrhythmias, specifically SVT/V-tach, Sinus bradycardia, AV block and IVCDs possible; however, may be normal.

- Arterial Line Values: CI <1.8 L/min, PCWP >18 mmHg, SBP <90, MAP <60, Increased CVP and PAP.

Treatment includes:

- Dobutamine IV to increase cardiac contractility.
- Norepinephrine IV if SBP <70.
- Morphine can be given for pain; while potential for hypotension, it will decrease SNS response and decrease HR and MVO_2.
- Treat underlying cause! (e.g., papillary rupture = valve replacement)
- Intra-aortic Balloon Pump (IABP): Increases cardiac blood flow.
- Re-vascularization if secondary to acute MI (CABG or PCI).

CARDIAC TAMPONADE

Cardiac tamponade occurs with pericardial effusion, causing pressure against the heart. It may be a complication of trauma, pericarditis, cardiac surgery, pneumothorax, or heart failure. About 50 mL of fluid normally circulates in the pericardial area to reduce friction, and a sudden increase in this volume or air in the pericardial sac can compress the heart, causing a number of cardiac responses:

- Increased end-diastolic pressure in both ventricles.
- Decrease in venous return.
- Decrease in ventricular filling.

Symptoms may include pressure or pain in the chest, dyspnea, and pulsus paradoxus >10 mmHg. Beck's triad (increased CVP, distended neck veins, muffled heart sounds, and hypotension) is common. A sudden decrease in chest tube drainage can occur as fluid and clots accumulate in the pericardial sac, preventing the blood from filling the ventricles and decreasing cardiac output and perfusion of the body, including the kidneys (resulting in decreased urinary output). X-ray may show change in cardiac silhouette and mediastinal shift (in 20%). Treatment includes pericardiocentesis with large bore needle or surgical repair to control bleeding and relieve cardiac compression. Risk factors include cardiac surgery, cardiac tumors, MI, and chest trauma.

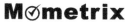

Cardiomyopathies

DILATED CARDIOMYOPATHY

Dilated cardiomyopathy (DCM) occurs when some precipitating factor leads to decreased cardiac perfusion. The resulting ischemic cardiac tissue is replaced with scar tissue, and the healthy cells are forced to over-compensate, causing hypertrophy and over stretching. Eventually, the muscle cells become stretched beyond compensation, and dilated and weak chamber results, unable to properly contract. This causes a decrease in stroke volume and cardiac output, with the end result being enlargement of the mitral and tricuspid valves and severe valve regurgitation. While DCM is the most common form of cardiomyopathy, causes include:

- **Vascular**: Cardiac ischemia, hypertension, atherosclerosis.
- **Metabolic:** Diabetes, uremia, thyrotoxicosis, and acromegaly, muscular dystrophy.
- **Genetics** (familial DCM), and childbirth (peripartum DCM).
- **Viral infections,** particularly adenovirus, Varicella zoster, HIV, and Hepatitis C may cause DCM.
- **Alcohol poisoning or cocaine addiction.**
- **Radiation or heavy metal poisoning**, specifically cobalt.

Signs/Symptoms: Dyspnea, SOB, tachycardia, S3/S4 heart sounds, holosystolic murmur, wheezes/crackles, pleural effusions, edema, JVD, ascites

Diagnosis: EKG (tachycardia/T wave changes), chest X-ray (cardiomegaly), 2D Echocardiogram (valve regurgitation/EF).

Treatment includes:

- Treat underlying cause if possible; supportive care.
- Heart transplant if candidate: damage is permanent.

HYPERTROPHIC CARDIOMYOPATHY

Hypertrophic cardiomyopathy (HCM) is a genetic disorder that causes idiopathic thickening of the heart muscle, primarily involving the ventricular septum and portions of the left ventricle. Patients with HCM produce abnormal sarcomeres and misalignment of muscle cells (myocardial disarray). Basically, HCM is characterized by ventricular hypertrophy, an asymmetrical septum, forceful systole, cardiac dysrhythmias, and myocardial disarray. Because the abnormal cells develop over time, it is common for HCM to remain undiagnosed until middle or late adulthood.

Signs/Symptoms: Exertional or atypical chest pain, dyspnea at rest, syncope, frequent palpitations (common due to reoccurring dysrhythmias).

Diagnosis: 2D echo (structure and EF), EKG (pathological Q waves and dysrhythmias), Xray (cardiomegaly), Family history (especially cardiac death, reoccurring dysrhythmias, or myocardial hypertrophy).

Treatment includes:

- **Surgery:** Septal myectomy is gold standard: high mortality (3-10%), but increases cardiac output and quality of life.
- **Alcohol-based septal ablation:** Ethanol 100% injected into a branch of the LAD, creating a controlled area of infarction and consequential thinning the septum.

25

RESTRICTIVE CARDIOMYOPATHY

Restrictive cardiomyopathy (RCM) occurs when the ventricles become stiff and noncompliant, resulting in decreased end-diastolic cardiac refill volume. The ventricular stiffening is caused by the infiltration of fibroelastic tissue into the cardiac muscle (such as in amyloidosis or sarcoidosis). Atrial enlargement can be seen in most cases of RCM as a result of the increased effort required to push blood from the atria into the ventricles. It is not uncommon for a patient to be in atrial fibrillation secondary to atrial enlargement. In advanced cases, ventricular dysrhythmias may also be seen.

Signs/Symptoms: Exercise intolerance/fatigue, edema, crackles, elevated CVP, S3/S4, murmur, SOB at rest.

Diagnosis: 2D echo (enlarged atria, decreased compliance of ventricle), hemodynamic monitoring (increased right atrial pressure and pulmonary wedge pressure, and SVR), X-Ray (cardiomegaly), EKG (atrial fibrillation), endomyocardial biopsy (to differentiate from constrictive pericarditis).

Treatment includes:

- **Medications**: β-blockers increase ventricular filling; antiarrhythmics may be ordered.
- **Surgical**: Heart transplant, if candidate.

Dysrhythmias

FIRST-DEGREE AV BLOCK

First-degree AV block occurs when the atrial impulses are conducted through the AV node to the ventricles at a rate that is slower than normal. While the P and QRS are usually normal, the PR interval is >0.20 seconds, and the P:QRS ratio is 1:1. A narrow QRS complex indicates a conduction abnormality only in the AV node, but a widened QRS indicates associated damage to the bundle branches as well. *Chronic* first-degree block may be caused by fibrosis/sclerosis of the conduction system related to coronary artery disease, valvular disease, cardiac myopathies and carries little morbidity, thus is often left untreated. *Acute* first-degree block, on the other hand, is of much more concern and may be related to digoxin toxicity, β-blockers, amiodarone, myocardial infarction, hyperkalemia, or edema related to valvular surgery.

Treatment: involves eliminating cause if possible, such as changing medications. Atropine 0.5-1.0 mg may be given IV if rate falls.

SECOND-DEGREE AV BLOCK

Second-degree AV block occurs when some of the atrial beats are blocked. Second-degree AV block is further subdivided according to the patterns of block.

TYPE I

Mobitz type I block (Wenckebach) occurs when each atrial impulse in a group of beats is conducted at a lengthened interval until one fails to conduct (the PR interval progressively increases), so there are more P waves than QRS complexes, but the QRS complex is usually of normal shape and duration. The sinus node functions at a regular rate, so the P-P interval is regular, but the R-R interval usually shortens with each impulse. The P:QRS ratio varies, such as 3:2, 4:3, 5:4. This type of block by itself usually does not cause significant morbidity unless associated with an inferior wall myocardial infarction.

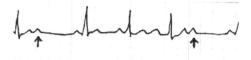

TYPE II AND 2:1 BLOCK

In second-degree AV block, **Mobitz type II,** only some of the atrial impulses are conducted unpredictably through the AV node to the ventricles, and the block always occurs below the AV node in the bundle of His, the bundle branches, or the Purkinje fibers. The PR intervals are the same if impulses are conducted, and QRS complex is usually widened. The P: QRS ratio varies 2:1, 3:1, and 4:1. Type II block is more dangerous than Type I because it may progress to complete AV block and may produce Stokes-Adams syncope. Additionally, if the block is at the Purkinje fibers, there is no escape impulse. Usually a transcutaneous cardiac pacemaker and defibrillator should be at bedside. **Symptoms** may include chest pain if the heart block is precipitated by myocarditis or myocardial ischemia.

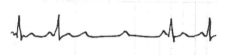

THIRD-DEGREE

With **third-degree AV block,** there are more P waves than QRS complexes, with no clear relationship between them. The atrial rate is 2-3 times the pulse rate, so the PR interval is irregular. If the SA node malfunctions, the AV node fires at a lower rate, and if the AV node malfunctions, the pacemaker site in the ventricles takes over at a bradycardic rate; thus, with complete AV block, the heart still contracts, but often ineffectually. With this type of block, the atrial P (sinus rhythm or atrial fibrillation) and the ventricular QRS (ventricular escape rhythm) are stimulated by different impulses, so there is AV dissociation. The heart may compensate at rest but can't keep pace with exertion. The resultant bradycardia may cause congestive heart failure, fainting, or even sudden death, and usually conduction abnormalities slowly worsen. **Symptoms** include dyspnea, chest pain, and hypotension, which are treated with IV atropine. Transcutaneous pacing may be needed. Complete persistent AV block normally requires implanted pacemakers, usually dual chamber.

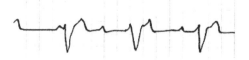

BUNDLE BRANCH BLOCKS

A **right bundle branch block** (RBBB) occurs when conduction is blocked in the right bundle branch that carries impulses from the Bundle of His to the ventricles. The impulse travels through the myocardium, but this causes a slight delay in contraction of the right ventricle. RBBB is characterized by normal P waves, but the QRS complex is widened and notched (rabbit-eared). PR interval is normal or prolonged, and the QRS interval is > 0.12 seconds. P: QRS ratio remains 1:1 with regular rhythms.

27

A **left bundle branch block** (LBBB) is characterized by normal P waves, but the QRS complex may be widened and notched (M-shaped) with interval of >0.12 seconds. The PR interval may be normal or prolonged. The P:QRS ratio is 1:1 and rhythm is regular.

In Lead I:

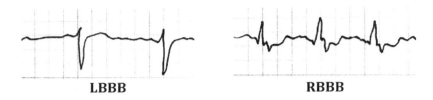

LBBB   RBBB

SINUS BRADYCARDIA

There are 3 primary types of **sinus node dysrhythmias**: sinus bradycardia, sinus tachycardia, and sinus arrhythmia. **Sinus bradycardia (SB)** is caused by a decreased rate of impulse from sinus node. The pulse and ECG usually appear normal except for a slower rate. SB is characterized by a regular pulse <50 to 60 bpm with P waves in front of QRS, which are usually normal in shape and duration. PR interval is 0.12 to 0.20 seconds, QRS interval 0.04 to 0.11 seconds, and P:QRS ratio of 1:1. SB may be caused by several factors:

- May be normal in athletes and older adults; generally not treated unless symptomatic.
- Conditions that lower the body's metabolic needs, such as hypothermia or sleep.
- Hypotension and decrease in oxygenation.
- Medications such as calcium channel blockers and β-blockers.
- Vagal stimulation that may result from vomiting, suctioning, defecating, or certain medical procedures (carotid stent placement, etc.).
- ↑Intracranial pressure.
- Myocardial infarction.

Treatment: involves eliminating cause if possible, such as changing medications. Atropine 0.5-1.0 mg may be given IV to block vagal stimulation or increase rate if symptomatic.

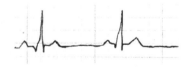

SINUS TACHYCARDIA

Sinus tachycardia (ST) occurs when the sinus node impulse increases in frequency. ST is characterized by a regular pulse >100 with P waves before QRS but sometimes part of the preceding T wave. QRS is usually of normal shape and duration (0.04 to 0.11 seconds) but may have consistent irregularity. PR interval is 0.12-0.20 seconds and P: QRS ratio of 1:1. The rapid pulse decreases diastolic filling time and causes reduced cardiac output with resultant hypotension. Acute pulmonary edema may result from the decreased ventricular filling if untreated. ST may be **caused** by a number of factors:

- Acute blood loss, shock, hypovolemia, anemia.
- Sinus arrhythmia, hypovolemic heart failure.
- Hypermetabolic conditions, fever, infection.

- Exertion/exercise, anxiety, stress.
- Medications, such as sympathomimetic drugs.

Treatment: eliminating precipitating factors, calcium channel blockers and β-blockers to reduce heart rate.

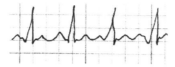

SUPRAVENTRICULAR TACHYCARDIA

Supraventricular tachycardia (SVT) (>100 BPM) may have a sudden onset and result in congestive heart failure. Rate may increase to 200 to 300 BMP, which will significantly decrease cardiac output due to decreased filling time. SVT originates in the atria rather than the ventricles, but is controlled by the tissue in the area of the AV node rather than the SA node. Rhythm is usually rapid but regular. The P wave is present but may not be clearly defined as it may be obscured by the preceding T wave, and the QRS complex appears normal. The PR interval is 0.12 to 0.20 seconds and QRS interval 0.04 to 0.11 seconds with P: QRS ratio of 1:1. SVT may be episodic with periods of normal heart rate and rhythm between episodes of SVT, so it is often referred to as paroxysmal SVT (PSVT).

Treatment: Adenosine, digoxin (Lanoxin®), Verapamil (Calan®, Verelan®), vagal maneuvers, cardioversion.

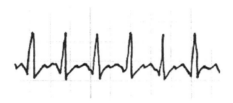

SINUS ARRHYTHMIA

Sinus arrhythmia (SA) results from irregular impulses from the sinus node, often paradoxical (increasing with inspiration and decreasing with expiration) because of stimulation of the vagal nerve during inspiration and rarely causes a negative hemodynamic effect. These cyclic changes in the pulse during respiration are quite common in both children and young adults and often lesson with age but may persist in some adults. Sinus arrhythmia can, in some cases, relate to heart or valvular disease and may be increased with vagal stimulation for suctioning, vomiting, or defecating. Characteristics of SA include a regular pulse 50-100 BPM, P waves in front of QRS with duration (0.4 to 0.11 seconds) and shape of QRS usually normal, PR interval of 0.12 to 0.20 seconds, and P: QRS ratio of 1:1.

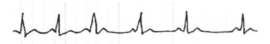

Treatment is usually not necessary unless it is associated with bradycardia.

PREMATURE ATRIAL CONTRACTIONS

There are 3 primary types of **atrial dysrhythmias**, including premature atrial contractions, atrial flutter, and atrial fibrillation. **Premature atrial contraction (PAC)** is essentially an extra beat

29

precipitated by an electrical impulse to the atrium before the sinus node impulse. The extra beat may be caused by alcohol, caffeine, nicotine, hypervolemia, hypokalemia, hypermetabolic conditions, atrial ischemia or infarction. Characteristics include an irregular pulse because of extra P waves, shape and duration of QRS is usually normal (0.04 to 0.11 seconds) but may be abnormal, PR interval remains between 0.12 to 0.20, and P: QRS ratio is 1:1. Rhythm is irregular with varying P-P and R-R intervals. PACs can occur in an essentially healthy heart and are not usually cause for concern unless they are frequent (>6 hr) and cause severe palpitations. In that case, atrial fibrillation should be suspected.

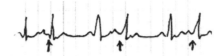

ATRIAL FLUTTER

Atrial flutter (AF) occurs when the atrial rate is faster, usually 250-400 beats per minute, than the AV node conduction rate so not all of the beats are conducted into the ventricles. The beats are effectively blocked at the AV node, preventing ventricular fibrillation although some extra ventricular impulses may pass though. AF is caused by the same conditions that cause A-fib: coronary artery disease, valvular disease, pulmonary disease, heavy alcohol ingestion, and cardiac surgery. AF is characterized by atrial rates of 250-400 with ventricular rates of 75-150, with ventricular rate usually being regular. P waves are saw-toothed (referred to as F waves), QRS shape and duration (0.4 to 0.11 seconds) are usually normal, PR interval may be hard to calculate because of F waves, and the P:QRS ratio is 2-4:1. Symptoms include chest pain, dyspnea, and hypotension.

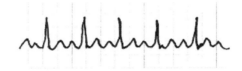

Treatment includes:

- Emergent cardioversion if condition is unstable.
- Medications to slow ventricular rate and conduction through AV node: non-dihydropyridine calcium channel blockers (Cardizem®, Calan®) and beta blockers.
- Medications to convert to sinus rhythm: Corvert®, Tikosyn, Amiodarone; also used in practice: Cardioquin®, Norpace®, Cordarone®.

ATRIAL FIBRILLATION

Atrial fibrillation (A-fib) is rapid, disorganized atrial beats that are ineffective in emptying the atria, so that blood pools in the chambers. This can lead to thrombus formation and emboli. The ventricular rate increases with a decreased stroke volume, and cardiac output decreases with increased myocardial ischemia, resulting in palpitations and fatigue. A-fib is caused by coronary artery disease, valvular disease, pulmonary disease, heavy alcohol ingestion, infection, and cardiac surgery; however, it can also be idiopathic. A-fib is characterized by very irregular pulse with atrial rate of 300-600 and ventricular rate of 120-200, shape and duration (0.4 to 0.11 seconds) of QRS is usually normal. Fibrillatory (F) waves are seen instead of P waves. The PR interval cannot be measured and the P: QRS ratio is highly variable.

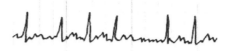

Treatment is the same as atrial flutter.

PREMATURE JUNCTIONAL CONTRACTIONS

The area around the AV node is the junction, and dysrhythmias that arise from that area are called junctional dysrhythmias. **Premature junctional contractions** (PJCs) occur when a premature impulse starts at the AV node before the next normal sinus impulse reaches the AV node. PJCs are similar to premature atrial contractions (PACs) and generally require no treatment although they may be an indication of digoxin toxicity. The ECG may appear basically normal with an early QRS complex that is normal in shape and duration (0.4 to 0.11 seconds). The P wave may be absent, precede, be part of, or follow the QRS with a PR interval of 0.12 seconds. The P: QRS ratio may vary from <1:1 to 1:1 (with inverted P wave). The underlying rhythm is usually regular at a heart rate of 60 to 100. Significant symptoms related to premature junctional contractions are rare.

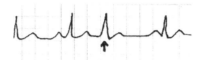

JUNCTIONAL RHYTHMS

Junctional rhythms occur when the AV node becomes the pacemaker of the heart. This can happen because the sinus node is depressed from increased vagal tone or a block at the AV node prevents sinus node impulses from being transmitted. While the sinus node normally sends impulses 60-100 beats per minute, the AV node junction usually sends impulses at 40-60 beats per minute. The QRS complex is of usual shape and duration (0.4 to 0.11 seconds). The P wave may be inverted and may be absent, hidden or after the QRS. If the P wave precedes the QRS, the PR interval is <0.12 seconds. The P:QRS ratio is <1:1 or 1:1. The junctional escape rhythm is a protective mechanism preventing asystole with failure of the sinus node. An **accelerated junctional rhythm** is similar, but the heart rate is 60 to 100. **Junctional tachycardia** occurs with heart rate of >100.

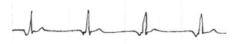

AV NODAL REENTRY TACHYCARDIA

AV nodal reentry tachycardia occurs when an impulse conducts to the area of the AV node, and is then sent in a rapidly repeating cycle back to the same area and to the ventricles, resulting in a fast ventricular rate. The onset and cessation are usually rapid. AV nodal reentry tachycardia (also known as paroxysmal atrial tachycardia or supraventricular tachycardia if no P waves) is characterized by atrial rate of 150-250 with ventricular rate of 75-250, P wave that is difficult to see or absent, QRS complex that is usually normal and a PR interval of <0.12 if a P wave is present. The P: QRS ratio is 1-2:1. Precipitating factors include nicotine, caffeine, hypoxemia, anxiety, underlying coronary artery disease and cardiomyopathy. Cardiac output may be decreased with a rapid heart rate, causing dyspnea, chest pain, and hypotension.

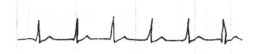

Treatment includes:

- Vagal maneuvers (carotid sinus massage, gag reflex, holding breath/bearing down).
- Medications (adenosine, verapamil, or diltiazem).
- Cardioversion if other methods unsuccessful.

PREMATURE VENTRICULAR CONTRACTIONS

Premature ventricular contractions (PVCs) are those in which the impulse begins in the ventricles and conducts through them prior to the next sinus impulse. The ectopic QRS complexes may vary in shape, depending upon whether there is one site (unifocal) or more (multifocal) that stimulates the ectopic beats. PVCs usually cause no morbidity unless there is underlying cardiac disease or an acute MI. PVCs are characterized by an irregular heartbeat, QRS that is ≥0.12 seconds and oddly shaped. PVCs are often not treated in otherwise healthy people. PVCs may be precipitated by electrolyte imbalances, caffeine, nicotine, or alcohol. Because PVCs may occur with any supraventricular dysrhythmia, the underlying rhythm must be noted as well as the PVCs. If there are more than six PVCs in an hour, that is a risk factor for developing ventricular tachycardia.

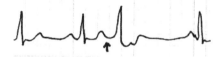

Treatment: Lidocaine (affects the ventricles, may cause CNS toxicity with nausea and vomiting), Procainamide (affects the atria and ventricles and may cause decreased BP and widening of QRS and QT); treat underlying cause.

VENTRICULAR TACHYCARDIA

Ventricular tachycardia (VT) is greater than 3 PVCs in a row with a ventricular rate of 100-200 beats per minute. Ventricular tachycardia may be triggered by the same factors as PVCs and often is related to underlying coronary artery disease. The rapid rate of contractions makes VT dangerous as the ineffective beats may render the person unconscious with no palpable pulse. A detectable rate is usually regular and the QRS complex is ≥0.12 seconds and is usually abnormally shaped. The P wave may be undetectable with an irregular PR interval if P wave is present. The P:QRS ratio is often difficult to ascertain because of absence of P waves.

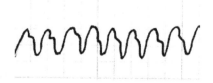

32

Treatment is as follows:

- With pulse: Synchronized cardioversion, adenosine.
- No pulse: Same as ventricular fibrillation.

NARROW COMPLEX AND WIDE COMPLEX TACHYCARDIAS

Tachycardias are classified as narrow complex or wide complex. Wide and narrow refer to the configuration of the QRS complex.

- **Wide complex tachycardia (WCT):** About 80% of cases of WCT are caused by ventricular tachycardia. WCT originates at some point below the AV node and may be associated with palpitations, dyspnea, anxiety, diaphoresis, and cardiac arrest. Wide complex tachycardia is diagnosed with more than 3 consecutive beats at a heart rate >100 BPM and QRS duration ≥0.12 seconds.
- **Narrow complex tachycardia:** NCT is associated with palpitations, dyspnea, and peripheral edema. NCT is generally supraventricular in origin. Narrow complex tachycardia is diagnosed with ≥3 consecutive beats at heart rate of >100 BPM and QRS duration of <0.12 seconds.

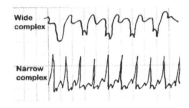

VENTRICULAR FIBRILLATION

Ventricular fibrillation (VF) is a rapid, very irregular ventricular rate >300 beats per minute with no atrial activity observable on the ECG, caused by disorganized electrical activity in the ventricles. The QRS complex is not recognizable as ECG shows irregular undulations. The causes are the same as for ventricular tachycardia and asystole. VF is accompanied by lack of palpable pulse, audible pulse, and respirations and is immediately life threatening without defibrillation.

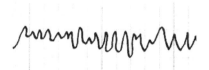

Treatment includes:

- Emergency defibrillation, the cause should be identified and treated.
- Epinephrine 1mg q3-5minutes then Amiodarone 300mg (2nd dose: 150mg) IV push.

IDIOVENTRICULAR RHYTHM

Ventricular escape rhythm (idioventricular) occurs when the Purkinje fibers below the AV node create an impulse. This may occur if the sinus node fails to fire or if there is blockage at the AV node so that the impulse does not go through. Idioventricular rhythm is characterized by a regular ventricular rate of 20-40 BPM. Rates >40 BPM are called accelerated idioventricular rhythm. The P wave is missing and the QRS complex has a very bizarre and abnormal shape with duration of ≥0.12 seconds. The low ventricular rate may cause a decrease in cardiac output, often making the patient lose consciousness. In other patients, the idioventricular rhythm may not be associated with reduced cardiac output.

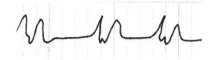

VENTRICULAR ASYSTOLE

Ventricular asystole is the absence of audible heartbeat, palpable pulse, and respirations, a condition often referred to as "cardiac arrest." While the ECG may show some P waves initially, the QRS complex is absent although there may be an occasional QRS "escape beat" (agonal rhythm). Cardiopulmonary resuscitation is required with intubation for ventilation and establishment of an intravenous line for fluids. Without immediate treatment, the patient will suffer from severe hypoxia and brain death within minutes. Identifying the cause is critical for the patient's survival. Consider the "Hs & Ts": hypovolemia, hypoxia, hydrogen ions (acidosis), hypo/hyperkalemia, hypothermia, tension pneumothorax, tamponade (cardiac), toxins, and thrombosis (pulmonary or coronary). Even with immediate treatment, the prognosis is poor and ventricular asystole is often a sign of impending death.

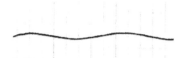

Treatment includes:

- CPR only; Asystole is not a shockable rhythm therefore defibrillation is not indicated.
- Epinephrine 1 mg q3-5 minutes.

SINUS PAUSE

Sinus pause occurs when the sinus node fails to function properly to stimulate heart contractions, so there is a pause on the ECG recording that may persist for a few seconds to minutes, depending on the severity of the dysfunction. A prolonged pause may be difficult to differentiate from cardiac arrest. During the sinus pause, the P wave, QRS complex and PR and QRS intervals are all absent. P: QRS ratio is 1:1 and the rhythm is irregular. The pulse rate may vary widely, usually 60 to 100 BPM. Patients with frequent pauses may complain of dizziness or syncope. The patient may need to undergo an electrophysiology study and medication reconciliation to determine the cause. If measures such as decreasing medication are not effective, a pacemaker is usually indicated (if symptomatic).

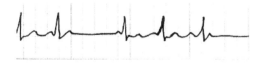

SYSTOLIC HEART FAILURE

Systolic heart failure is the typical "left-sided" failure and reduces the amount of blood ejected from the ventricles during contraction (decreased ejection fraction). This stimulates the SNS to produce catecholamines to support the myocardium, which eventually causes down regulation, the destruction of beta and adrenergic receptor sites, and ultimately further myocardial damage. Because of reduced perfusion, the R-A-A pathway (renin, angiotensin I&II, aldosterone) is initiated

34

by the kidneys, causing sodium and fluid retention. The end result of these processes is increased preload and afterload, thus increased workload on the ventricles. They begin to lose contractibility and blood begins to pool inside, stretching the myocardium (ventricular remodeling). The heart compensates by thickening the muscle (hypertrophy) without an adequate increase in capillary blood supply, leading to ischemia.

Symptoms: Activity intolerance, dyspnea/orthopnea (sleeping in a recliner is classic symptom), cough (frothy sputum), edema, heart sounds S3 and S4, hepatomegaly, JVD, LOC changes, and tachycardia.

Treatment includes:

- Medication
- **Surgery**: Heart transplant (if a candidate).
- **Lifestyle modification**: Low-sodium diet, supplemental oxygen, daily weights (report >3 lb/day or 5 lb/week weight gain to physician).

DIASTOLIC HEART FAILURE

Diastolic heart failure may be difficult to differentiate from systolic heart failure based on clinical symptoms, which are similar. With diastolic heart failure, the myocardium is unable to sufficiently relax to facilitate filling of the ventricles. This may be the end result of systolic heart failure as myocardial hypertrophy stiffens the muscles, and the causes are similar. Diastolic heart failure is more common in females >75. Typically, intra-cardiac pressures at rest are within normal range but increase markedly on exertion. Because the relaxation of the heart is delayed, the ventricles do not expand enough for the fill-volume, and the heart cannot increase stroke volume during exercise, so symptoms (dyspnea, fatigue, pulmonary edema) are often pronounced on exertion. Ejection fractions are usually >40-50% with increase in left ventricular end-diastolic pressure (LVEDP) and decrease in left ventricular end-diastolic volume (LVEDV).

The major goal with all types of heart failure is to prevent further damage and remodeling, prevent exacerbations, and improve the patient's long-term prognosis.

ACUTE HEART FAILURE

Acute decompensated heart failure occurs when the body cannot compensate for the heart's inability to provide adequate perfusion. Cardiac output is no longer sufficient to meet the metabolic demands of the body. Acute heart failure occurs suddenly and can be precipitated by dysrhythmias, illness, noncompliance with medications, acute ischemia, fluid overload or hypertensive crisis. Acute heart failure is most commonly related to left ventricular systolic or diastolic dysfunction. It requires immediate treatment to restore adequate perfusion and is often life-threatening.

Signs and symptoms: Dyspnea, cough, edema, ascites and elevated jugular venous pressure, fatigue, cool extremities, hypotension and altered mental status.

Diagnostic testing: Chest X-ray, electrocardiogram, physical exam; labs—basic metabolic panel, BUN, creatinine and B-natriuretic peptide (BNP).

Treatment: Rapid assessment and stabilization of the patient. The physical assessment should include a thorough evaluation of the patient's respiratory status and supplemental oxygen and potentially ventilator support may be necessary. Medications: Diuretics to decrease fluid volume; vasodilators to decrease pulmonary congestion. Cardiac monitoring, urine output monitoring, sodium restriction, and venous thromboembolism prophylaxis may also be utilized.

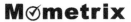

Hypertensive Crises, Conduction System Abnormalities, Papillary Muscle Rupture, and Pericarditis

HYPERTENSIVE CRISES

Hypertensive crises are marked elevations in blood pressure that can cause severe organ damage if left untreated. Hypertensive crises may be caused by endocrine/renal disorders (pheochromocytoma), dissection of an aortic aneurysm, pulmonary edema, subarachnoid hemorrhage, stroke, eclampsia, and medication noncompliance. There are 2 classifications:

- **Hypertensive emergency** occurs when acute hypertension (1.5 x the 95th percentile), usually >220 systolic and 120 mmHg diastolic, must be treated immediately to lower blood pressure in order to prevent damage to vital organs.
- **Hypertensive urgency** occurs when acute hypertension must be treated within a few hours but the vital organs are not in immediate danger. Blood pressure is lowered more slowly to avoid hypotension, ischemia of vital organs, or failure of autoregulation.
  - o 1/3 reduction in 6 hours.
  - o 1/3 reduction in next 24 hours.
  - o 1/3 reduction over days 2-4.

Symptoms: Basilar HA, blurred vision, chest pain, N/V, SOB, seizures, ruddy pallor, and anxiety.

Diagnostics: ECG, Chest x-ray, CBC, BMP, Urinalysis (+ blood and casts).

Treatment includes:

- Medications: Vasodilators (Cardene, Nitro, etc.) & diuretics.
- Nursing Interventions: Raise HOB to 90°, supplemental O_2, frequent neuro checks, teach concerning medication compliance.

MYOCARDIAL CONDUCTION SYSTEM ABNORMALITIES
PROLONGED QT INTERVAL

The normal **QT interval** is 400 to 460 ms in females and 400 to 440 ms in males. QT interval value greater than 500 ms increases risk of cardiac abnormalities. If the QT interval extends greater than half the RR, it is prolonged. Long QT syndrome occurs when depolarization and repolarization is prolonged between beats and can result in torsades de points or VT. "R-on-T" phenomenon can trigger these dangerous arrhythmias, and is a serious risk with long QT intervals, as the chance of a PVC (specifically the ventricular depolarization of the PVC) falling on the t-wave is what induces the arrhythmia. The longer the QT interval, the greater the chance of this phenomenon occurring. Long QT syndrome may be a genetic condition or may be acquired and associated with electrolyte imbalances, some medications (antidepressants, diuretics, antibiotics), and some conditions (anorexia nervosa). Continuous QT interval monitoring measures from the QRS complex (depolarization) to the end of the T wave (repolarization). Indications (AHA recommendations) include patients:

- Newly diagnosed with bradyarrhythmia.
- Receiving anti-arrhythmic drugs or other drugs associated with torsade de pointes (a life-threatening dysrhythmia).
- Overdosing on agents or receiving antipsychotics or drugs that may cause arrhythmias.

- With electrolyte imbalances (hypokalemia, hypomagnesemia) that may cause arrhythmias.
- With acute neurological events, such as stroke.

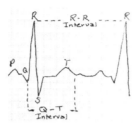

WOLFF-PARKINSON-WHITE SYNDROME

The **Wolff-Parkinson-White syndrome** (a preexcitation syndrome) is characterized by a short P-R interval and a delta wave, which appears as a slurred upstroke into the QRS complex, so the PR interval is missing. The QRS complex is prolonged because of the delta wave. The rhythm is very irregular and the rate is often 250 to 300 bpm. The delta wave is produced because of premature depolarization of part of the ventricles. With preexcitation syndromes, electrical stimulation of the ventricles occurs through an accessory (in this case Kent's bundle) pathway while the impulse also travels through the AV node, and this can lead to rapid paroxysmal tachyarrhythmias (usually AV reentry tachycardia—AVRT). About 40% develop atrial fibrillation. Medications, such as amiodarone and sotalol may be used to slow conduction, but cardioversion may be necessary. WPW syndrome is most common in children and young adults.

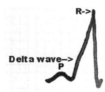

PAPILLARY MUSCLE RUPTURE

Papillary muscle rupture is a rare but often deadly complication of myocardial ischemia/infarct. It most commonly occurs with inferior infarcts. The papillary muscles are part of the cardiac wall structure; attached to the lower portion of the ventricles, they are responsible for the opening and closing of the tricuspid and mitral valve and preventing prolapse during systole. Rupture of the papillary muscle can occur with myocardial infarct or ischemia in the area of the heart surrounding the papillary muscle. Since the papillary muscles support the mitral valve, rupture will cause severe mitral regurgitation that may result in cardiogenic shock and subsequent death. Rupture of the papillary muscle may be partial or complete and is considered a life-threatening emergency.

Signs and symptoms: Acute heart failure, pulmonary edema, and cardiogenic shock (tachycardia, diaphoresis, loss of consciousness, pallor, tachypnea, mental status changes, weak or thready pulse, and decreased urinary output).

Diagnosis: Transesophageal echocardiography (TEE) to visualize the papillary muscles, color flow Doppler, echocardiogram and physical assessment. In patients with papillary muscle rupture, a holosystolic murmur starting at the apex and radiating to the axilla may be present.

Treatment: Emergent surgical intervention to repair the mitral valve.

In the cases of complete rupture, patients often experience the rapid development of cardiogenic shock and subsequent death.

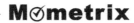

ACUTE PERICARDITIS

Pericarditis is inflammation of the pericardial sac with or without increased pericardial fluid. It may be an isolated process or the effect of an underlying disease. If the underlying cause is autoimmune or related to malignancy of some sort, the patient usually presents with symptoms that relate to that disorder. However, most cases are related to a viral etiology, and therefore usually present with flu-like symptoms. Patients that have idiopathic pericarditis or viral pericarditis have a good prognosis with medication alone.

Signs/Symptoms: Sharp chest pain, worsened with inspiration and relieved by leaning forward or sitting up (most common symptom; "Mohammad's Sign"), pericardial effusion, respiratory distress, auscultated friction rub, ST elevation/PR depression (progresses to flattened T, inverted T, then return to normal); risk of pericardial effusion.

Diagnosis: Echocardiogram, ECG, pericardiocentesis or pericardial biopsy, cardiac enzymes (may be mildly elevated), WBC/ESR/CRP all elevated.

Treatment includes:

- **Medications**: NSAIDs for pain / inflammation, Colchicine 0.5 mg twice a day for six months is often prescribed in adjunct to NSAID therapy, as it decreases the incidence of recurrence.
- **Surgery**: Pericardiectomy only in extreme cases.

Structural Heart Defects

MITRAL STENOSIS

Mitral stenosis is a narrowing of the mitral valve that allows blood to flow from the left atrium to the left ventricle. Pressure in the left atrium increases to overcome resistance, resulting in enlargement of the left atrium and increased pressure in the pulmonary veins and capillaries of the lung (pulmonary hypertension). Mitral stenosis can be caused by infective endocarditis, calcifications, or tumors in the left atrium.

Signs/Symptoms: Exertional dyspnea, orthopnea/nocturnal dyspnea, right-sided heart failure, loud S_1 and S_2, and mid-diastolic murmur.

Diagnosis: Cardiac catheterization, chest XRAY, echocardiogram, ECG.

Treatment includes:

- **Medications**: Antiarrhythmic, anticoagulant, and antihypertensive medications.
- **Surgical**: Open/closed commissurotomy, balloon valvuloplasty, and mitral valve replacement.

MITRAL VALVE INSUFFICIENCY

Mitral valve insufficiency occurs when the mitral valve fails to close completely so that there is backflow into the left atrium from the left ventricle during systole, decreasing cardiac output. It may occur with mitral stenosis or independently. Mitral valve insufficiency can result from damage caused by rheumatic fever, myxomatous degeneration, infective endocarditis, collagen vascular

38

disease (Marfan's syndrome), or cardiomyopathy/ left heart failure. There are 3 phases of the disease:

- **Acute:** May occur with rupture of a chordae tendineae or papillary muscle causing sudden left ventricular flooding and overload.
- **Chronic compensated:** Enlargement of the left atrium to decrease filling pressure, and hypertrophy of the left ventricle.
- **Chronic decompensated:** Left ventricle fails to compensate for the volume overload; ↓stroke volume & ↓ cardiac output.

Symptoms: Orthopnea/dyspnea, split $S_2/S_3/S_4$ heart sounds, systolic murmur, palpitations, right-sided heart failure, fatigue, angina (rare).

Diagnosis: Cardiac catheterization, chest XRAY, echocardiogram, ECG.

Treatment includes:

- **Medications**: Antiarrhythmic, anticoagulant, and antihypertensive medications.
- **Surgical**: Annuloplasty or valvuloplasty, and mitral valve replacement.

AORTIC STENOSIS

Aortic stenosis is a stricture (narrowing) of the aortic valve that controls the flow of blood from the left ventricle. This causes the left ventricular wall to thicken as it increases pressure to overcome the valvular resistance, increasing afterload and increasing the need for blood supply from the coronary arteries. This condition may result from a birth defect or childhood rheumatic fever, and tends to worsen over the years as the heart grows.

Symptoms: Angina, exercise intolerance, dyspnea, split S_1 and S_2, systolic murmur at base of carotids, hypotension on exertion, syncope, left-sided heart failure; sudden death can occur.

Diagnosis: Cardiac catheterization, chest XRAY, echocardiogram, ECG.

Treatment includes:

- **Medications**: Antiarrhythmic, anticoagulant, and antihypertensive medications.
- **Surgical**: Balloon valvuloplasty, and aortic valve replacement.

PULMONIC STENOSIS

Pulmonic stenosis is a stricture of the pulmonary blood that controls the flow of blood from the right ventricle to the lungs, resulting in right ventricular hypertrophy as the pressure increases in the right ventricle and decreased pulmonary blood flow. The condition may be asymptomatic or symptoms may not be evident until adulthood, depending upon the severity of the defect. Pulmonic stenosis may be associated with a number of other heart defects.

Symptoms: May be asymptomatic; dyspnea on exertion, systolic heart murmur, right-sided heart failure.

Diagnosis: Cardiac catheterization, chest XRAY, echocardiogram, ECG.

Treatment includes:

- **Medications**: Antiarrhythmic, anticoagulant, and antihypertensive medications.
- **Surgical**: Balloon valvuloplasty, valvotomy, valvectomy with or without transannular patch, and pulmonary valve replacement.

CARDIAC SURGICAL OPTIONS FOR REPAIR OF CARDIAC VALVES

There are a number of different surgical options for **repair of cardiac valves**:

- **Valvotomy/ Valvuloplasty** is usually done through cardiac catheterization. A valvotomy/valvuloplasty involves releasing valve leaflet adhesions or opening a stenosed valve. In balloon valvuloplasty, a catheter with an inflatable balloon is positioned in the stenotic valve and inflated and deflated a number of times to dilate the opening. Risks include stroke from broken-off calcified valve and worsened valvular insufficiency/rupture.
- **Aortic valve replacement** is an open-heart procedure with cardiopulmonary bypass. Aortic valves are tricuspid (3 leaflets) and repair is usually not possible, so defective valves must be replaced with either mechanical (metal, plastic, or pyrolytic carbon) or biological (porcine or bovine) grafts.
- **Aortic homograft** uses part of a donor's aorta with the aortic valve attached to replace the recipient's faulty aortic valve and part of the ascending aorta.
- **Ross procedure** uses the patient's pulmonary artery with the pulmonary valve to replace the aortic valve and part of the aorta and then uses a donor graft to replace the pulmonary artery.

CONGENITAL HEART DEFECTS SEEN IN ADULTHOOD

Congenital heart defects are often identified in infancy or early childhood; however, diagnosis may be delayed until adulthood due to the lack of signs and symptoms. Atrial septal and ventricular septal defects are common congenital anomalies that can present at any age. An atrial septal defect occurs when part of the atrial septum does not form properly, leaving a hole in the septum. A ventricular septal defect results from a hole in the septum separating the ventricles. Patent ductus arteriosus, coarctation of the aorta and Ebstein's anomaly are other types of congenital defects that are less commonly diagnosed in adulthood.

Signs and symptoms: Murmurs, cyanosis, clubbing of the fingernails, shortness of breath, fatigue, syncope, palpitations and edema. Heart failure and endocarditis may also occur.

Diagnosis: Physical assessment, EKG, Chest X-ray, transesophageal echocardiogram, CT, and MRI.

Treatment: Treatment options depend on the size and location of the defect. Most commonly the anomaly will be corrected by open surgical repair; however percutaneous intervention may be an option in some patients.

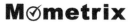

Cardiovascular Medication Management

FIBRINOLYTIC (THROMBOLYTIC) INFUSIONS

Fibrinolytic infusion is indicated for acute myocardial infarction under these conditions:

- Symptoms of MI, <6-12 hours since onset of symptoms.
- ≥1 mm elevation of ST in ≥2 contiguous leads.
- No contraindications and no cardiogenic shock.

Fibrinolytic agents should be administered as soon as possible, within 30 minutes is best. All agents convert plasminogen to plasmin, which breaks down fibrin, dissolving clots:

- Streptokinase & anistreplase (1st generation).
- Alteplase or tissue plasminogen activator (tPA) (second generation).
- Reteplase & tenecteplase (3rd generation).

Relative Contraindications: Active peptic ulcer, >10 minutes of CPR,

advanced renal or hepatic disease, pregnancy, anticoagulation therapy, acute uncontrolled hypertension/chronic poorly controlled hypertension, recent (2-4 weeks) internal bleeding, noncompressible vascular punctures.

Absolute Contraindications: Present or recent bleeding or history of severe bleeding, history of intracranial hemorrhage, history of stroke (<3 months unless within 3 hours), aortic dissection, pericarditis, intracranial/ intraspinal surgery or trauma within 3 months, neoplasm, aneurysm, or AVM.

MAXIMIZING PERFUSION IN PERIPHERALLY VASCULAR DISEASE

The primary focus of **pharmacologic measures to maximize perfusion** in peripheral vascular disease is to reduce the risk of thromboses/acute vascular occlusion:

- **Antiplatelet agents,** such as aspirin, Ticlid®, and Plavix®, which interfere with the function of the plasma membrane, reducing clotting of the blood. These agents are ineffective to treat clots but prevent clot formation.
- **Vasodilators** may divert blood from already ischemic areas, but some may be indicated, such as Pletal®, which dilates arteries and decreases clotting, and is used for control of intermittent claudication.
- **Antilipemic,** such as Zocor® and Questran®, slow progression of atherosclerosis.
- **Hemorrheologics,** such as Trental®, reduce fibrinogen, reducing blood viscosity and rigidity of erythrocytes; however, clinical studies show limited benefit. It may be used for intermittent claudication.
- **Analgesics** may be necessary to improve quality of life. Opioids may be needed in some cases.
- **Thrombolytics** may be injected into a blocked artery under angiography to dissolve clots.
- **Anticoagulants,** such as Coumadin® and Lovenox®, prevent blood clots from forming.

41

Copyright © Mometrix Media. You have been licensed one copy of this document for personal use only. Any other reproduction or redistribution is strictly prohibited. All rights reserved.

ANTICOAGULANTS

Anticoagulants are used to prevent thromboemboli. All pose risk of bleeding:

- **Aspirin:** Often used prophylactically to prevent clots and poses less danger of bleeding than other drugs. Do not give to adolescents or younger (risk of Reyes syndrome).
- **Warfarin (Coumadin®):** Blocks utilization of vitamin K and decreases production of clotting factors. Oral medications for those at risk of developing blood clots, such as those with mechanical heart valves, atrial fibrillation, and clotting disorders. Antidote: Vitamin K.
- **Heparin:** The primary intravenous anticoagulant and increases the activity of antithrombin III. It is used for those with MI and those undergoing PCI or other cardiac surgery, as well as patients with active clots. Monitored by aPTT or AntiXa; monitor for signs of heparin-induced thrombocytopenia (HIT), an allergic response to heparin that causes a platelet count drop <150,000, usually to 30-50% of baseline, usually occurring 5-14 days after beginning heparin.
- **Dalteparin (Fragmin®) & Enoxaparin (Lovenox®):** Low-molecular weight heparins that increase activity of antithrombin III used for DVT prophylaxis, unstable angina, MI, and cardiac surgery.
- **Bivalirudin (Angiomax®):** Direct thrombin inhibitors used for unstable angina, PCI, and for prophylaxis and treatment of thrombosis in heparin-induced thrombocytopenia (HIT).

GLYCOPROTEIN IIB/IIIA INHIBITORS

Glycoprotein IIB/IIIA Inhibitors are drugs that are used to inhibit platelet binding and prevent clots prior to and following invasive cardiac procedures, such as angioplasty and stent placement. These medications are used in combination with anticoagulant drugs, such as heparin and aspirin for the following:

- Acute coronary syndromes (ACS), such as unstable angina or myocardial infarctions.
- Percutaneous coronary intervention (PCI), such as angioplasty and stent placement.

These medications are contraindicated in those with a low platelet count or active bleeding:

- **Abciximab (ReoPro®):** Used with both heparin and aspirin for ACS and PCI and affects platelet binding for 48 hours after administration.
- **Eptifibatide (Integrilin®):** Used with both heparin and aspirin for ACS and PCI and affects platelet binding for 6-8 hours after administration. Should not be used in patients with renal problems.
- **Tirofiban (Aggrastat®):** Used with heparin for PCI patients, with reduced dosage for those with renal problems, and affects platelet blinding for only 4-8 hours after administration.

MEDICATIONS FOR HEART FAILURE

Medications for heart failure are as follows:

- **ACE inhibitors:** Captopril (Capoten®), enalapril (Vasotec®), and lisinopril (Prinivil®): Decrease afterload/preload and reverse ventricular remodeling; also prevent neuropathy in DM. Contraindicated with renal insufficiency, renal artery stenosis, and pregnancy. Side effects include cough (most common), hyperkalemia, hypotension, angioedema, dizziness, and weakness.

- **Angiotensin receptor blockers (ARBs):** Losartan (Cozaar®) and valsartan (Diovan®): Decrease afterload/preload and reverse ventricular remodeling, causing vasodilation and reducing blood pressure. They are used for those who cannot tolerate ACE inhibitors. Side effects include cough (less common than with ACE inhibitors), hyperkalemia, hypotension, headache, dizziness, metallic taste, and rash.
- **β-Blockers:** Metoprolol (Lopressor®), carvedilol (Coreg®) and esmolol (Brevibloc®) Slow the heart rate, reduce hypertension, prevent dysrhythmias, and reverse ventricular remodeling. Contraindicated in bradyarrhythmias, decompensated HF, uncontrolled hypoglycemia/ diabetes mellitus, and airway disease (such as asthma). Side effects: Bradycardia, hypotension, bronchospasm, may mask signs of hypoglycemia.
- **Aldosterone antagonists: Spironolactone (Aldactone®):** Decreases preload and myocardial hypertrophy and reduces edema and sodium retention but may increase serum potassium.
- **Furosemide (Lasix®)** is used for the control of congestive heart failure as well as renal insufficiency. It is used after surgery to decrease preload and to reduce the inflammatory response caused by cardiopulmonary bypass (post-perfusion syndrome).

SMOOTH MUSCLE RELAXANTS AND CALCIUM CHANNEL BLOCKERS

Smooth muscle relaxants decrease peripheral vascular resistance and may cause hypotension and headaches:

- Sodium nitroprusside (Nipride®) dilates both arteries and veins; rapid-acting and used for reduction of hypertension and afterload reduction for heart failure.
- Nitroglycerin (Tridil®) primarily dilates veins and is used sublingual or IV to reduce preload for acute heart failure, unstable angina, and acute MI. Nitroglycerin may also be used prophylactically after PCIs to prevent vasospasm.
- Hydralazine (Apresoline®) dilates arteries and is given intermittently to reduce hypertension.

Calcium channel blockers are primarily arterial vasodilators that may affect the peripheral and/or coronary arteries. Side effects include lethargy, flushing, edema, ascites, and indigestion.

- Nifedipine (Procardia®) and nicardipine (Cardene®) are primarily arterial vasodilators, used to treat acute hypertension.
- Diltiazem (Cardizem®) and Verapamil (Calan®, Isoptin®) dilate primarily coronary arteries and slow the heart rate, thus are used for angina, atrial fibrillation, and SVT.
- Nifedipine (Procardia®) should be avoided in older adults due to increased risk of hypotension and myocardial ischemia.

B-TYPE NATRIURETIC PEPTIDES

B-type natriuretic peptide (BNP) (Nesiritide—Natrecor®) are described below:

- A type of vasodilator (non-inotropic), which is a recombinant form of a peptide of the human brain.
- It decreases filling pressure, vascular resistance, and increases U/O.
- May cause hypotension, headache, bradycardia, and nausea. It is used short term for worsening decompensated CHF; contraindicated in SBP<90, cardiogenic shock, constrictive pericarditis, or valve stenosis.

ALPHA-ADRENERGIC BLOCKERS

Alpha-adrenergic blockers are described below:

- Blocks alpha receptors in arteries and veins, causing vasodilation.
- May cause orthostatic hypotension and edema from fluid retention.
- Labetalol (Normodyne®) is a combination peripheral alpha-blocker and cardiac β-blocker and is used to treat acute hypertension, acute stroke, and acute aortic dissection. Phentolamine (Regitine®) is a peripheral arterial dilator that reduces afterload. It is used for HTN crisis in patients with pheochromocytoma, as well as a subcutaneous injection for extravasation of vesicants.

SELECTIVE SPECIFIC DOPAMINE DA-1 RECEPTOR AGONISTS

Selective specific dopamine DA-1-receptor agonists are described below:

- Fenoldopam (Corlopam®): A peripheral dilator affecting renal and mesenteric arteries and can be used for patients with renal dysfunction or those at risk of renal insufficiency.

INOTROPIC AGENTS

Inotropic agents are drugs used to increase cardiac output and improve contractibility. IV inotropic agents may increase the risk of death, but may be used when other drugs fail. Oral forms of these drugs are less effective than intravenous. Inotropic agents include:

- **β-Adrenergic agonists:**
  - *Dobutamine* improves cardiac output, treats cardiac decompensation, and increases blood pressure. It helps the body to utilize norepinephrine. Side effects include increased or labile blood pressure, increased heart rate, PVCs, N/V, and bronchospasm.
  - *Dopamine* improves cardiac output, blood pressure, and blood flow to the renal and mesenteric arteries. Side effects include tachycardia or bradycardia, palpitations, BP changes, dyspnea, nausea and vomiting, headache, and gangrene of extremities.
- **Phosphodiesterase III inhibitors:**
  - *Milrinone* (Primacor®) increases strength of contractions and causes vasodilation. Side effects include ventricular arrhythmias, hypotension, and headaches.
- **Digoxin** (Lanoxin®):
  - Increases contractibility and cardiac output and prevents arrhythmias.

DIGOXIN (LANOXIN®)

Digitalis drugs, most commonly administered in the form of digoxin (Lanoxin®), are derived from the foxglove plant and are used to increase myocardial contractility, left ventricular output, and slow conduction through the AV node, decreasing rapid heart rates and promoting diuresis. Digoxin does not affect mortality, but increases tolerance to activity and reduces hospitalizations for heart failure. Therapeutic levels (0.5-2.0 ng/mL) should be maintained to avoid digitalis toxicity, which can occur even if digoxin levels are within therapeutic range, so observation of symptoms is critical. Because patients with heart failure are often on diuretics which decrease potassium levels, they are at increased risk for toxicity.

Symptoms of toxicity are as follows:

- *Early signs*: Increasing fatigue, lethargy, depression, and nausea and vomiting; progress to severe diarrhea, blurred vision/ yellow or green halos around lights, fatigue/weakness.
- Arrythmias: SA or AV block, VT/VF, PVCs, and bradycardia.

Treatment consists of the following:

- Monitor serum levels and symptoms.
- Digoxin immune FAB (Digibind®) may be used to bind to digoxin and inactivate it if necessary.

ANTIDYSRHYTHMICS

Antidysrhythmics include a number of drugs that act on the conduction system, the ventricles and/or the atria to control dysrhythmias. There are 4 classes of drugs that are used as well as some that are unclassified:

- **Class I:** 3 subtypes of sodium channel blockers (quinidine, lidocaine, procainamide).
- **Class II:** β-receptor blockers (esmolol, propranolol).
- **Class III:** Slows repolarization (amiodarone, ibutilide).
- **Class IV**: Calcium channel blockers (diltiazem, verapamil).
- **Unclassified** (Adenosine).

Cardiovascular Assessment and Monitoring

MIXED VENOUS GASES/SvO2

Mixed venous gases (MVG), especially venous oxygen saturation (SvO$_2$), are monitored for indications of respiratory failure, reduced oxygenation, anemia, and changes in cardiac output. Mixed venous gas refers to venous blood that has returned to the heart from the superior and inferior vena cava and the coronary sinus. Obtaining a sample from the right atrium may reflect primarily blood from the superior vena cava, which usually has a lower saturation (70%) than the blood from the inferior vena cava (80%) or the coronary sinus (56%). The blood in the right ventricle and pulmonary artery is completed "mixed" and the saturation averaged. MVG are usually measured by sampling through a PA catheter, but can pulled from a central line. Normal values:

- **PCO$_2$:** 40-50 mmHg (venous partial pressure of CO$_2$); 35-45 mmHg (arterial partial pressure of CO$_2$).
- **PvO$_2$:** 30-40 mmHg (venous partial pressure of oxygen); 75-100 mmHg (arterial partial pressure of CO$_2$).
- **SvO$_2$:** 60-80% (venous oxygen saturation.).

If there is a decrease in SvO$_2$, then the oxygenation is not sufficient for tissue needs.

ASSESSMENT OF HEART SOUNDS

Auscultation of **heart sounds** can help to diagnose different cardiac disorders. Areas to auscultate include the aortic area, pulmonic area, Erb's point, tricuspid area, and the apical area. The normal heart sounds represent closing of the valves. The first heart sound (S1) "lub" is closure of the mitral and tricuspid valves (heard at apex/left ventricular area of the heart). The second heart sound (S2) "dub" is closure of the aortic and pulmonic valves (heard at the base of the heart).

Additional heart sounds are listed and described below:

- **Gallop rhythms:** *S3* commonly occurs after S2 in children and young adults but may indicate heart failure or left ventricular failure in older adults (heard with patient lying on left side). *S4* occurs before S1, during the contracting of the atria when there is ventricular hypertrophy, found in coronary artery disease, hypertension, or aortic valve stenosis.
- **Opening snap:** Unusual high-pitched sound occurring after S2 with stenosis of mitral valve from rheumatic heart disease.
- **Ejection click:** Brief high-pitched sound after S1; aortic stenosis.
- **Friction rub:** Harsh, grating holosystolic sound; pericarditis.
- **Murmur:** Sound caused by turbulent blood flow from stenotic or malfunctioning valves, congenital defects, or increased blood flow. Murmurs are characterized by location, timing in the cardiac cycle, intensity (rated from Grade I to Grade VI), pitch (low to high-pitched), quality (rumbling, whistling, blowing) and radiation (to the carotids, axilla, neck, shoulder, or back).

JUGULAR VENOUS PRESSURE

Jugular venous pressure (neck-vein) is used to assess the cardiac output and pressure in the right heart as the pulsations relate to changes in pressure in the right atrium. This procedure is usually not accurate if pulse rate is >100. This is a non-invasive estimation of central venous pressure and waveform. Measurement should be done with the internal jugular if possible; if not, the external jugular may be used.

- Elevate the patient's head to 45° (and to 90° if necessary) with patient's head turned to the right.
- Position light at an angle to illuminate veins and shadows.
- Measure the height of the jugular vein pulsation above the sternal joint, using a ruler.
  - Normal height is ≤ 4 cm above sternal angle
  - Increased pressure (> 4 cm) indicates increased pressure in right atrium and possible right-sided heart failure. It may also indicate pericarditis or tricuspid stenosis. Laughing or coughing may trigger the Valsalva response and also cause an increase in pressure.

ELECTROCARDIOGRAM (PQRSTU)

The **electrocardiogram** records and shows a graphic display of the electrical activity of the heart through a number of different waveforms, complexes, and intervals:

- P wave: Start of electrical impulse in the sinus node and spreading through the atria, muscle depolarization.
- QRS complex: Ventricular muscle depolarization and atrial repolarization.
- T wave: Ventricular muscle repolarization (resting state) as cells regain negative charge.
- U wave: Repolarization of the Purkinje fibers.

A modified lead II ECG is often used to monitor basic heart rhythms and dysrhythmias:

- Typical placement of leads for 2-lead ECG is 3 to 5 cm inferior to the right clavicle and left lower ribcage. Typical placement for 3-lead ECG is (RA) right arm near shoulder, (LA) V_5 position over 5th intercostal space, and (LL) left upper leg near groin.

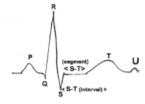

ADMINISTRATION OF 12 LEAD ECG

The **electrocardiogram** provides a continuous graphic representation of the electrical activity of the heart. It is indicated for chest pain, dyspnea, syncope, acute coronary syndrome, pulmonary embolism, and possible MI. The standard 12 lead ECG gives a picture of electrical activity from 12 perspectives through placement of 10 body leads:

- 4 limb leads are placed distally on the wrists and ankles (but may be placed more proximally if necessary).
- Precordial leads:
  - V1: right sternal border at 4th intercostal space.
  - V2: left sternal border at 4th intercostal space.
  - V3: Midway between V2 and V4.
  - V4: Left midclavicular line at 5th intercostal space.
  - V5: Horizontal to V4 at left anterior axillary line.
  - V6: Horizontal to V5 at left mid-axillary line.

In some cases, additional leads may be used:

- Right-sided leads are placed on the right in a mirror image of the left leads, usually to diagnose right ventricular infarction through ST elevation.

CARDIAC MONITORING

Cardiac monitoring includes evaluation of different intervals and segments on the electrocardiogram:

- **QT interval:** This is the complete time of ventricular depolarization and repolarization, which being with the QRS segment and ends when the Y wave is completed. Typically, duration usually ranges from 0.36 to 0.44 seconds, but this may vary depending on the heart rate. If the heat rate is rapid, the duration is shorter and vice versa.
- **ST segment:** This is an isoelectric period when the ventricles are in a plateau phase, completely depolarized and beginning recovery and repolarization. Deflection is usually isoelectric, but may range from -0.5 to +1mm. If the ST segment is ≥0.5 mm below the baseline, it is considered depressed and may be an indication of myocardial ischemia. Depression may also indicate digitalis toxicity. If the ST segment is elevated ≥1 mm above baseline, this is an indication of myocardial injury.

CARDIAC OUTPUT

Cardiac output (CO) is the amount of blood pumped through the ventricles, usually calculated in liters per minute.

- *Normal value at rest: 4-6 L/min.*

CARDIAC INDEX

Cardiac index (CI) is the cardiac output (CO) divided by the body surface area (BSA). This is essentially a measure of cardiac output tailored to the individual, based on height and weight, measured in liters/min per square meter of BSA.

- *Normal value: 2.2-4.0 L/min/m².*

STROKE VOLUME

Stroke volume (SV) is the amount of blood pumped through the left ventricle with each contraction, minus any blood remaining inside the ventricle at the end of systole.

- *Normal values: 60-70 mL.*

Formula:

$$\left(CO \ in \ \frac{L}{min}\right) \times (heart \ rate \ per \ minute) \times (1000) = SV \ in \ mL.$$

PULMONARY VASCULAR RESISTANCE

Pulmonary vascular resistance (PVR) is the resistance in the pulmonary arteries and arterioles against which the right ventricle has to pump during contraction. It is the mean pressure in the pulmonary vascular bed divided by blood flow. If PVR increases, SV decreases.

- *Normal value: 1.2-3.0 units or 100-250 dynes/sec/cm⁵.*

Ejection Fraction (EF) is the percentage of the total blood volume of the heart that is pumped out with each beat.

- *Normal value: 60-70%.*

CARDIAC OUTPUT

Cardiac output (CO) is the amount of blood pumped through the ventricles during a specified period. Normal cardiac output is about 5 liters per minutes at rest for an adult. Under exercise or stress, this volume may multiply 3 or 4 times with concomitant changes in the heart rate (HR) and stroke volume (SV). The basic formulation for calculating cardiac output is the heart rate (HR) per minute multiplied by the stroke volume (SR), which is the amount of blood pumped through the ventricles with each contraction. The stroke volume is controlled by preload, afterload, and contractibility.

$$CO = HR \times SV$$

The heart rate is controlled by the autonomic nervous system. Normally, if the heart rate decreases, stroke volume increases to compensate. The exception to this would be cardiomyopathies, so bradycardia results in a sharp decline in cardiac output.

PRELOAD AND AFTERLOAD

Preload refers to the amount of elasticity in the myocardium at the end of diastole when the ventricles are filled to their maximum volume and the stretch on the muscle fibers is the greatest. The preload value is based on the volume in the ventricles. The amount of preload (stretch) affects stroke volume because as stretch increases, the resultant contraction also increases (Frank-Starling Law). Preload may decrease because of dehydration, diuresis, or vasodilation. Preload may increase because of increased venous return, controlling fluid loss, transfusion, or intravenous fluids.

Afterload refers to the amount of systemic vascular resistance to left ventricular ejection of blood and pulmonary vascular resistance to right ventricular ejection of blood. Determinants of afterload include the size and elasticity of the great vessels and the functioning of the pulmonic and aortic valves. Afterload increases with hypertension, stenotic valves, and vasoconstriction.

MINIMALLY INVASIVE/NON-INVASIVE HEMODYNAMIC MONITORING

Hemodynamic monitoring and evaluation of cardiac function is an important component of the care of the critically ill patient. **Minimally or non-invasive alternatives** to traditional invasive means of hemodynamic monitoring (such as the use of a pulmonary artery catheter) include esophageal Doppler, arterial pressure based cardiac output monitoring, and impedance cardiography:

- **Esophageal Doppler** is a minimally invasive option used in surgical patients to monitor descending aortic blood flow and estimate cardiac output. A probe is inserted into the esophagus and then connected to a monitor, where waveform shapes produced by aortic blood flow are displayed.
- **Arterial pressure based cardiac output** monitors (APCO's) use an algorithm to estimate cardiac output through the analysis of the arterial pressure waveform. The radial or femoral artery is accessed using a standard arterial catheter and no external calibration is needed.
- **Impedance cardiography** is a non-invasive method of hemodynamic monitoring in which sensors placed on the body use electrical signals to measure the level of change in impedance in the thoracic fluid. A waveform is generated and is then used to calculate cardiac output and stroke volume, as well as ten additional hemodynamic parameters.

CENTRAL VENOUS ACCESS IN HEMODYNAMIC MONITORING AND MAINTENANCE

Central venous pressure (CVP), the pressure in the right atrium or vena cava, is used to assess function of the right ventricles, preload, and flow of venous blood to the heart. Central lines may be placed into the internal jugular vein (right preferred), subclavian vein, or femoral vein (usually avoided) to help determine hemodynamic therapy. Indications include hypovolemic shock, post-operative monitoring, and confirmation of right-sided heart failure. CVP is no longer used to determine fluid replacement needs. CVP can be monitored manually with a manometer or electronically with a transducer that displays a continuous waveform on a monitor. Normal pressure ranges from 2-6 mmHg but may be elevated after cardiac surgery to 6-8 mmHg. Incorrect catheter placement or malfunctioning can affect readings.

- **Increased CVP** is related to overload of intravascular volume caused by decreased function, hypertrophy, or failure of the right ventricle; increased right ventricular afterload, tricuspid valve stenosis, regurgitation, or thrombus obstruction; or shunt from left ventricle to right atrium. It can also be caused by arrhythmias or cardiac tamponade and fluid overload.
- **Decreased CVP** is related to low intravascular volume, decreased preload, vasodilation, and distributive shock.

MAP

The **MAP** (mean arterial pressure) is most commonly used to evaluate perfusion as it shows pressure throughout the cardiac cycle. Systole is one-third and diastole two-thirds of the normal cardiac cycle. The MAP for a blood pressure of 120/60 (Normal range 70-100 mmHg):

$$MAP = \frac{\text{Diastole} \times 2 + \text{Systole} \times 1}{3}$$

Example: Blood pressure 120/60

$$MAP = \frac{60 \times 2 + 120 \times 1}{3} = \frac{240}{3} = 80$$

HEMODYNAMIC MONITORING AND OXYGEN SATURATION

Hemodynamic monitoring includes monitoring **oxygen saturation** levels, which must be maintained for proper cardiac function. The central venous catheter often has an oxygen sensor at the tip to monitor oxygen saturation in the right atrium. If the catheter tip is located near the renal veins, this can cause an increase in right atrial oxygen saturation; and near the coronary sinus, a decrease.

- Increased oxygen saturation may result from left atrial to right atrial shunt, abnormal pulmonary venous return, increased delivery of oxygen or decrease in extraction of oxygen.
- Decreased oxygen saturation may be related to low cardiac output with an increase in oxygen extraction or decrease in arterial oxygen saturation with normal differences in the atrial and ventricular oxygen saturation.

INTRAARTERIAL BLOOD PRESSURE MONITORING

Intraarterial blood pressure monitoring uses a catheter to measure systolic, diastolic, and mean arterial pressures (MAP) continuously. Before catheter insertion, collateral circulation must be assessed by Doppler or the Allen test (radial). Complications include arterial vasospasm, hematoma formation, hemorrhage (accidental disconnect), catheter occlusion, compartment syndrome, retroperitoneal bleed (femoral site), and thrombus/embolus.

Set up: The line should be connected to the monitor as well as a pressure bag set at 300mHg with no longer than 3 feet of stiff, noncompliant tubing to ensure accuracy. The transducer is leveled at the phlebostatic axis of the patient. The line should be kept free of any air or bubbles, and re-zeroed every four hours and with a change of patient position.

Waveform: A normal ABP waveform should be smooth and regular, with a dicrotic notch. To test, perform a "square-wave" or "Fast Flush" test; flush the line while watching the monitor. There should be a square shape, followed by two oscillations and a return to normal waves. A missing dicrotic notch indicates a blockage of some kind (thrombus, plaque, and vasospasm) or low pressure in the bag. Too many oscillations or an increased sharpness of the wave indicates under dampening and is caused by increased SVR or too long of tubing.

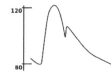

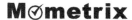

Cardiovascular Procedures and Interventions

POSTOPERATIVE CARE FOR CARDIAC SURGERY

The **recovery period** is discussed below:

- 2:1 Nursing ratio; monitor hemodynamics closely (VS q5-15 minutes)
- Warm patient according to policy; monitor ECG closely for arrhythmias during rewarming.
- Maintain MAP between 70-110 mm/hg to prevent inadequate perfusion or graft rupture/hemorrhage; urine output should be >30 mL/hr.
- Patient will have multiple chest tubes; ensure output is not excessive (>200 mL/hr = hemorrhage) and does not suddenly stop/decrease.
- Auscultate heart sounds, evaluate extremities frequently to assess perfusion; hourly urine output should be 30 mL/hr OR 1mL/kg/hr (gold standard).
- Monitor ABGS (may be q2-4h during recovery); adjust ventilator settings accordingly.
- Close blood sugar control (will probably be on insulin drip) and prophylactic cephalosporin to prevent infection.
- Monitor CMP and replace electrolyte imbalances as ordered.

Monitor for the following complications:

- Cardiac Tamponade: bleeding from graft sites into pericardial sac
- Hypotension/shock: decreased cardiac output
- Arrhythmias: due to blood flow changes and cardioplegic solution – be prepared for epicardial pacing and defibrillation if needed
- Stroke (clots from grafts), infection (surgical site), etc.

Nursing considerations are as follows:

- Educate patient: recovery, possibility of Dressler's Syndrome and post- operative depression; adequate pain management and splinting.

TAVR

Transcatheter aortic valve replacement (TAVR) is usually reserved for patients with advanced symptomatic stenosis of the aortic valve and who are unable to tolerate open-heart surgery or at high risk with the procedure. Symptoms of aortic stenosis include chest pain, peripheral edema, dyspnea, fainting, weakness, and heart failure. With a TAVR, patients generally receive a general anesthesia, and a catheter is inserted, usually transfemoral (most common), transaortic, or transapical. Two types of replacement valves are available in the US: a balloon expandable valve (Sapien XT®) or a self-expanding valve (CoreValue®). Once the catheter with a balloon device and the replacement valve attached is in place in the aortic valve, the balloon is inflated to secure the replacement valve, then the balloon deflated, and the catheter removed. With the self-expanding valve, the valve is attached to catheter and expanded when it is in place in the stenotic valve and the catheter removed.

PERICARDIOCENTESIS

Pericardiocentesis is done with ultrasound guidance to diagnose pericardial effusion or with ECG and ultrasound guidance to relieve cardiac tamponade. Pericardiocentesis may be done as treatment for cardiac arrest or with presentation of PEA with increased jugular venous pressure. Non-hemorrhagic tamponade may be relieved in 60-90% of cases, but hemorrhagic tamponade requires thoracotomy, as blood will continue to accumulate until the cause of the hemorrhage is corrected. Resuscitation equipment must be available, including a defibrillator, intravenous line in place, and cardiac monitoring:

The **procedure** is as follows:

- Elevate chest 45° to bring heart closer to chest wall, pre-medicate with atropine and insert nasogastric tube if indicated.
- Cleanse skin with chlorohexidine or other appropriate cleanser
- After insertion of the needle using ultrasound guidance, the obturator is removed and a syringe attached for aspiration.
- The needle can often be replaced with a catheter after removal for drainage.
- Post procedure chest x-ray should be done to check for pneumothorax.

Possible Complications: Pneumo/hemothorax, coronary artery rupture, hepatic injury, dysrhythmias, false negative/positive aspiration.

TRANSCUTANEOUS PACING

Transcutaneous pacing is used temporarily in an emergency situation to treat symptomatic bradydysrhythmias that don't respond to medications (atropine) and results in hemodynamic instability. Generally, the patient provided oxygen and some sort of mild sedation before the pacing. The placement of pacing pads is usually one pacing pad (negative) is placed on the left chest, inferior to the clavicle, and the other (positive) on the left back, inferior to the scapula, so the heart is sandwiched between the two. Lead wires attach the pads to the monitor. The rate of pacing is usually set around 80 BPM. Current is increased slowly until capture occurs—a spiking followed by QRS sequence, then the current is readjusted downward if possible just to maintain capture, keeping it 5-10mA above the pacing threshold. Both demand and fixed modes are available, but demand mode is preferred. Patient should be warned that the shocks may induce pain.

EPICARDIAL PACING

Epicardial pacing wires may be attached directly to the exterior atria, ventricles, or both at the conclusion of surgery for CPB or valve repair in the event that postoperative pacing support is required or for those with risk of AV block because of medications used to control atrial fibrillation. Cold cardioplegia may precipitate transient sinus node or AV node dysfunction. While some surgeons avoid placing epicardial pacing wires because of concerns about bleeding and cardiac tamponade on removal, recommendations include placing at least one ventricular pacing wire. A typical configuration for pacing wires is atrial pacing wires placed in a plastic disk that is sutured low on the right atrium. The two ventricular wires are attached over the right ventricular wall. Atrial pacing wires may be used to record atrial activity and, and with standard ECG, can help to distinguish atrial and junctional arrhythmias and ventricular arrhythmias. Pacing wires can also be used therapeutically to increase the heart rate to about 90 bpm in order to achieve optimal hemodynamics. The epicardial leads are intended for use of 7 days or less and may be less reliable if used for extended periods. The wires are removed by applying gentle traction.

TEMPORARY TRANSVENOUS PACEMAKERS

Transvenous pacemakers, comprised of a catheter with a lead at the end, may be used prophylactically or therapeutically on a temporary basis to treat symptomatic bradycardias or heart blocks when other methods have failed. The catheter has a balloon tip that must be checked for leaks prior to insertion – this is usually done by inflating the catheter tip while submersed in normal saline and checking for bubbles. After the balloon's integrity is verified, the catheter is inserted through the femoral or jugular vein and the balloon is inflated. The catheter is then attached to an external pulse generator, and the settings are adjusted to achieve capture. The balloon is then deflated, and placement can be verified via ultrasound or chest x-ray.

Complications are similar to those of PCI and permanent pacemaker insertion, including infection, hemorrhage, perforation, embolism, thrombosis, and pacemaker syndrome.

PROBLEMS RELATED TO TRANSVENOUS PACING

With **transvenous pacing** (usually per a pulse generator connected to a pacing cable and a pacing wire, which is inserted into the right internal jugular to the right ventricle for ventricular pacing and right atrium for atrial pacing), sensing refers to the ability to detect electrical activity of the heart. Capture occurs when an artificial stimulus (the pulse generator) depolarizes the heart, indicated by a pacer spike followed by the QRS complex. Problems include:

- **Undersensing:** The sensitivity is too low to detect cardiac depolarizations and triggers unneeded contractions, competing with patient's native rhythm. This may be related to dislodging of lead, incorrect positioning of lead, or low-amplitude cardiac signal.
- **Oversensing:** The sensitivity is too high and misinterprets artifacts (such as muscle contractions) and non-depolarization events as contractions and fails to trigger, resulting in decreased cardiac output because of interruption in contractions. This may result from damage or disconnection of lead.
- **Non-capture:** The pacemaker does not trigger contractions. This may be related to settings, lead disconnection, low battery, or metabolic changes. This is represented by a pacer spike that is not followed by a QRS.

TRANSVENOUS PACER SETTINGS

Temporary **transvenous pacing** utilizes bipolar leads with two tails: positive/proximal and negative/distal, and these must be connected properly to the pulse generator with the distal end of the pacing lead to the negative terminal and the proximal end to the positive terminal. Once the transvenous pacing wire is inserted and leads connected to the pulse generator, it must be set to the patient's needs:

- **Rate**: The beats per minute are usually set between 70 and 80 (allowable range generally 50 to 90) but this may vary according to individual needs.
- **Sensitivity**: The myocardial voltage needed for the pacing electrode to detect P or R waves. The sensitivity is usually set a 2 mV and then adjusted as needed to ensure capture. Most pacemakers can sense 0.3 to 10 mV from the atria and 0.8 to 29 mV from the ventricles, but setting it relatively low prevents oversensing.
- **Output**: The current or pulse produced by the pulse generator is usually set at 5mA. The current is delivered rapidly, in about 0.6 ms.

PACEMAKER COMPLICATIONS

Pacemakers, transvenous and permanent, are invasive foreign bodies and as such can cause a number of different **complications**:

- Infection, bleeding, or hematoma may occur at the entry site of leads for temporary pacemakers or at the subcutaneous area of implantation for permanent generators.
- Puncture of the subclavian vein or internal mammary artery may cause a hemothorax.
- The endocardial electrode may irritate the ventricular wall, causing ectopic beats or tachycardia.

- Dislodgement of transvenous lead may lead to malfunction or perforation of the myocardium. This is one of the most common early complications.
- Dislocation of leads may result in phrenic nerve or muscle stimulation (which may be evidenced by hiccupping).
- Cardiac tamponade may result when epicardial wires of temporary pacing are removed.
- General malfunctioning of pacemaker may indicate dislodgement, dislocation, interference caused by electromagnetic fields, and the need for new batteries or generator.
- Pacemaker syndrome.

PACEMAKER SYNDROME

Pacemaker syndrome can occur with any type of pacemaker if there is inadequate synchronicity between the contractions of the atria and ventricles, resulting in a decrease in cardiac output and inadequate atrial contribution to the filling of the ventricles. Total peripheral vascular resistance may increase to maintain blood pressure, but hypotension occurs after decompensation.

- **Mild:**
  o Pulsations evident in neck and abdomen.
  o Cardiac palpitations.
  o Headache and feeling of anxiety.
  o General malaise and unexplained weakness.
  o Pain or "fullness" in jaw, chest.
- **Moderate:**
  o Increasing dyspnea on exertion with accompanying orthopnea.
  o Dizziness, vertigo, increasing confusion.
  o Feeling of choking.
- **Severe:**
  o Increasing pulmonary edema with dyspnea even at rest
  o Crackling rales.
  o Syncope.
  o Heart failure.

CLOSURE DEVICES WITH PCI

Percutaneous catheter intervention (PCI) is often the treatment choice for patients with symptomatic coronary artery disease. Percutaneous transluminal coronary angioplasty (PTCA), arthrectomy, and stent insertion are common types of percutaneous catheter intervention procedures. While historically, manual compression has been utilized to achieve hemostasis after PCI, different types of devices exist to assist in achieving hemostasis post-procedure. Passive devices such as hemostasis pads and compression devices help to enhance hemostasis. Active devices are used at the femoral access site after the sheath used for the procedure is removed. There are different types of active devices including percutaneous suture mediated devices that use needles and sutures to suture the artery closed after the procedure. Collagen plugs are another type of closure, where collagen is injected into the supra-arterial space until hemostasis is achieved. These devices may be used independently or in combination. Clip devices such as implantable clips can be used to pull the edges of the arteriotomy together for closure. Active devices shorten the time to achieve hemostasis as well as the time the patient must remain hospitalized post-procedure.

Complications: Persistent coronary artery spasms, dissection of the coronary artery, thrombosis, bleeding and hematoma formation. Other complications may arise depending on the type of closure

54

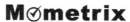

device utilized. For example, the use of clip devices may result in arterial laceration, occlusion of the artery or arterial stenosis.

PTCA AND STENT INSERTION

Percutaneous transluminal coronary angioplasty (PTCA) is a procedure done to reperfuse coronary arteries blocked by plaque or an embolus. Cardiac catheterization is done with a hollow catheter (sheath), usually inserted into the femoral vein or artery and fed through the vessels to the coronary arteries. When the atheroma is verified by fluoroscopy, a balloon-tipped catheter is fed over the sheath and the balloon is inflated with a contrast agent, to a specified pressure to compress the atheroma. The balloon may be inflated a number of times to ensure that residual stenosis is <20%. Laser angioplasty using the excimer laser is also used to vaporize plaque. **Stents** may be inserted during the angioplasty to maintain patency. Stents may be flexible plastic or wire mesh and are typically placed over the catheter, which is inflated to expand the stent against the arterial wall. All patients with a stent must be discharged on aspirin, an antiplatelet, and a statin.

Complications include:

- **Intraoperative**: Perforation/dissection of the coronary artery, arrythmias, vasospasm.
- **Postoperative**: Hemorrhage/hematoma at insertion site, thrombus/embolus, arteriovenous fistula/pseudoaneurysm, retroperitoneal bleed, and failure of angioplasty.

INTRAAORTIC BALLOON PUMP

The intra-aortic balloon pump (IABP) is a catheter with an inflatable balloon at the tip which is inserted through the femoral artery and threaded into the descending thoracic aorta. The balloon inflates during diastole to increase circulation to the coronary arteries, and then deflates during systole to decrease afterload. It is indicated in patients in cardiogenic/septic shock, acute heart failure, unstable angina, and papillary or ventricular septal rupture.

Contraindications: Aortic valve stenosis and large aortic aneurysms.

Complications: Stroke, peripheral ischemia, renal injury, air embolus, arrhythmias.

Nursing considerations are as follows:

- **Placement:**
  o Too High: Occludes the left subclavian artery: dizziness & decreased radial pulse.
  o Too Low: Occludes the renal artery: flank pain & sudden decrease in urine output.
  o Prevention: patient cannot bend his knee, sit up/flex his hips ≥ 45°.
- **Timing:** In ECG mode, the balloon should inflate in the T-wave and deflate with the R. Do site checks, I&O, neuro-checks, and vascular checks every hour.

NOTE: If a gas-leak alarm sounds OR you see blood in the catheter, this indicates balloon rupture/damage to the catheter. Immediately shut down the machine and place patient in Trendelenburg, notify physician.

Weaning: Decrease balloon volume/frequency to wean. Use flutter function to prevent embolus while the catheter is still in place. After removal, the physician will allow bleeding for five seconds to eject clots.

CABG

Coronary artery bypass graft (CABG) is a surgical procedure for treatment of angina that does not respond to medical treatment, unstable angina, blockage of >60% in left main coronary artery, blockage of multiple coronary arteries that include the proximal left anterior descending artery, left ventricular dysfunction, and previous unsuccessful PCIs. The surgery is performed through a midsternal incision that exposes the heart, which is chilled and placed on cardiopulmonary bypass with blood going from the right atrium to the machine and back to the body while the aorta is clamped to keep the surgical field free of blood. Bypass grafts are sutured into place to bypass areas of occluded coronary arteries. Grafts may be obtained from various sites: gastroepiploic artery, internal mammary artery, radial artery, saphenous vein (commonly used, especially for emergency procedures).

Complications: Arrythmias, infection, cardiac tamponade, cardiogenic shock, embolus/stroke, renal or pulmonary dysfunction

MIDCAB AND PORT ACCESS CORONARY ARTERY BYPASS GRAFT

Minimally-invasive direct coronary artery bypass (MIDCAB) applies a bypass graft through a 10 cm incision in the mid chest, without using cardiopulmonary bypass. Because the incision must be over the bypass area, this procedure is suitable only for bypass of one or two coronary arteries, usually on the left side of the heart. A small portion or rib is removed to allow access to the heart and the internal mammary artery is used for grafting. Special instruments, such as a heart stabilizer, are used to limited movement of the heart during suturing. Surgery usually takes 2-3 hours and recovery time is decreased as patients have less pain. Because anastomosis is difficult on a beating heart, complications such as ischemia may occur during surgery so a cardiopulmonary bypass machine must be available.

Port access coronary artery bypass graft is an alternative form of CABG that utilizes a number of small incisions (ports) along with cardiopulmonary bypass (CPB) and cardioplegia to do a video-assisted surgical repair. Usually 3 or more incisions are required, with one in the femoral area to allow access to the femoral artery for a multipurpose catheter that is threaded through to the ascending aorta to return blood from the CPB, block the aorta with a balloon, provide cardioplegic solution, and vent air. Another catheter is threaded through the femoral vein to the right atrium to carry blood to the CPB. An incision is also needed for access to the jugular vein for catheters to the pulmonary artery and the coronary sinus. One to three thoracotomy incisions are made for insertion of video imaging equipment and instruments. While the midsternal incision is avoided, multiple incisions pose the potential for possible increased morbidity.

CARDIOVERSION

Cardioversion is a timed electrical stimulation to the heart to convert a tachydysrhythmia (such as atrial fibrillation) to a normal sinus rhythm. Usually anticoagulation therapy is done for at least 3 weeks prior to elective cardioversion to reduce the risk of emboli and digoxin is discontinued for at least 48 hours prior. During the procedure, the patient is usually sedated and/or anesthetized. Electrodes in the form of gel-covered paddles or pads are placed in the anteroposterior position, and then connected by leads to a computerized ECG and cardiac monitor with a defibrillator. The defibrillator is synchronized with the ECG so that the electrical current is delivered during ventricular depolarization (QRS). The timing must be precise in order to prevent ventricular tachycardia or ventricular fibrillation. Sometimes, drug therapy is used in conjunction with cardioversion; for example, antiarrhythmics (Cardizem®, Cordarone®) may be given before the procedure to slow the heart rate.

Arrythmia: Beginning Monophasic Shock/Beginning Biphasic Shock

- **A fib:** 50-100 J/ 25 J.
- **A flutter:**25-50 J/ 15 J.
- **Vtach** (monomorphic asymptomatic):100-200 J / 50 J.

EMERGENCY DEFIBRILLATION

Emergency defibrillation is non-synchronized shock which is given to treat acute ventricular fibrillation, pulseless ventricular tachycardia, or polymorphic ventricular tachycardia with a rapid rate and decompensating hemodynamics. Defibrillation can be given at any point in the cardiac cycle. It causes depolarization of myocardial cells, which can then repolarize to regain a normal sinus rhythm. Defibrillation delivers an electrical discharge through pads/paddles. In an acute care setting, the preferred position to place the pads is the anteroposterior position. In this position one pad is placed to the right of the sternum, about the second to third intercostal space and the other pad is placed between the left scapula and the spinal column. This decreases the chances of damaging implanted devices, such as pacemakers, and this positioning has also been shown to be more effective for external cardioversion (if indicated at some point during resuscitation). There are two main types of defibrillator shock waveforms, monophasic and biphasic. Biphasic defibrillators deliver a shock one direction for half of the shock, and then in the return direction for the other half, making them more effective, and able to be used at lower energy levels. Monophasic defibrillation is given at 200-360 J and biphasic defibrillation is given at 100-200 J.

Respiratory

Pulmonary Embolism

ACUTE PULMONARY EMBOLISM

Acute pulmonary embolism occurs when a pulmonary artery or arteriole is blocked, cutting off blood supply to the pulmonary vessels and subsequent oxygenation of the blood. While most pulmonary emboli are from thrombus formation, other causes may be air, fat, or septic embolus (from bacterial invasion of a thrombus). Common originating sites for thrombus formation are the deep veins in the legs, the pelvic veins, and the right atrium. Causes include stasis related to damage to endothelial wall and changes in blood coagulation factors. Atrial fibrillation poses a serious risk because blood pools in the right atrium, forming clots that travel directly through the right ventricle to the lungs. The obstruction of the artery/arteriole causes an increase in alveolar dead space in which there is ventilation but impairment of gas exchange because of the ventilation/perfusion mismatching or intrapulmonary shunting. This results in hypoxia, hypercapnia, and the release of mediators that cause bronchoconstriction. If more than 50% of the vascular bed becomes excluded, pulmonary hypertension occurs.

SYMPTOMS AND DIAGNOSIS

Clinical manifestations of **acute pulmonary embolism** (PE) vary according to the size of the embolus and the area of occlusion.

Symptoms include:

- Dyspnea with tachypnea.
- Cyanosis; may turn grey/blue from nipple line up (massive PE).
- Anxiety and restlessness – "feeling of doom."
- Chest pain, tachycardia – may progress to arrhythmias (PEA).
- Fever.
- Rales.
- Cough (sometimes with hemoptysis).
- Hemodynamic instability.

Diagnostic tests are as follows:

- ABG analysis may show hypoxemia (decreased PaO_2), hypocarbia (decreased $PaCO_2$) and respiratory alkalosis (increased pH).
- D-dimer (will show elevation with PE but is not definitively diagnostic without a CT scan).
- ECG may show sinus tachycardia or other abnormalities.
- Echocardiogram can show emboli in the central arteries and can assess the hemodynamic status of the right side of the heart.
- Spiral CT may provide definitive diagnosis.
- V/Q scintigraphy can confirm diagnosis.
- Pulmonary angiograms also can confirm diagnosis.

MEDICAL MANAGEMENT

Medical management of **pulmonary embolism** starts with preventive measures for those at risk, including leg exercises, elastic compression stockings, and anticoagulation therapy. Most

58

pulmonary emboli present as medical emergencies, so the immediate task is to stabilize the patient. Medical management may include:

- **Oxygen** to relieve hypoxemia.
- **Intravenous infusions:** Dobutamine (Dobutrex®) or dopamine (Intropin®) to relieve hypotension.
- **Cardiac monitoring** for dysrhythmias and issues due to right sided heart failure.
- **Medications** as indicated: digitalis glycosides, diuretic, and antiarrhythmics.
- Intubation and mechanical ventilation may be required.
- **Analgesia** (such as morphine sulfate) or sedation to relieve anxiety.
- **Anticoagulants** to prevent recurrence (although it will not dissolve clots already present), including heparin and warfarin (Coumadin®).
- **Placement of percutaneous venous filter** (Greenfield) in the inferior vena cava to prevent further emboli from entering the lungs may be done if anticoagulation therapy is contraindicated.
- **Thrombolytic therapy,** recombinant tissue-type plasminogen activator (rt-PA) or streptokinase, for those severely compromised, but these treatments have limited success and pose the danger of bleeding.

Asphyxia

TRAUMATIC ASPHYXIA

Asphyxia may relate to a number of different injuries:

- **Traumatic asphyxia** most commonly involves a crush injury of the thorax, and traumatic injuries to multiple organs may be present. Crush injuries are characterized by petechiae in the area of compression although tight-fitting clothing, such as a woman's bra, may prevent petechiae from forming.
- **Manual strangulation** may involve crush injuries to the throat, such as hyoid fracture. Often the face appears cyanotic while the rest of the body does not. Petechiae may be present on the face as well. Bruising may be noted about the throat.
- **Ligature strangulation** is similar to manual although throat markings are different, with an indented area surrounding the neck.
- **Hanging** produces a V-shaped marking on the throat and does not encircle the neck.
- **Choking** obstructs the airway. (May require bronchoscopy to remove foreign object).

In all cases, immediate establishment of airway, breathing, and circulation (ABCs) takes precedence. Surgical intervention may be needed for traumatic crush injuries.

NEAR-DROWNING ASPHYXIA

Submersion asphyxiation can cause profound damage to the central nervous system, pulmonary dysfunction related to aspiration, cardiac hypoxia with life-threatening arrhythmias, fluid and electrolyte imbalances, and multi-organ damage, so treatment can be complex. Hypothermia related to near drowning has some protective affect because blood is shunted to the brain and heart. Treatment includes:

- Immediate establishment of airway, breathing and circulation (ABCs).
- NG tube and gastric decompression to reduce risk of aspiration.
- Neurological evaluation.

- Pulmonary management includes monitoring for ≥72 hours for respiratory deterioration. Ventilation may need positive-end expiratory pressure (PEEP), but this poses danger to cardiac output and can cause barotrauma, so use should be limited.
- In patients that are symptomatic but do not yet need intubation, use supplemental oxygen to keep $SpO_2 > 94\%$.
- Monitoring of cardiac output and function.
- Neurological care to reduce cerebral edema and increased intracranial pressure, and prevent secondary injury.
- Rewarming if necessary (0.5 to 1 °C/hr).

ARDS

ACUTE LUNG INJURY

Acute lung injury (ALI) comprises a syndrome of respiratory distress culminating in **acute respiratory distress syndrome (ARDS)**, a rare complication of cardiac surgery. ALI and ARDS usually occur more than 24 hours postoperatively. ARDS is characterized by damage to the vascular endothelium and an increase in the permeability of the alveolar–capillary membrane when damage to the lung results from toxic substances (e.g., gastric fluids, bacteria, chemicals, toxins emitted by neutrophils as part of the inflammatory-mediated response); these substances reduce surfactant and cause pulmonary edema as the alveoli fill with blood and protein-rich fluid and then collapse (atelectasis). This decrease in surfactant also leads to decreased lung compliance (sometimes referred to as stiffening). The fluid in the alveoli becomes a medium for infection. Because there is neither adequate ventilation nor perfusion, the result is increasing hypoxemia and tachypnea as the body tries to compensate to maintain a normal partial pressure of carbon dioxide. Untreated, the condition results in respiratory failure, MODS, and a mortality rate of 5-30%. Symptoms: #1 – refractory hypoxemia (hypoxemia not responding to increasing levels of oxygen), crackling rales/wheezing in lungs, ↓ in pulmonary compliance which results in ↑ tachypnea with expiratory grunting, cyanosis/skin mottling, hypotension and tachycardia, symptoms associated with volume overload are missing (3rd heart sound or JVD), respiratory alkalosis initially but replaced as the disease progresses with hypercarbia and respiratory acidosis, and normal X-ray initially but then diffuse infiltrates in both lungs, but the heart and vessels appear normal.

MANAGEMENT

The management of **acute respiratory distress syndrome (ARDS)** involves providing adequate gas exchange and preventing further damage to the lung from forced ventilation.

Treatment includes:

- Mechanical ventilation is often required to maintain oxygenation and ventilation.
- Corticosteroids (may increase mortality rates in some patient populations, though this is the most common given), nitrous oxide, inhaled surfactant, and anti-inflammatory medications.
- Treatment of the underlying condition is the only proven treatment, especially identifying and treating with appropriate antibiotics any infection, as sepsis is most common etiology for ARDS, but prophylactic antibiotics are not indicated.
- Conservative fluid management is indicated to reduce days on the ventilator, but does not reduce overall mortality.

Pharmacologic preventive care: Enoxaparin 40 mg subcutaneously QD, sucralfate 1 g NGT four times daily or omeprazole 40 mg IV QD, and enteral nutrition support within 24 hours of ICU admission or intubation.

VENTILATION MANAGEMENT

Ventilation management in ARDS consists of the following:

- O_2 therapy by nasal prongs/cannula or mask may be sufficient in very mild cases to maintain oxygen saturation above 90%. Oxygen should be administered at 100% because of the mismatch between ventilation (V) and perfusion (Q), which can result in hypoxia on position change.
- ARDS oxygenation goal is PaO_2 55-80 mmHg or SpO_2 88-95%.
- Many times, endotracheal intubation may be needed if SpO_2 falls or CO_2 levels rise.
- The ARDS Network recommends low tidal volumes (6 mL/kg) and higher PEEP (12 cmH$_2$O or more).
- The low tidal volume ventilation described above is referred to as lung protective ventilation, and it has been shown to reduce mortality in patients with ARDS.
- For patients with severe ARDS, trials placing patient in prone position 18-24 hours/day with chest and pelvis supported and abdomen unsupported allows the diaphragm to move posteriorly, increasing functional residual capacity (FRC) in many patients.

Acute Respiratory Failure

CARDINAL SIGNS

The **cardinal signs of respiratory failure** include:

- Tachypnea.
- Tachycardia.
- Anxiety and restlessness.
- Diaphoresis.

Symptoms may vary according to the cause. An obstruction may cause more obvious respiratory symptoms than other disorders. Early signs may include changes in the depth and pattern of respirations with flaring nares, sternal retractions, expiratory grunting, wheezing, and extended expiration as the body tries to compensate for hypoxemia and increasing levels of carbon dioxide. Cyanosis may be evident. Central nervous depression, with alterations in consciousness occurs with decreased perfusion to the brain. As the hypoxemia worsens, cardiac arrhythmias, including bradycardia, may occur with either hypotension or hypertension. Dyspnea becomes more pronounced with depressed respirations. Eventually stupor, coma, and death can occur if the condition is not reversed.

HYPOXEMIC AND HYPERCAPNIC RESPIRATORY FAILURE

Hypoxemic respiratory failure occurs suddenly when gaseous exchange of oxygen for carbon dioxide cannot keep up with demand for oxygen or production of carbon dioxide:

- PaO_2 <60 mmHg.
- $PaCO_2$ >40 mmHg.
- Arterial pH <7.35.

Hypoxemic respiratory failure can be the result of low inhaled oxygen, as at high elevations or with smoke inhalation. The following ventilatory mechanisms may be involved:

- Alveolar hypotension.
- Ventilation-perfusion mismatch (the most common cause).
- Intrapulmonary shunts.
- Diffusion impairment.

Hypercapnic respiratory failure results from an increase in $PaCO_2$ >45-50 mmHg associated with respiratory acidosis and may include:

- Reduction in minute ventilation, total volume of gas ventilated in one minute (often related to neurological, muscle, or chest wall disorders, drug overdoses, obstruction of upper airway.)
- Increased dead space with wasted ventilation (related to lung disease or disorders of chest wall, such as scoliosis).
- Increased production of CO_2 (usually related to infection, burns, or other causes of hypermetabolism).
- Oxygen saturation may be normal or below normal.

UNDERLYING CAUSES

There are a number of underlying causes for **respiratory failure:**

- **Airway obstruction:** Obstruction may result from an inhaled object or from an underlying disease process, such as cystic fibrosis, asthma, pulmonary edema, or infection.
- **Inadequate respirations:** This is a common cause among adults, especially related to obesity and sleep apnea. It may also be induced by an overdose of sedation medications such as opioids.
- **Neuromuscular disorders:** Those disorders that interfere with the neuromuscular functioning of the lungs or the chest wall, such as muscular dystrophy or spinal cord injuries can prevent adequate ventilation.
- **Pulmonary abnormalities:** Those abnormalities of the lung tissue, found in pulmonary fibrosis, burns, ARDS, and reactions to drugs, can lead to failure.
- **Chest wall abnormalities:** Disorders that impact lung parenchyma, such as severe scoliosis or chest wounds can interfere with lung functioning.

Nursing interventions to help prevent respiratory issues: turn, position, ambulate, cough, deep breathe, vibration and percussion treatments, hydrate the patient to help hydrate the airway secretions, and incentive spirometry.

MANAGEMENT

Respiratory failure must be **treated** immediately before severe hypoxemia causes irreversible damage to vital organs.

- **Identifying and treating** the underlying cause should be done immediately because emergency medications or surgery may be indicated. Medical treatments will vary widely depending upon the cause; for example, cardiopulmonary structural defects may require surgical repair, pulmonary edema may require diuresis, inhaled objects may require surgical removal, and infections may require aggressive antimicrobials.
- **Intravenous lines/ central lines** are inserted for testing, fluids and medications.

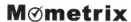

- **Oxygen therapy** should be initiated to attempt to reverse hypoxemia; however, if refractory hypoxemia occurs, then oxygen therapy alone will not suffice. Oxygen levels must be titrated carefully.
- **Intubation and mechanical ventilation** are frequently required to maintain adequate ventilation and oxygenation. Positive end expiratory pressure (PEEP) may be necessary with refractory hypoxemia and collapsed alveoli.
- **Respiratory status** must be monitored constantly, including arterial blood gases and vital signs.

Pneumonia/Aspiration

PNEUMONIA

Pneumonia is inflammation of the lung parenchyma, filling the alveoli with exudate. It is common throughout childhood and adulthood. Pneumonia may be a primary disease or may occur secondary to another infection or disease, such as lung cancer. Pneumonia may be caused by bacteria, viruses, parasites, or fungi. Common causes for community-acquired pneumonia (CAP) include:

- *Streptococcus pneumoniae.*
- *Legionella* species.
- *Haemophilus influenzae.*
- *Staphylococcus aureus.*
- *Mycoplasma pneumoniae.*
- Viruses.

Pneumonia may also be caused by chemical damage. Pneumonia is characterized by location:

- Lobar involves one or more lobes of the lungs. If lobes in both lungs are affected, it is referred to as "bilateral" or "double" pneumonia.
- Bronchial/lobular involves the terminal bronchioles and exudate can involve the adjacent lobules. Usually the pneumonia occurs in scattered patches throughout the lungs.
- Interstitial involves primarily the interstitium and alveoli where white blood cells and plasma fill the alveoli, generating inflammation and creating fibrotic tissue as the alveoli are destroyed.

HOSPITAL-ACQUIRED PNEUMONIA

Hospital-acquired pneumonia (HAP) is defined as pneumonia that did not appear to already be present on admission that occurs at least 48 hours after admission to a hospital. **Healthcare-associated pneumonia (HCAP)** is defined as pneumonia that occurs in a patient within 90 days of being hospitalized for 2 or more days at an acute care hospital or LTAC. **Ventilator-associated pneumonia (VAP)** is one type of hospital acquired pneumonia that a patient acquires more than 48 hours after having an ETT placed. The most common way that the patient is infected is via aspiration of bacteria that is colonized in the upper respiratory tract. It is estimated that close to 75% of patients that are critically ill will be colonized with multidrug resistant bacteria within 48 hours of entering an ICU. Aspiration occurs at a rate of about 45% in patients with no health problems and the rate is much higher in the ill. Combining this with the colonization of the critically ill, leads to high rates of HAP, HCAP, and VAP. The frequency of patients developing these types of pneumonia is increasing, with those at highest risk being those with immunosuppression, septic shock, currently hospitalized for more than five days, and those who have had antibiotics for

63

another infection within the previous three months. These types of pneumonia should be considered if a patient already hospitalized has purulent sputum or a change in respiratory status such as deoxygenating, in combination with a worsening or new chest x-ray infiltrate.

Treatment includes:

- Antibiotic therapy.
- Using appropriate isolation and precautions with infected patients.
- Preventive measures include maintaining ventilated patients in 30° upright positions, frequent oral care for vent patients, and changing ventilator circuits as per protocol.

Antibiotic treatment options for HAP, HCAP, and VAP should take into account many factors, including culture data (when available), patient's comorbidities, flora in the unit, any recent antibiotics by the patient, and whether the patient is at high risk for having multidrug resistant bacteria. As most critical care patients are at high risk, due to factors such as being in an ICU setting, ventilators, and comorbidities, antibiotic recommendations to follow are for coverage for patients with risk factors for multidrug resistant bacteria.

One of the following:

- Ceftazidime 2 g q 8 hours IV **OR**
- Cefepime 2 g q 8 hours IV **OR**
- Imipenem 500 mg q 6 hours IV **OR**
- Piperacillin-tazobactam 4.5 g q 6 hours IV

AND:

- Ciprofloxacin 400 mg q 8 hours IV **OR**
- Levaquin 750 mg QD IV

ASPIRATION PNEUMONITIS/PNEUMONIA

Aspiration pneumonitis/pneumonia may occur as the result of any type of aspiration, including foreign objects. The aspirated material creates an inflammatory response, with the irritated mucous membrane at high risk for bacterial infection secondary to the aspiration, causing pneumonia. Gastric contents and oropharyngeal bacteria are commonly aspirated. Gastric contents can cause a severe chemical pneumonitis with hypoxemia, especially if the pH is <2.5. Acidic food particles can cause severe reactions. With acidic damage, bronchospasm and atelectasis occur rapidly with tracheal irritation, bronchitis, and alveolar damage with interstitial edema and hemorrhage. Intrapulmonary shunting and V/Q mismatch may occur. Pulmonary artery pressure increases. Non-acidic liquids and food particles are less damaging, and symptoms may clear within 4 hours of liquid aspiration or granuloma may form about food particles in 1-5 days. Depending upon the type of aspiration, pneumonitis may clear within a week, ARDS or pneumonia may develop, or progressive acute respiratory failure may lead to death.

There are a number of risk factors that can lead to **aspiration pneumonitis/pneumonia:**

- Altered level of consciousness related to illness or sedation.
- Depression of gag, swallowing reflex.
- Intubation or feeding tubes.
- Ileus or gastric distention.
- Gastrointestinal disorders, such as gastroesophageal reflux disorders (GERD).

64

Diagnosis is based on clinical findings, ABGs showing hypoxemia, infiltrates observed on x-ray, and ↑ WBC if infection present.

Symptoms: similar to other pneumonias:

- Cough often with copious sputum
- Respiratory distress, dyspnea.
- Cyanosis.
- Tachycardia.
- Hypotension.

Treatment includes:

- Suctioning as needed to clear upper airway.
- Supplemental oxygen.
- Antibiotic therapy as indicated after 48 hours if symptoms not resolving.
- Symptomatic respiratory support.

FOREIGN BODY ASPIRATION

Foreign body aspiration can cause obstruction of the pharynx, larynx or trachea, leading to acute dyspnea or asphyxiation and the object may be drawn distally into the bronchial tree. With adults, most foreign bodies migrate more readily down the right bronchus. Food is the most frequently aspirated, but other small objects, such as coins or needles, may also be aspirated. Sometimes the object causes swelling, ulceration, and general inflammation that hampers removal.

Symptoms include:

- *Initial:* Severe coughing, gagging, sternal retraction, wheezing. Objects in the larynx may cause inability to breathe or speak and lead to respiratory arrest. Objects in the bronchus cause cough, dyspnea, and wheezing.
- *Delayed:* Hours, days, or weeks later, an undetected aspirant may cause an infection distal to the aspirated material. Symptoms depend on the area and extent of the infection.

Treatment includes:

- Removal with laryngoscopy or bronchoscopy (rigid is often better than flexible).
- Antibiotic therapy for secondary infection.
- Surgical bronchotomy (rarely required).
- Symptomatic support.

CHRONIC BRONCHITIS

Chronic bronchitis is a pulmonary airway disease characterized by severe cough with sputum production for at least 3 months a year for at least 2 consecutive years. Irritation of the airways (often from smoke or pollutants) causes an inflammatory response, increasing the number of mucus-secreting glands and goblet cells while ciliary function decreases so that the extra mucus plugs the airways. Additionally, the bronchial walls thicken and alveoli near the inflamed bronchioles become fibrotic, and alveolar macrophages cannot function properly, increasing susceptibility to infections. Chronic bronchitis is most common in those >45 years old and occurs twice as frequently in females as males.

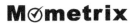

Symptoms include:

- Persistent cough with increasing sputum.
- Dyspnea.
- Frequent respiratory infections.

Treatment includes:

- Bronchodilators.
- Long term continuous oxygen therapy or supplemental oxygen during exercise may be needed.
- Pulmonary rehabilitation to improve exercise and breathing.
- Antibiotics during infections.
- Corticosteroids may be used for acute episodes.

Chronic Conditions

EMPHYSEMA

Emphysema, the primary component of COPD, is characterized by abnormal distention of air spaces at the ends of the terminal bronchioles, with destruction of alveolar walls so that there is less and less gaseous exchange and increasing dead space with resultant hypoxemia and hypercapnia and respiratory acidosis. The capillary bed is damaged as well, altering pulmonary blood flow and raising pressure in the right atrium (cor pulmonale) and pulmonary artery, leading to cardiac failure. Complications include respiratory insufficiency and failure. There are 2 primary types of emphysema (and both forms may be present):

- **Centrilobular** (the most common form) involves the central portion of the respiratory lobule, sparing distal alveoli and usually affects the upper lobes. Typical symptoms include abnormal ventilation-perfusion ratios, hypoxemia, hypercapnia, and polycythemia with right-sided heart failure.
- **Panlobular** involves enlargement of all air spaces, including the bronchiole, alveolar duct, and alveoli, but there is minimal inflammatory disease. Typical symptoms include hyperextended rigid barrel chest, marked dyspnea, weight loss, and active expiration.

CHRONIC ASTHMA

The 3 primary symptoms of **chronic asthma** are cough, wheezing, and dyspnea. In cough-variant asthma, a severe cough may be the only symptom, at least initially. Chronic asthma is characterized by recurring bronchospasm and inflammation of the airways resulting in airway obstruction. Asthma affects the bronchi and not the alveoli. While no longer considered part of COPD because airway obstruction is not constant and is responsive to treatment, over time fibrotic changes in the airways can result in permanent obstruction, especially if asthma is not treated adequately. Symptoms of chronic asthma include nighttime coughing, exertional dyspnea, tightness in the chest, and cough. Acute exacerbations may occur, sometimes related to triggers, such as allergies, resulting in increased dyspnea, wheezing, cough, tachycardia, bronchospasm, and rhonchi. Treatment of chronic asthma includes chest hygiene, identification and avoidance of triggers, prompt treatment of infections, bronchodilators, long-acting β-2 agonists, and inhaled glucocorticoids.

COPD

STAGES

Functional dyspnea, body mass index (BMI), and spirometry are used to assess the **stages of chronic obstructive pulmonary disease (COPD)**. Spirometry measures used are the ratio of forced expiratory volume in the first by second of expiration (FEV_1) after full inhalation to total forced vital capacity (FVC). Normal lung function decreases after age 35; so normal values are adjusted for height, weight, gender, and age:

- **Stage I** (mild): Minimal dyspnea with/without cough and sputum. FEV_1 is ≥80% of predicted rate and FEV_1: FVC = <70%
- **Stage 2** (moderate): Moderate to severe chronic exertional dyspnea with/without cough and sputum. FEV_1 is 50-80% of predicted rate and FEV_1: FVC = <70%.
- **Stage 3** (severe): As stage 2 but repeated episodes with increased exertional dyspnea and condition impacting quality of life. FEV_1 is 30-50% of predicted rate and FEV_1: FVC = <70%.
- **Stage 4** (very severe): Severe dyspnea and life-threatening episodes that severely impact quality of life. FEV_1 is 30% of predicted rate or <50% with chronic respiratory failure and FEV_1: FVC = <70%.

MANAGEMENT

COPD is not reversible, so management aims at slowing progressing, relieving symptoms, and improving quality of life:

- Smoking cessation is the primary means to slow progression and may require smoking cessation support in the form of classes or medications, such as Zyban®, nicotine patches or gum, clonidine, or nortriptyline.
- Bronchodilators, such as albuterol (Ventolin®) and salmeterol (Serevent), relieve bronchospasm and airway obstruction.
- Corticosteroids, both inhaled (Pulmicort®, Vanceril®) and oral (prednisone) may improve symptoms but are used most for associated asthma.
- Oxygen therapy may be long term continuous or used during exertion.
- Bullectomy (for bullous emphysema) to remove bullae (enlarged airspaces that do not ventilate).
- Lung volume reduction surgery may be done if involvement in lung is limited; however, mortality rates are high.
- Lung transplantation is a definitive high-risk option.
- Pulmonary rehabilitation includes breathing exercises, muscle training, activity pacing, and modification of activities.

CHRONIC VENTILATORY FAILURE

Chronic ventilatory failure occurs when alveolar ventilation fails to increase in response to increasing levels of carbon dioxide, usually associated with chronic pulmonary diseases, such as asthma and COPD, drug overdoses, or diseases that impair respiratory effort, such as Guillain-Barré and myasthenia gravis. Normally, the ventilatory system is able to maintain PCO_2 and pH levels within narrow limits, even though PO_2 levels may be more variable, but with ventilatory failure, the body is not able to compensate for the resultant hypercapnia, and pH falls, resulting in respiratory acidosis. Symptoms include increasing dyspnea with tachypnea, gasping respirations, and use of accessory muscles. Patients may become confused as hypercapnia causes increased intracranial pressure. If pH is <7.2, cardiac arrhythmias, hyperkalemia, and hypotension can occur as pulmonary arteries constrict and the peripheral vascular system dilates. Diagnosis is per symptoms, ABGs consistent with respiratory acidosis (PCO_2 >50 and pH <7.35), pulse oximetry, and chest x-ray. Treatment can include non-invasive PPV (BiPAP), endotracheal mechanical ventilation, corticosteroids, and bronchodilators.

Pleural Space Abnormalities

AIR LEAK SYNDROMES

Air leak syndromes may result in significant respiratory distress. Leaks may occur spontaneously or secondary to some type of trauma (accidental, mechanical, iatrogenic) or disease. As pressure increases inside alveoli, the alveolar wall pulls away from the perivascular sheath and subsequent alveolar rupture allows air to follow the perivascular planes and flow into adjacent areas. There are two categories

- **Pneumothorax:**
  o Air in the pleural space causes a lung to collapse.
- **Barotrauma/volutrauma** with air in the interstitial space (usually resolve over time):
  o Pneumoperitoneum is air in the peritoneal area, including the abdomen and occasionally the scrotal sac of male infants.
  o Pneumomediastinum is air in the mediastinal area between the lungs.
  o Pneumopericardium is air in the pericardial sac that surrounds the heart.
  o Subcutaneous emphysema is air in the subcutaneous tissue planes of the chest wall.
  o Pulmonary interstitial emphysema (PIE) is air trapped in the interstitium between the alveoli.

PNEUMOTHORAX

Pneumothorax occurs when there is a leak of air into the pleural space, resulting in complete or partial collapse of a lung.

Symptoms: Vary widely depending on the cause and degree of the pneumothorax and whether or not there is underlying disease: Acute pleuritic pain (95%), usually on the affected side, decreased breath sounds. In a *tension pneumothorax,* symptoms include tracheal deviation and hemodynamic compromise.

Diagnosis: Clinical findings; radiograph: 6-foot upright posterior-anterior; ultrasound may detect traumatic pneumothorax.

Treatment: Chest-tube thoracostomy with underwater seal drainage is the most common treatment for all types of pneumothorax.

- Tension pneumothorax: Immediate needle decompression and chest tube thoracostomy.
- Small pneumothorax, patient stable: Oxygen administration and observation for 3-6 hours. If no increase shown on repeat x-ray, patient may be discharged with another x-ray in 24 hours.
- Primary spontaneous pneumothorax: Catheter aspiration or chest tube thoracostomy.

PLEURAL EFFUSION AND EMPYEMA

Pleural effusion is accumulation of fluid in the pleural space, usually secondary to other disease processes, such as heart failure, TB, neoplasms, nephrotic syndrome, and viral respiratory infections. The fluid may be serous, bloody, or purulent (empyema) and transudative or exudative.

Signs and symptoms depend on underlying condition but includes dyspnea, from mild to severe. Tracheal deviation away from affected side may be evident. Diagnosis includes chest x-ray, lateral decubitus x-ray, CT, thoracentesis, and pleural biopsy. Treatment includes treating underlying cause, thoracentesis to remove fluid, insertion of chest tube, pleurodesis, or pleurectomy or pleuroperitoneal shunt (primarily with malignancy).

Empyema is a pleural effusion in which the collection of pleural fluid is thick and purulent, usually as a result of bacterial pneumonia or penetrating chest trauma. Empyema may also occur as a complication of thoracentesis or thoracic surgery. Signs and symptoms include acute illness with fever, chills, pain, cough, and dyspnea. Diagnosis is per chest CT and thoracentesis with culture and sensitivity. Treatment includes antibiotics and drainage of pleural space per needle aspiration, tube thoracostomy, or open chest drainage with thoracotomy.

Pulmonary Fibrosis, Pulmonary Hypertension, and Status Asthmaticus

PULMONARY FIBROSIS

Pulmonary fibrosis is a progressive disease of the lungs in which scarring of the tissue causes the lining of the lungs to thicken. This thickening prevents adequate oxygen exchange from occurring. The cause of pulmonary fibrosis is unknown, however environmental toxins such as asbestos, infections, smoking and occupational exposure to wood or metal dust may be contributing factors. The disease is more prevalent in males and the average age at the time of diagnosis is between 40 and 70. There may also be a genetic predisposition in the development of pulmonary fibrosis. The median survival for patients diagnosed with pulmonary fibrosis is less than five years.

Signs and symptoms: Shortness of breath, dry cough, fatigue, weight loss, and clubbing of the finger tips and nails

Diagnosis: Physical assessment, chest x-ray and/or computed tomography, pulmonary function tests, arterial blood gases and lung biopsy.

Treatment: There is no cure for pulmonary fibrosis and treatment options are minimal. Anti-inflammatory medications such as corticosteroids may be used for symptom management as well as supplemental oxygen therapy. Lung transplantation may be an option for some patients based on age and advancement of disease. Some patients may be eligible for participation in a clinical trial, as there are research efforts focused on treatment options to halt the progression of the disease.

PULMONARY HYPERTENSION AND PULMONARY ARTERIAL HYPERTENSION

Pulmonary arterial hypertension (PAH) is a progressive disease of the pulmonary arteries that can severely compromise cardiovascular patients. It may involve multiple processes. Usually the pulmonary vasculature adjusts easily to accommodate blood volume from the right ventricle. If there is increased blood flow, the low resistance causes vasodilation and vice versa. However, sometimes the pulmonary vascular bed is damaged or obstructed, and this can impair the ability to handle changing volumes of blood. In that case, an increase in flow will increase the pulmonary arterial pressure, increasing pulmonary vascular resistance (PVR). This in turn, increases pressure on the right ventricle (RV) with increased RV workload, and eventual RV hypertrophy with displacement of the intraventricular septum and tricuspid regurgitation (cor pulmonale). Over time, this leads to right heart failure and death. Pulmonary hypertension is usually diagnosed by right-sided heart catheterization and is indicated by systolic pulmonary artery pressure >30 mmHg and mean pulmonary artery pressure >25 mmHg. Non-invasive testing may include echocardiogram to look for cardiac changes.

TYPES

Pulmonary hypertension or pulmonary arterial hypertension (PAH) may be classified as primary (idiopathic) or secondary.

- **Primary (idiopathic) PAH** may result from changes in immune responses, pulmonary emboli, sickle cell disease, collagen diseases, Raynaud's, and the use of contraceptives. The cause may be unknown or genetic.
- **Secondary PAH** may result from pulmonary vasoconstriction brought on by hypoxemia related to COPD, sleep-disordered breathing, kyphoscoliosis, obesity, smoke inhalation, altitude sickness, interstitial pneumonia, and neuromuscular disorders. It may also be caused by a decrease in pulmonary vascular bed of 50-75%, which may result from pulmonary emboli, vasculitis, tumor emboli, and interstitial lung disease, such as sarcoidosis). Primary cardiac disease, such as congenital defects in infants, and acquired disorders, such as rheumatic valve disease, mitral stenosis, and left ventricular failure may also contribute to PAH.

TREATMENT OPTIONS FOR PAH

Medical treatment for **pulmonary arterial hypertension (PAH)** aims to identify and treat any underlying cardiac or pulmonary disease, control symptoms, and prevent complications:

- **Oxygen therapy** may be needed, especially supplemental oxygen during exercise.
- **Calcium channel blockers** may provide vasodilation for some patients.
- **Pulmonary vascular dilators**, such as IV epoprostenol (Flolan®) and subcutaneous treprostinil sodium (Remodulin®) and oral bosentan (Tracleer®) help to control symptoms and prolong life.
- **Anticoagulants**, such as warfarin (Coumadin®) are an important part of therapy because of recurrent pulmonary emboli. Studies have shown that anticoagulation increases survival rates.
- **Diuretics**, such as furosemide (Lasix®) may be needed to relieve edema and restrict fluids, especially with right ventricular hypertrophy.

In some patients who cannot be managed adequately through medical treatment, a heart-lung transplant may be considered as the only effective treatment for long-term survival.

STATUS ASTHMATICUS

PATHOPHYSIOLOGY

Status asthmaticus is a severe acute attack of asthma that does not respond to conventional therapy. An acute attack of asthma is precipitated by some stimulus, such as an antigen that triggers an allergic response, resulting in an inflammatory cascade that causes edema of the mucous membranes (swollen airway), contraction of smooth muscles (bronchospasm), increased mucus production (cough and obstruction), and hyperinflation of airways (decreased ventilation and shunting). Mast cells and T lymphocytes produce cytokines, which continue the inflammatory response through increased blood flow coupled with vasoconstriction and bronchoconstriction, resulting in fluid leakage from the vasculature. Epithelial cells and cilia are destroyed, exposing nerves and causing hypersensitivity. Sympathetic nervous system receptors in the bronchi stimulate bronchodilation.

Clinical Symptoms

The person with **status asthmaticus** will often present in acute distress, non-responsive to inhaled bronchodilators. Symptoms include:

- Signs of airway obstruction.
- Sternal and intercostal retractions.
- Tachypnea and dyspnea with increasing cyanosis.
- Forced prolonged expirations.
- Cardiac decompensation with ↑ left ventricular afterload and increased pulmonary edema resulting from alveolar-capillary permeability. Hypoxia may trigger and ↑ in pulmonary vascular resistance with ↑ right ventricular afterload.
- Pulsus paradoxus (decreased pulse on inspiration and increased on expiration) with extra beats on inspiration detected through auscultation but not detected radially. Blood pressure normally decreases slightly during inspiration, but this response is exaggerated. Pulsus paradoxus indicates increasing severity of asthma.
- Hypoxemia (with impending respiratory failure).
- Hypocapnia followed by hypercapnia (with impending respiratory failure).
- Metabolic acidosis.

Thoracic Trauma

Management of Pulmonary Trauma
Pulmonary Hemorrhage

Pulmonary hemorrhage is an acute life-threatening injury that often results in death prior to arrival at the hospital; however, those presenting with traumatic pulmonary hemorrhage, as from a blunt or penetrating injury, requires immediate surgical repair. Even with immediate surgery, survival after serious injury to a major pulmonary vessel is rare. It is important that a large bore IV be immediately inserted and fluid replacement begun while blood is typed and cross matched. The patient should be evaluated for shock and treatment, including colloid solutions, crystalloids, or blood, provided as indicated. Pulmonary hemorrhage may result in hemothorax. In some cases, pneumothorax may also be present, resulting in mediastinal shift that increases the difficulty of identifying and repairing the bleeding vessel. If the patient is stabilized, computed tomography may provide accurate diagnosis to isolate the area of hemorrhage.

Tracheal Perforation/Injury

Tracheal perforation/injury may result from external injury, such as from trauma from a vehicle accident or from an assault, such as a gunshot or knife wound or in some cases a laceration as a complication of percutaneous dilation tracheostomy (PDT) or other endotracheal tubes. In some cases, an inhaled foreign object may become lodged in the trachea and eventually erode the tissue. If the injury is severe, respiratory failure may cause death in a very short period of time, so rapid diagnosis and treatment is critical.

Symptoms include:

- Severe respiratory distress.
- Hemoptysis.
- Strider with progressive dysphonia.
- Pneumothorax, pneumomediastinum.
- Subcutaneous emphysema from air leaking from the pleural space into the tissues of the chest wall, neck, face, and even into the upper extremities.

Treatment includes:

- Intubation and non-surgical healing for small lacerations.
- Surgical repair for larger wounds or severe respiratory distress.

MANAGEMENT OF THORACIC TRAUMA

PULMONARY CONTUSION

Pulmonary contusion is the result of direct force to the lung, resulting in parenchymal injury and bleeding and edema that impact the capillary-alveoli juncture, resulting in intrapulmonary shunting as the alveoli and interstitium fill with fluid. Parenchymal injury reduces compliance and impairs ventilation. Diagnosis may be more difficult if other injuries, such as fractured ribs or pneumothorax are also present because they may all contribute to respiratory distress. CT scans provide the best diagnostic tool.

Symptoms vary widely depending upon the degree of injury:

- Mild dyspnea/
- Severe progressive dyspnea.
- Hemoptysis.
- Acute respiratory failure.

Treatment varies according to the injury:

- Close monitoring of arterial blood gases and respiratory status.
- Supplemental oxygen.
- Intubation and mechanical ventilation with positive-end expiratory pressure (PEEP) for more severe respiratory distress.
- Fluid management and diuretics to control pulmonary edema.
- Respiratory physiotherapy to clear secretions.

FRACTURED RIBS

Fractured ribs are usually the result of severe trauma, such as blunt force from a motor vehicle accident or physical abuse. Underlying injuries should be expected according to the area of fractures:

- Upper 2 ribs: Injuries to trachea, bronchi, or great vessels.
- Right-sided ≥ rib 8: Trauma to liver.
- Left-sided ≥ rib 8: Trauma to spleen.

Pain, often localized or experienced on respirations or compression of chest way may be the primary symptom of rib fractures, resulting in shallow breathing that can lead to atelectasis or pneumonia.

Diagnosis: Chest x-ray or CT scan.

Treatment is primarily supportive as rib fractures usually heal in about 6 weeks: however, preventing pulmonary complications (pneumothorax, hemothorax) often necessitates adequate pain control. Underlying injuries are treated according to the type and degree of injury:

- Supplemental oxygen.
- Analgesia may include NSAIDs, intercostal nerve blocks, and narcotics.
- Pulmonary physiotherapy.
- Rib Belts
- Surgical fixation (ORIF) is usually done only in those requiring thoracotomy for underlying injuries.
- Splinting

FLAIL CHEST

Flail chest is a more common injury in adults and older teens than children. It occurs when at least 3 adjacent ribs are fractured, both anteriorly and posteriorly, so that they float free of the rib cage. There may be variations, such as the sternum floating with ribs fractured on both sides. Flail chest results in a failure of the chest wall to support changes in intrathoracic pressure so that paradoxical respirations occur with the flail area contracting on inspiration and expanding on expiration. The lungs are not able to expand properly, decreasing ventilation, but the degree of respiratory distress may relate to injury to underlying structures more than the flail chest alone. **Treatment**:

- Initial stabilization with tape, one side only, don't wrap chest.
- Analgesia for pain relief.
- Respiratory physiotherapy to prevent atelectasis.
- Mechanical ventilation is usually not indicated unless needed for underlying injuries.
- Surgical fixation is usually done only in those requiring thoracotomy for underlying injuries.

HEMOTHORAX

Hemothorax occurs with bleeding into the pleural space, usually from major vascular injury such as tears in intercostal vessels, lacerations of great vessels, or trauma to lung parenchyma. A small bleed may be self-limiting and seal, but a tear in a large vessel can result in massive bleeding, followed quickly by hypovolemic shock. The pressure from the blood may result in inability of the lung to ventilate and a mediastinal shift. Often a hemothorax occurs with a pneumothorax, especially in severe chest trauma. Further symptoms include severe respiratory distress, decreased breath sounds, and dullness on auscultation.

Treatment includes placement of a chest tube to drain the hemothorax, but with large volumes, the pressure may be preventing exsanguination, which can occur abruptly as the blood drains and pressure is reduced, so a large bore intravenous line should be in place before placement of the chest tube and typed and cross-matched blood immediately available. Autotransfusion may be used, contraindicated if wound is older than three hours, possibility of bowel/stomach contamination, liver failure, and malignancy. Thoracotomy may be indicated after chest tube insertion if there is still hemodynamic instability, tension hemothorax, more than 1500 mL blood initially on insertion, or bleeding continues at a rate of >300 mL/hr.

Pulmonary Medication Management

PHARMACOLOGICAL AGENTS USED FOR ASTHMA

Numerous **pharmacological agents** are used for control of asthma, some long acting to prevent attacks and others that are short-acting to provide relief for acute episodes. Listed with each are the standard med and dosage used for urgent care:

- **β-Adrenergic agonists** include both long-acting and short-acting preparations used for relaxation of smooth muscles and bronchodilation, reducing edema and aiding clearance of mucus. Medications include salmeterol (Serevent), sustained release albuterol (Volmax ER®) and short-acting albuterol (Proventil®) and levalbuterol (Xopenex®). Albuterol 2.5 to 5 mg q 20 minutes x 3 doses by nebulizer.
- **Anticholinergics** aid in preventing bronchial constriction and potentiate the bronchodilating action of β-Adrenergic agonists. The most-commonly used medication is ipratropium bromide (Atrovent®) 500 mcg q 20 minutes x 3 doses by nebulizer.
- **Corticosteroids** provide anti-inflammatory action by inhibiting immune responses, decreasing edema, mucus, and hyper-responsiveness. Because of numerous side effects, glucocorticosteroids are usually administered orally or parenterally for ≤5 days (prednisone, prednisolone, methylprednisolone) and then switched to inhaled steroids. If a person receives glucocorticoids for more than 5 days, then dosages are tapered. Methylprednisolone 60 to 125 mg IV is the standard dose for respiratory failure. The Global Initiative for Asthma (GINA) recommends daily inhaled corticosteroids for all individuals with severe asthma to reduce the risk of exacerbations.
- **Methylxanthines** are used to improve pulmonary function and decrease need for mechanical ventilation. Medications include aminophylline and theophylline.
- **Magnesium sulfate** is used to relax smooth muscles and decrease inflammation. If administered intravenously, it must be given slowly to prevent hypotension and bradycardia. Inhaled, it potentiates the action of albuterol. Standard dosage: 2 g (8 mmol) IV x 1 dose over 20 minutes.
- **Heliox** (helium-oxygen) is administered to decrease airway resistance with airway obstruction, thereby decreasing respiratory effort. Heliox improves oxygenation of those on mechanical ventilation.
- **Leukotriene inhibitors** are used to inhibit inflammation and bronchospasm for long-term management. Medications include montelukast (Singulair®).

PULMONARY PHARMACOLOGY

There are a wide range of agents used for **pulmonary pharmacology**, depending upon the type and degree of pulmonary disease. Agents include:

- **Opioid analgesics:** Used to provide both pain relief and sedation for those on mechanical ventilation to reduce sympathetic response. Medications may include fentanyl (Sublimaze®) or morphine sulfate (MS Contin®).
- **Neuromuscular blockers:** Used for induced paralysis of those who have not responded adequately to sedation, especially for intubation and mechanical ventilation. Medications may include pancuronium (Pavulon®) and vecuronium (Norcuron®). However, there is controversy about the use as induced paralysis has been linked to increased mortality rates, sensory hearing loss (pancuronium), atelectasis, and ventilation-perfusion mismatch.
- **Human B-type natriuretic peptides:** Used to reduce pulmonary capillary wedge pressure. Medications include nesiritide (Natrecor®).

- **Surfactants**: Reduces surface tension to prevent collapse of alveoli. Beractant (Survanta®) is derived from bovine lung tissue and calfactant (Infasurf®) from calf lung tissue. They are administered as inhalants.
- **Alkalinizers**: Used to treat metabolic acidosis and ↓ pulmonary vascular resistance by achieving an alkaline pH. Medications include sodium bicarbonate and tromethamine (THAM).
- **Pulmonary vasodilator (inhaled nitric oxide):** Used to relax the vascular muscles and produce pulmonary vasodilation. Some studies show it reduces need for extracorporeal membrane oxygenation (ECMO).
- **Methylxanthines:** Used to stimulate muscle contractions of chest and stimulate respirations. Medications include aminophylline (Aminophylline®), caffeine citrate (Cafcit®), and doxapram (Dopram®).
- **Diuretics**: Used to reduce pulmonary edema. Medications include loop diuretics such as furosemide (Lasix®) and metolazone (Mykrox®).
- **Nitrates**: Used for vasodilation to reduce preload and afterload to reduce myocardial need for oxygen. Medications include nitroglycerin (Nitro-Bid®) and nitroprusside sodium (Nitropress®).
- **Antibiotics**: Used for treatment of respiratory infections, including pneumonia. Medications are used according to the pathogenic agent and may include macrolides, such as azithromycin (Zithromax®), erythromycin (E-Mycin®).
- **Antimycobacterials**: Used for treatment of TB and other mycobacterial diseases. Medications include isoniazid (Laniazid®, Nydrazid®), ethambutol (Myambutol®), rifampin (Rifadin®), streptomycin sulfate, and pyrazinamide.
- **Antivirals**: Used to inhibit replication of virus early in a viral infection. Effectiveness decreases as time passes because replication process has already begun. Medications include ribavirin (Virazole®) and zanamivir (Relenza®).

Pulmonary Diagnostics, Assessment, and Management

DIAGNOSTIC PROCEDURES AND TOOLS FOR ASSESSMENT OF PULMONARY TRAUMA/DISEASE

The **diagnostic procedures** and tools used during assessment of **pulmonary and thoracic trauma/disease** will vary according to the type and degree of injury/disease, but may include:

- **Thorough physical examination** including cardiac and pulmonary status, assessing for any abnormalities.
- **Electrocardiogram** to assess for cardiac arrhythmias.
- **Chest x-ray** should be done for all those with injuries to check for fractures, pneumothorax, major injuries, and placement of intubation tubes. X-rays can be taken quickly and with portable equipment so they can be completed quickly during the initial assessment.
- **Computerized tomography** may be indicated after initial assessment, especially if there is a possibility of damage to the parenchyma of the lungs.
- **Oximetry and atrial blood gases** as indicated.
- **12-lead electrocardiogram** may be needed if there are arrhythmias for more careful observation.
- **Echocardiogram** should be done if there is apparent cardiac damage.

BRONCHOSCOPY

Bronchoscopy utilizes a thin flexible fiberoptic bronchoscope to inspect the larynx, trachea, and bronchi for diagnostic purposes. It is also used to collect specimens, obtain biopsies, remove foreign bodies or secretions, treat atelectasis, and to excise lesions. The patient is in supine position during the procedure. The Mallampati classification may be used to determine difficulty of airway. The patient receives local anesthesia to the nares (lidocaine gel) and oropharynx (lidocaine gel, spray, or nebulizer), and usually receives a benzodiazepine (commonly midazolam or lorazepam), an opioid (fentanyl or meperidine), or propofol. Medications are usually given in small incremental doses through the procedure and may be combined. Oversedation may cause physiologic depression, but undersedation may result in recall and agitation with sympathetic activation. The tube is advanced through the nares and down the trachea to the bronchi. Airway patency, respiratory rate, and oxygen saturation must be constantly monitored. Complications can include bleeding, arrhythmias, obstruction, laryngospasm, and respiratory failure.

ARTERIAL BLOOD GASES

Arterial blood gases (ABGs) are monitored to assess effectiveness of oxygenation, ventilation, and acid-base status, and to determine oxygen flow rates. Partial pressure of a gas is that exerted by each gas in a mixture of gases, proportional to its concentration, based on total atmospheric pressure of 760 mmHg at sea level. Normal values include:

- **Acidity/alkalinity (pH)**: 7.35-7.45.
- **Partial pressure of carbon dioxide ($PaCO_2$)**: 35-45 mmHg.
- **Partial pressure of oxygen (PaO_2)**: ≥80 mg Hg.
- **Bicarbonate concentration (HCO_3^-)**: 22-26 mEq/L.
- **Oxygen saturation (SaO_2)**: ≥95%.

The relationship between these elements, particularly the $PaCO_2$ and the PaO_2 indicates respiratory status. For example, $PaCO_2$ >55 and the PaO_2 <60 in a patient previously in good health indicates respiratory failure. There are many issues to consider. Ventilator management may require a higher $PaCO_2$ to prevent barotrauma and a lower PaO_2 to reduce oxygen toxicity.

CAPNOGRAPHY WITH END-TIDAL CO_2 DETECTOR

Capnometry utilizes an **end-tidal CO_2 (ETCO) detector** that measures the concentration of CO_2 in expired air, usually through pH sensitive paper that changes color (commonly purple to yellow). Typically, the capnometer is attached to the ETT and a bag-valve-mask (BVM) ventilator attached. The capnogram provides data in the shape of a waveform that represents the partial pressure of exhaled gas. It is often used to confirm placement of endotracheal tubes as clinical assessment is not always sufficient, and it is a noninvasive mode of monitoring carbon dioxide in the respiratory cycle. Information provided by the capnogram includes:

- $PaCO_2$ level.
- Type and degree of bronchial obstruction, such as COPD (waveform changes from rectangular to a fin-like).
- Air leaks in the ventilation system.
- Rebreathing precipitated by need for new CO_2 absorber.
- Cardiac arrest.
- Hypothermia or reduced metabolism.

AIRWAY CLEARANCE

Airway clearance, the ability to move secretions/foreign particles from the upper airway and prevent aspiration, depends on an intact and functioning mucociliary system and the ability to cough effectively. Mucous provides barrier protection to the tissue, and the cilia mechanically move mucous and particles upward. Inflammation, asthma, COPD, CF, and mechanical ventilation can alter the viscosity of the mucous and impair its effectiveness. CF, lung transplantation, mechanical irritation, and smoking can damage cilia. Patients with tracheostomies and/or mechanical ventilation tend to retain secretions, impairing the exchange of oxygen and increasing the effort required to breathe, leading to increased inflammation and infection that further impairs lung function. Both increased and retained secretions lead to decreased FEV1 and higher mortality rates. Cough is impaired by mechanical ventilation as well as restrictive and obstructive respiratory diseases. Airway clearance measures include:

- Directed cough, chest physiotherapy (if not on ventilator).
- Positioning with head of bed elevated.
- Suctioning as needed (limited to 5 seconds in duration).
- Antibiotics for infection.
- Bronchodilators.
- Airway clearance devices.

AIRWAY DEVICES

OROPHARYNGEAL, NASOPHARYNGEAL, AND TRACHEOSTOMY TUBES

Airways are used to establish a patent airway and facilitate respirations:

- **Oropharyngeal**: This plastic airway curves over the tongue and creates space between the mouth and the posterior pharynx. It is used for anesthetized or unconscious patients to keep tongue and epiglottis from blocking the airway.
- **Nasopharyngeal** (trumpet): This smaller flexible airway is more commonly used in conscious patients and is inserted through one nostril, extending to the nasopharynx. It is commonly utilized in patients who need frequent suctioning.
- **Tracheostomy tubes**: Tracheostomy may be utilized for mechanical ventilation. Tubes are inserted into the opening in the trachea to provide a conduit and maintain the opening. The tube is secured with ties around the neck. Because the air entering the lungs through the tracheostomy bypasses the warming and moistening effects of the upper airway, air is humidified through a room humidifier or through delivery of humidified air through a special mask or mechanical ventilation. If the tracheostomy is going to be long-term, eventually a stoma will form at the site and the tube can be removed.

LARYNGEAL MASK AIRWAY

The **laryngeal-mask airway** (LMA) is an intermediate airway allowing ventilation but not complete respiratory control. The LMA consists of an inflatable cuff (the mask) with a connecting tube. It may be used temporarily before tracheal intubation or when tracheal intubation can't be done. It can also be a conduit for later blind insertion of an endotracheal tube. The head and neck must be in neutral position for insertion of the LMA. If the patient has a gag reflex, conscious sedation or topical anesthesia (deep oropharyngeal) is required. The LMA is inserted by sliding along the hard palate, using the finger as a guide, into the pharynx, and the ring is inflated to create a seal about the opening to the larynx, allowing ventilation with mild positive-pressure. The ProSeal® LMA has a modified cuff that extends onto the back of the mask to improve seal. LMA is

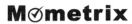

contraindicated in morbid obesity, obstructions or abnormalities of oropharynx, and non-fasting patients, as some aspiration is possible even with the cuff seal inflated.

ESOPHAGEAL-TRACHEAL COMBITUBE®

The **esophageal tracheal Combitube®** (ETC) is an intermediate airway that contains two lumens and can be inserted into either the trachea or the esophagus (≤91%). The twin-lumen tube has a proximal cuff providing a seal of the oropharynx and a distal cuff providing a seal about the distal tube. Prior to insertion, the Combitube® cuffs should be checked for leaks (15 mL of air into distal and 85 mL of air into proximal). The patient should be non-responsive and with absent gag reflex with head in neutral position. The tube is passed along the tongue and into the pharynx, utilizing markings on the tube (black guidelines) to determine depth by aligning the ETC with the upper incisors or alveolar ridge. Once in place the distal cuff is inflated (10-15 mL) and then placement in the trachea or esophagus should be determined, so the proper lumen for ventilation can be used. The proximal cuff is inflated (usually to 50-75 mL) and ventilation begun. Capnogram should be used to confirm ventilation.

CHEST TUBES

Chest tubes with a closed drainage system are usually left in place after thoracic surgery or pneumothorax to drain air or fluid. Nursing interventions during insertion include ensuring the patient receives adequate pain control, attending to sterile technique, assisting physician with suturing as needed, attaching the tube to the chest tube drainage device, placing an occlusive dressing, and confirming placement.

Chest tube drainage systems have 3 major parts: suction control, water seal, and a chamber for collection. The system should have no bubbling in the water seal area (such would indicate a leak), but a subtle rise and fall of the water seal corresponding with respirations, and gentle bubbling in the suction control chamber.

Nursing interventions after chest tube is in place: In most circumstances, report drainage >100 mL/hr, assess tubing after position changes for occlusion, maintain sterile dressing, avoid stripping the tubing, and assessing the insertion site for drainage or crepitus, the tubing, the patency of the entire system, and the output (including color, amount, and any other traits). The nurse should be knowledgeable about specimen collection, replacing the system, and dealing with clots.

Non-Invasive Ventilation

NASAL CANNULA

A **nasal cannula** can be used to deliver supplemental oxygen to a patient, but it is only useful for flow rates ≤6 L/min as higher rates are drying of the nasal passages. As it is not an airtight system, some ambient air is breathed in as well so oxygen concentration ranges from about 24-44%. The nasal cannula does not allow for control of respiratory rate, so the patient must be able to breathe independently.

NON-REBREATHER MASK

A **non-rebreather mask** can be used to deliver higher concentrations (60-90%) of oxygen to those patients who are able to breathe independently. The mask fits over the nose and mouth and is secured by an elastic strap. A 1.5 L reservoir bag is attached and connects to an oxygen source. The bag is inflated to about 1 liter at a rate of 8-15 L/min before the mask is applied as the patient breathes from this reservoir. A one-way exhalation valve prevents most exhaled air from being rebreathed.

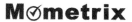

NON-INVASIVE POSITIVE PRESSURE VENTILATORS

Non-invasive positive pressure ventilators provide air through a tight-fitting nasal or facemask, usually pressure cycled, avoiding the need for intubation and reducing the danger of hospital-acquired infection and mortality rates. It can be used for acute respiratory failure and pulmonary edema. There are 2 types of non-invasive positive pressure ventilators:

- **CPAP (Continuous positive airway pressure)** provides a steady stream of pressurized air throughout both inspiration and expiration. CPAP improves breathing by decreasing preload for patients with congestive heart failure. It reduces the effort required for breathing by increasing residual volume and improving gas exchange.
- **Bi-PAP (Bi-level positive airway pressure)** provides a steady stream of pressurized air as CPAP but it senses inspiratory effort and increases pressure during inspiration. Bi-PAP pressures for inspiration and expiration can be set independently. Machines can be programmed with a backup rate to ensure a set number of respirations per minute.

*NEVER place a patient in wrist restraints while wearing these devices. If the patient vomits, they need to be able to remove the mask to prevent aspiration.

FACEMASK

Ensuring that a **facemask** (Ambu bag) is the correct fit and type is important for adequate ventilation, oxygenation, and prevention of aspiration. Difficulties in management of facemask ventilation relate to risk factors: >55 years, obesity, beard, edentulous, and history of snoring. In some cases, if dentures are adhered well, they may be left in place during induction. The facemask is applied by lifting the mandible (jaw thrust) to the mask and avoiding pressure on soft tissue. Oral or nasal airways may be used, ensuring that the distal end is at the angle of the mandible. There are a number of steps to prevent mask airway leaks:

- Increasing or decreasing the amount of air to the mask to allow better seal.
- Securing the mask with both hands while another person ventilates.
- Accommodating a large nose by using the mask upside down.
- Utilizing a laryngeal mask airway if excessive beard prevents seal.

HIGH AND LOW FLOW OXYGEN DELIVERY

High flow oxygen delivery devices provide oxygen at flow rates higher than the patient's inspiratory flow rate at specific medium to high FIO_2, up to 100%. However, a flow of 100% oxygen actually provides only 60 to 80% FIO_2 to the patient because the patient also breathes in some room air, diluting the oxygen. The actual amount of oxygen received depends on the type of interface or mask. Additionally, the flow rate is actually less than the inspiratory flow rate upon actual delivery. High flow oxygen delivery is usually not used in the sleep center. Humidification is usually required because the high flow is drying.

Low flow oxygen delivery devices provide 100% oxygen at flow rates lower than the patient's inspiratory flow rate, but the oxygen mixes with room air, so the FIO_2 varies. Humidification is usually only required if flow rate is >3L/min. Much oxygen is wasted with exhalation, so a number of different devices to conserve oxygen are available. Interfaces include transtracheal catheters and cannulae with reservoirs.

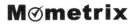

Mechanical Ventilation

INDICATIONS FOR MECHANICAL VENTILATION FOR STATUS ASTHMATICUS

Mechanical ventilation (MV) for status asthmaticus should be avoided if possible because of the danger of increased bronchospasm as well as barotrauma and decreased circulation. However, there are some absolute indications for the use of intubation and ventilation and a number of other indications that are evaluated on an individual basis.

The following are **absolute indications for MV**:

- Cardiac and/or pulmonary arrest.
- Markedly depressed mental status (obtundation).
- Severe hypoxia and/or apnea.

The following are **relative indications for MV**:

- Exhaustion/muscle fatigue from exertion of breathing.
- Sharply diminished breath sounds and no audible wheezing.
- Pulse paradoxus >20-40 mmHg; absent = imminent respiratory arrest.
- PaO_2 <70 mmHg on 100% oxygen.
- Dysphonia.
- Central cyanosis.
- Increased hypercapnia.
- Metabolic/respiratory acidosis: pH <7.20.

In this patient population, ventilator goal is to minimize airway pressures while oxygenating the patient. Vent settings include: low tidal volume (6-8 mL/kg), low respiratory rate (10-14 respirations/minute), and high inspiratory flow rate (80-100 L/min).

> **Review Video: Medical Ventilators**
> Visit mometrix.com/academy and enter code: 679637

ENDOTRACHEAL INTUBATION

Endotracheal intubation is often necessary with respiratory failure for control of hypoxemia, hypercapnia, hypoventilation, and/or obstructed airway. Equipment should be assembled and tubes and connections checked for air leaks with a 10 mL syringe. The mouth and/or nose should be cleaned of secretions and suctioned if necessary. The patient should be supine with the patient's head level with the lower sternum of the clinician. With orotracheal/endotracheal intubation, the clinician holds the laryngoscope (in left hand) and inserts it into right corner of mouth, the epiglottis is lifted and the larynx exposed. A thin flexible intubation stylet may be used and the endotracheal tube (ETT) (in right hand) is inserted through the vocal cords and into the trachea, cuff inflated to minimal air leak (10 mL initially until patient stabilizes), and placement confirmed through capnometry or esophageal detection devices. The correct depth of insertion is verified: 21 cm (female), 23 cm (male). After insertion, the tube is secured.

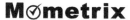

CONFIRMING CORRECT PLACEMENT OF ENDOTRACHEAL TUBES

There are a number of methods to confirm correct placement of **endotracheal tubes**. Clinical assessment alone is not adequate.

- **Capnometry** utilizes an end-tidal CO_2 (ETCO$_2$) detector that measures the concentration of CO_2 in expired air, usually through pH sensitive paper that changes color (commonly purple to yellow). The capnometer is attached to the ETT and a bag-valve-mask (BVM) ventilator attached. The patient is provided 6 ventilations and the CO_2 concentration checked.
- **Capnography** is attached to the ETT and provides a waveform graph, showing the varying concentrations of CO_2 in real time throughout each ventilation (with increased CO_2 on expiration) and can indicate changes in respiratory status.
- **Esophageal detection devices** fit over the end of the ETT so that a large syringe can be used to attempt to aspirate. If the ETT is in the esophagus, the walls collapse on aspiration and resistance occurs whereas the syringe fills with air if the ETT is in the trachea. A self-inflating bulb (Ellick® device) may also be used.
- **Chest X-ray** provides visual confirmation of placement.

VENTILATOR MANAGEMENT

There are many types of ventilators now in use, and the specific directions for use of each type must be followed carefully, but there are general principles that apply to all **ventilator management.** The following should be monitored:

- **Type of ventilation:** Volume-cycled, pressure-cycled, negative-pressure, HFJV, HFOV, CPAP, Bi-PAP.
- **Control mode**: Controlled ventilation, assisted ventilation, synchronized intermittent mandatory [allows spontaneous breaths between ventilator-controlled inhalation/exhalation], positive-end expiratory pressure (PEEP) [positive pressure at end of expiration], CPAP, Bi-PAP.
- **Tidal volume** (TV) range should be set in relation to respiratory rate.
- **Inspiratory-expiratory ratio** (I: E) usually ranges from 1:2-1:5, but may vary.
- **Respiratory rate** will depend upon TV and PaCO$_2$ target.
- **Fraction of inspired oxygen** (FiO$_2$) [percentage of oxygen in the inspired air], usually ranging from 21-100%, usually maintained <40% to avoid toxicity.
- **Sensitivity** determines the effort needed to trigger inspiration.
- **Pressure** controls the pressure exerted in delivering TV.
- **Rate of flow** controls the L/min speed of TV.

HIGH FREQUENCY JET VENTILATION

High frequency jet ventilation (HFJV) (Life Pulse®) directs a high velocity stream of air into the lungs in a long spiraling spike that forces carbon dioxide against the walls, penetrating dead space and providing gas exchange by using small tidal volumes of 1-3 mL/kg, much smaller than with conventional mechanical ventilation. Because the jet stream technology is effective for short distances, the valve and pressure transducer must be placed by the person's head. Inhalation is controlled while expiration is passive, but the rate of respiration is up to 11 per second ("panting" respirations). HFJV may be used in conjunction with low-pressure conventional ventilation to increase flow to alveoli. HFJV reduces barotrauma because of the low tidal volume and low pressure. HFJV is used for numerous conditions, including evolving chronic lung disease, pulmonary interstitial emphysema, bronchopulmonary dysplasia, and hypoxemic respiratory

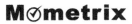

failure. It reduces mean airway pressure (MAP) and the oxygenation index. Treatment with HFJV may reduce the need for ECMO.

HIGH FREQUENCY OSCILLATORY VENTILATION

High frequency oscillatory ventilation (HFOV) provides pressurized ventilation with tidal volumes approximately equal to dead space at about 150 breaths per minutes (BPM). Pressure is usually higher with HFOV than HFJV in order to maintain expansion of the alveoli and to keep the airway open during gas exchange. Oxygenation is regulated separately. HFOV has both an active inspiration and expiration, so the respiratory cycle is completely controlled. HFOV reduces pulmonary vascular resistance and improves ventilation-perfusion matching and oxygenation without injuring the lung, reducing the risk of barotrauma. HFOV is used for respiratory distress syndrome, persistent pulmonary hypertension, more commonly for infants and children, but there is increasing interest in using HFOV with adults because of the smaller tidal volume that prevents overinflation of the lungs and atelectasis of those with ARDS.

POSITIVE PRESSURE VENTILATORS

Positive pressure ventilators assist respiration by applying pressure directly to the airway, inflating the lungs, forcing expansion of the alveoli, and facilitating gas exchange. Generally, endotracheal intubation or tracheostomy is necessary to maintain positive pressure ventilation for extended periods. There are 3 basic kinds of positive pressure ventilators:

- **Pressure cycled:** This type of ventilation is usually used for short-term treatment in adolescents or adults. The IPPB machine is the most common type. This delivers a flow of air to a preset pressure and then cycles off. Airway resistance or changes in compliance can affect volume of air and may compromise ventilation.
- **Time cycled**: This type of ventilation regulates the volume of air the patient receives by controlling the length of inspiration and the flow rate.
- **Volume cycled**: This type of ventilation provides a preset flow of pressurized air during inspiration and then cycles off and allows passive expiration, providing a fairly consistent volume of air.

VENTILATION-INDUCED LUNG INJURY

Ventilation-induced lung injury (VILI) is damage caused by mechanical ventilation. It is common in acute distress syndrome (ARDS) but can affect any mechanically ventilated patient. VILI comprises 4 interrelated elements:

- **Barotrauma**: Damage to the lung caused by excessive pressure.
- **Volutrauma**: Alveolar damage related to high tidal volume ventilation.
- **Atelectotrauma**: Injury caused by repetitive forced opening and closing of alveoli.
- **Biotrauma**: Inflammatory response.

In VILI, essentially the increased pressure and tidal volume over-distends the alveoli, which rupture, and air moves into the interstitial tissue resulting in pulmonary interstitial emphysema. With continued ventilation, the air in the interstitium moves into the subcutaneous tissue and may result in pneumopericardium and pneumomediastinum, or rupture the pleural sac which can cause tension pneumothorax and mediastinal shift, which can cause respiratory failure and cardiac arrest. VILI has caused a change in ventilation procedures with lower tidal volumes and pressures used as well as newer forms of ventilation, HFJV and HFOV, preferred to traditional mechanical ventilation for many patients.

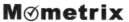

PREVENTING COMPLICATIONS FROM VENTILATORS

Methods to **prevent complications from mechanical ventilation ("ventilator bundle")** include:

- Elevate patient's head and chest to 30° to prevent aspiration and ventilation-associated pneumonia.
- Reposition patient every 2 hours.
- Provide DVT prophylaxis, such as external compression support and/or heparin (5000 u sq 2-3 times daily).
- Administer famotidine or pantoprazole PO/IV daily to prevent gastrointestinal stress-ulcers / bleeding.
- Decrease and eliminate sedation/analgesia as soon as possible – regular sedation vacations to assess neurological status.
- Follow careful protocols for pressure settings to prevent barotrauma. Tidal volumes are usually maintained at 8 to 12 mL/kg PBW (per AACN guidelines), but in incidences of high probability of ARDS, volumes should be less (6 mL/kg) to avoid lung injury.
- Monitor for pneumothorax or evidence of barotrauma.
- Conduct nutritional assessment (including lab tests) to prevent malnutrition.
- Monitor intake and output carefully and administer IV fluids to prevent dehydration.
- Do daily spontaneous breathing trials and discontinue ventilation as soon as possible.

VENTILATOR WEANING

Ventilator weaning has 3 phases: Changing settings of the ventilator to allow the patient to demonstrate the ability to breath on their own (standby mode), extubation, and finally removal of supportive oxygen. Criteria for ventilator weaning include:

- Vital capacity 10 to 15 mL/kg.
- Maximum (negative) inspiratory pressure of at least -20 cmH$_2$O.
- Tidal volume (TV) of 7 to 9 mL/kg.
- Minute ventilation of about 6L/min (Respiratory rate x TV).
- Rapid shallow breath index <100 breaths/m/L.
- PaO$_2$ >60 mmHg.
- FiO$_2$ <40%.

If these criteria are met and the patient passes a spontaneous breathing trial (SBT), then extubation can be done. Various protocols are followed in weaning patients off of ventilators, including the use of intermittent mandatory ventilation (IMV) and synchronized intermittent mandatory ventilation (SIMV), which can be used with pressure support ventilation (PSV). **Criteria for oxygen weaning**:

- FiO$_2$ reduced until PaO$_2$ 70 to 100 mmHg on room air.
- Supplemental O$_2$ necessary with PaO$_2$ < 70 mmHg (Medicare requires PaO$_2$ 55 mmHg for reimbursement for home oxygen use).

SPONTANEOUS BREATHING TRIAL AS PREPARATION FOR EXTUBATION

A **spontaneous breathing trial** (SBT) is when a patient is taken off mechanical ventilation while remaining intubated (usually by changing the ventilator settings to CPAP) for a short period of time to assess readiness to extubate. SBT should be used prior to extubating a patient if the patient is not agitated and has no evidence of myocardial ischemia or increased ICP. The patient should exhibit some spontaneous triggering of respirations and should not be receiving large doses of vasopressor or inotropic agent. SpO$_2$ should be ≥88% with FiO$_2$ of 0.50 and PEEP at 7.5 cmH$_2$O prior to the SBT.

The SBT should be done in the morning for a prescribed period (usually 30 to 120 minutes). The ventilator rate is adjusted to 0 and pressure support decreased to 0 to 7. The SBT should be discontinued if the following occur:

- Respiratory rate >35 or <8 for >5 minutes.
- Mental status changes.
- SpO_2 <88% for >15 minutes.
- Respiratory distress (HR >130 BPM or <60 BPM, marked dyspnea, diaphoresis, increased use of accessory respiratory muscles, respiratory arrest).

Patients who pass the SBT have an 85-90% chance of breathing successfully after extubation. Patients who repeatedly fail daily SBT may require tracheostomy.

FAILURE TO WEAN FROM MECHANICAL VENTILATION

Failure to wean from mechanical ventilation can occur in approximately 20-30% of ventilated patients. Many factors affect a patient's ability to wean from mechanical ventilation including physical, psychological and situational factors. Before discontinuation of ventilation can be considered, the patient must be able to protect his/her airway, be hemodynamically stable and have resolution of the clinical problem that initiated the need for mechanical ventilation. Weaning protocols use clinical criteria such as oxygen saturation, blood pressure, respiratory rate, and tidal volume to determine the patient's tolerance of lessening mechanical ventilator support. Weaning failure is defined as the inability to pass a spontaneous breathing trial or reintubation within 48 hours of extubation. Failure to resolve the clinical problem(s) that initiated mechanical ventilation, insufficient ventilator drive, respiratory muscle weakness, co-morbidities, and/or the development of new clinical problems (e.g., infection) may contribute to the inability to wean.

Signs and symptoms: Decreased tidal volume, increased respiratory rate, increased $PaCO_2$, oxygen desaturation, anxiety, diaphoresis, fatigue, changes in blood pressure or heart rate, mental status changes, and hemodynamic changes.

Treatment: The initial treatment strategy for patients who experience a dysfunctional ventilator weaning response is identification and treatment of the underlying cause(s) of the weaning failure. In addition, other treatment strategies may include psychological preparation of the patient for further weaning attempts, readiness testing and respiratory muscle training.

SEDATION/ANALGESIA WITH MECHANICAL VENTILATION

Patients intubated for mechanical ventilation are usually given **sedation and/or analgesia** initially, but medications should be reduced and given in boluses rather than with continuous IV drip with a goal of stopping sedation as it prolongs ventilation time. Typical sedatives include midazolam, propofol, and lorazepam. Narcotic analgesics include fentanyl and morphine sulfate. Uses of sedation include:

- Controlling agitation and excessive movement that may interfere with ventilation.
- Reduce pain and discomfort associated with ventilation.
- Control respiratory distress.

Triglyceride levels must be checked periodically if propofol is administered for >24-48 hours. Neuromuscular blocking agents are rarely used because they may cause long-term weakness and increase length of ventilation although they may be indicated in some cases, such as with excessive shivering or cardiac arrest. Many patients are able to tolerate mechanical ventilation without sedation, and sedation should always be decreased to the minimal amount necessary as excess

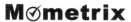

sedation may delay extubation. An ideal level of sedation will keep the patient calm and compliant with the ventilator but still alert and able to follow commands.

CONSCIOUS SEDATION

Conscious sedation is used to decrease sensations of pain and awareness caused by a surgical or invasive procedure, such a biopsy, chest tube insertion, fracture repair, and endoscopy. It is also used during presurgical preparations, such as insertion of central lines, catheters, and use of cooling blankets. Conscious sedation uses a combination of analgesia and sedation so that patients can remain responsive and follow verbal cues but have a brief amnesia preventing recall of the procedures. The patient must be monitored carefully, including pulse oximetry, during this type of sedation. The most commonly used drugs include:

- Midazolam (Versed®): This is a short-acting water-soluble sedative, with onset of 1-5 minutes, peaking in 30, and duration usually about 1 hour (up to 6 hours).
- Fentanyl: This is a short-acting opioid with immediate onset, peaking in 10-15 minutes and with duration of about 20-45 minutes. Monitor respiratory function.

The fentanyl/midazolam combination provides both sedation and pain control. Conscious sedation usually requires 6 hours fasting prior to administration.

THERAPEUTIC GASES

Carbon dioxide is a potent stimulator of respirations, but it is rarely used therapeutically because it can depress respirations if hypercarbia or respiratory acidosis is present. CO_2 may be administered at times as part of anesthesia, but it is most commonly used for insufflation for laparoscopic/endoscopic procedures.

Nitric oxide (NO) is used as a pulmonary vessel dilator to improve oxygenation by decreasing pulmonary artery pressure and pulmonary vascular resistance. NO is FDA-approved for use for neonatal PPH but is sometimes used for adults, although studies have not shown it an effective treatment for ARDS. NO should be delivered at 0.1 to 50 ppm to avoid toxicity that can occur over 50 ppm. Toxic reactions include methemoglobinemia and platelet inhibition with resultant bleeding.

Heliox is helium mixed with oxygen that is used to reduce airway resistance during mechanical ventilation and for pulmonary function tests. Heliox may also be used to treat respiratory obstruction and is used during laser surgery on the airway because it readily conducts heat away from the surgical site, reducing tissue damage. Heliox is sometimes used for COPD patients as it increases hyperventilation and reduces carbon dioxide levels.

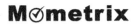

Procedures and Interventions

THORACENTESIS

A **thoracentesis** (aspiration of fluid or air from pleural space) is done to make a diagnosis, relieve pressure on the lung caused by pleural effusion, or instill medications. A chest x-ray is done prior to the procedure. A sedative may be given. The patient is in sitting position, leaning onto a padded bedside stand, straddling a chair with head supported on the back of the chair, or lying on the opposite side with the head of the bed elevated 30-45° to ensure that fluid remains at the base. The patient should avoid coughing or moving during the procedure. The chest x-ray or ultrasound determines needle placement. After a local anesthetic is administered, a needle (with an attached 20-mL syringe and 3-way stopcock with tubing and a receptacle) is advanced intercostally into the pleural space. Fluid is drained, collected, examined, and measured. The needle is removed and a pressure dressing applied. A chest x-ray is done to ensure there is no pneumothorax. The patient is monitored for cough, dyspnea, and hypoxemia.

TRACHEOSTOMY

Tracheostomy, surgical tracheal opening, may be utilized for mechanical ventilation. Tracheostomy tubes are inserted directly into an opening in the trachea to provide a conduit and maintain the opening. Tracheostomy tubes are usually silastic or plastic, and may have permanent of disposable inner cannulas. The tube is secured with ties around the neck. Because the air entering the lungs through the tracheostomy bypasses the warming and moistening effects of the upper airway, air is humidified through a room humidifier or through delivery of humidified air through a special mask or mechanical ventilation. The patient with a tracheostomy must have continuous monitoring of vital signs and respiratory status to ensure patency of tracheostomy. The inner cannula should be cleaned/replaced regularly (every 8-24 hours and PRN). Regular suctioning is needed, especially initially, to remove secretions:

- Suction catheter should be 50% the size of the tracheostomy tube to allow ventilation during suctioning.
- Vacuum pressure: 80-100 mmHg.
- Catheter should only be inserted ≤ 0.5 cm beyond tube to avoid damage to tissues or perforation,
- Catheter should be inserted without suction and intermittent suction on withdrawal.

THORACIC SURGERY

LUNG VOLUME REDUCTION

Lung volume reduction surgery (LVRS) usually involves removing about 20-35% of lung tissue that is not functioning adequately in order to reduce the lung size so that the lungs work more effectively. This procedure is most commonly used with adult emphysematous COPD patients. In adults, surgery is usually bilateral; however, some patients are not candidates for bilateral surgery because of cardiac disease or emphysema affecting only one lung. Unilateral surgery has been shown to be effective. Surgical removal of part of the lung improves ventilation and gas exchange and does not require the immunosuppressant therapy required for lung transplantation. Studies have shown that those with low risk for the surgery and with emphysematous changes in the upper lobes can benefit from the surgery, but high-risk patients with more widespread emphysematous changes have increased mortality rates. The surgery may be done through an open-chest thoracotomy or through a less invasive video-assisted thoracotomy.

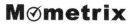

PNEUMONECTOMY

Pneumonectomy is surgical removal of one of the lungs. There are 2 surgical procedures:

- **Simple**: removal of just the lung
- **Extrapleural**: removal not only of the lung but also part of the diaphragm on the affected side and the pericardium on that same side.

During the operative procedure, much care must be taken to prevent contamination of the remaining lung, including the use of bronchus blockers or prone position during surgery.

Removal of the lung is indicated for a number of conditions, including:

- Cancerous lesions (the most common reason for surgery).
- Severe bronchiectasis from chronic suppurative pneumonia, resulting in dilation of terminal bronchioles.
- Severe hypoplasia.
- Unilateral lung destruction with pulmonary hypertension.
- Pulmonary hemorrhage.
- Lobar emphysema.
- Chronic pulmonary infections with destruction of lung tissue.

Because the lung capacity is reduced, persistent shortness of breath may occur with exertion even many months after surgery.

LOBECTOMY AND OTHER PROCEDURES TO REMOVE PARTIAL LUNG TISSUE

Lobectomy removes one or more lobes of a lung (which has 2 on the left and 3 on the right) and is usually done for lesions or trauma that is confined to one lobe, such as tubercular lesions, abscesses or cysts, cancer (usually non-small cell in early stages), traumatic injury, or bronchiectasis. Surgery is usually done through an open thoracotomy or video-assisted thoracotomy. Complications can include hemorrhage, post-operative infection with or without abscess formation, and pneumothorax. Usually 1-2 chest tubes are left in place in the immediate post-surgical period to remove air and/or fluid.

- **Segmental resection** removes a bronchovascular segment and is used for small lesions in the periphery, bronchiectasis or congenital cysts or blebs.
- **Wedge resection** removes a small wedged-shape portion of the lung tissue and is used for small peripheral lesions, granulomas, or blebs.
- **Bronchoplastic (sleeve) reconstruction** removes part of bronchus and lung tissue with reanastomosis of bronchus and is used for small lesions of the carina or bronchus.

Important Terms

Alveolar Hypoventilation: Alveolar hypoventilation occurs when effectiveness of alveolar gas exchange reduces so PaO_2 and $PaCO_2$ both increase. The failure to eliminate carbon dioxide displaces oxygen in the alveolar sacs.

Physiologic Shunting: Physiologic shunting is venous blood in the lung bypassing the alveoli and re-entering the arterial system. This normally occurs with 2-3% of venous blood but may increase with alveolar congestion related to pulmonary edema, atelectasis, or other disorder.

Intrapulmonary Shunting: Intrapulmonary shunting involves alveolar perfusion without ventilation, so the oxygenated blood reaches the alveolus but cannot exchange for carbon dioxide because the alveolus is damaged or diseased.

Refractory Hypoxemia: Refractory hypoxemia occurs when there is so much loss of alveoli that oxygen administration is unable to correct the hypoxemia.

Dead Space: Dead space occurs when a well-ventilated alveolus cannot be perfused because of blockage by an embolus, capillary compression, or other damage in the pulmonary capillaries.

Ventilation-Perfusion (V/Q) Mismatch: Ventilation-perfusion mismatch (V/Q) occurs when well-ventilated alveoli lack adequate perfusion (creating partial dead space) or poorly-ventilated alveoli have adequate perfusion (creating partial shunts).

Endocrine

Diabetes Insipidus and Diabetes Mellitus

DIABETES INSIPIDUS

Diabetes insipidus (DI) is caused by a deficiency of the antidiuretic hormone (ADH), or vasopressin. DI may develop secondary to head trauma, primary brain tumor, meningitis, encephalitis, or surgical ablation or irradiation of the pituitary gland, or metastatic tumors. This is different from congenital nephrogenic diabetes insipidus, in which production of ADH is normal but the renal tubules do not respond.

Symptoms: Polydipsia & polyuria, may drink in excess of 2-20 liters a day; withholding fluids results in dehydration but polyuria continues (water deprivation test); urine output will exceed 250 cc/hr.

Diagnosis: Diagnostic tests include serum sodium levels, increased BUN, serum ADH level, and increased serum osmolality. Expect elevated serum sodium and decreased urine osmolality (less than 200 mOsm/kg) and urine specific gravity (<1.005).

Treatment includes:

- Vasopressin tannate is available in injectable (*IM* or SQ) or nasal spray. Injectable forms may last up to 72 hours.
- Desmopressin acetate is available as a nasal spray or oral medication and is usually taken twice daily. Water intoxication can occur with overdose – watch neurological status closely.
- Correct fluid deficits with hypotonic solutions; treat slowly (want decrease of 1 mEq/hr), watch for signs/symptoms of cerebral edema.

DIABETES MELLITUS TYPES 1 AND 2

Diabetes mellitus is the most common metabolic disorder. Over 6% of adults have diabetes, but only two-thirds are diagnosed. Insulin resistance tends to increase in older adults, so there is less ability to handle glucose. Type II is more common in older adults, with incidence increasing with age.

- **Type I:** Immune-mediated form with insufficient insulin production because of destruction of pancreatic beta cells
  - o **Symptoms** include pronounced polyuria and polydipsia, short onset, obesity or recent weight loss, and ketoacidosis present on diagnosis.
  - o **Treatment** includes insulin as needed to control blood sugar, glucose monitoring 1-4 times daily, diet with carbohydrate control, and exercise.
- **Type II:** Insulin resistant form with defect in insulin secretion
  - o **Symptoms** include long onset, obesity with no weight loss or significant weight loss, mild or absent polyuria and polydipsia, ketoacidosis or glycosuria without ketonuria, androgen-mediated problems such as hirsutism and acne (adolescents), and hypertension.
  - o **Treatment** includes diet and exercise, glucose monitoring, and oral medications.

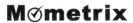

DIABETIC KETOACIDOSIS

Ketoacidosis is a complication of type 1 diabetes mellitus, usually related to noncompliance with treatment, stress, illness, or lack of awareness of having diabetes (this event often being the first time that diabetes is diagnosed). Inadequate production of insulin results in glucose being unavailable for metabolism, so lipolysis (breakdown of fat) produces free fatty acids (FFAs) as an alternate fuel source. Glycerol is converted to ketone bodies which are used for cellular metabolism less efficiently than glucose. Excess ketone bodies are excreted in the urine (ketonuria) or exhalations. Acidosis of any type causes potassium in cells to shift to the serum. The ketone bodies lower serum pH, leading to ketoacidosis.

Symptoms include:

- Kussmaul respirations: "ketone breath." – fruity smelling breath; progresses to CNS depression with loss of airway.
- Fluid imbalance, including loss of potassium and other electrolytes from cellular death, resulting in dehydration and diuresis with excess thirst.
- Dangerous cardiac arrhythmias, related to potassium loss; hypotension, chest pain, tachycardia.
- GI: Nausea/vomiting, abdominal pain, loss of appetite.
- Neurological: malaise, confusion/lethargy progressing to coma.

Diagnosis is based on:

- Labs: Blood glucose >250 mg/dL, ↓Na/↑K (switches after treatment), elevated beta-hydroxybutyrate (byproduct of ketones).
- ABG: pH <7.3, HCO_3 <18 mEq/L.
- Urine: + glucose, ketones.

TREATMENT AND POTENTIAL COMPLICATIONS

Treatment of DKA:

- **Fluids:** Priority is fluid resuscitation with 1-2 liters of isotonic fluids given in the first hour, up to 8 liters in the first 24 hours. Potassium will be added to the fluids when levels begin to fall.
- **Insulin:** Continuous drip IV, with/without loading dose. Will usually begin @ 0.1 unit/kg/ hour (5-7 units an hour generally), with a goal of decreasing blood glucose 50-75 mg/dL an hour. Blood glucose is checked every hour, and when levels are < 200 mg/dL, add dextrose to IV fluids to prevent rebound hypoglycemia.
- **Potassium:** Watch carefully, as fluids and insulin will cause rapid fall in serum levels. When K <5 mEq/L, it should be added to the IV fluids (Per liter: 20 mEq for K 4-5, 40 mEq for K 3-4). If potassium falls below 3, stop insulin drip and give 10-20 an hour until >3.5.
- **Sodium & Magnesium**: Na has an inverse relationship with potassium, and will increase as potassium falls. If sodium levels rise above 150 mEq, switch fluids to 0.45 NS. Low magnesium levels prevent potassium uptake, so replace as necessary.
- Continue to monitor electrolytes and anion gap during ICU stay. When ABG and electrolytes normalized, transition to SQ insulin.

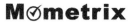

Potential complications include:

- Sudden electrolyte shifts (potassium) leading to catastrophic arrythmias, cerebral edema, and other complications.
- Vomiting and decreased LOC leading to aspiration/ARDS.
- Mechanical ventilation = stops respiratory alkalosis = ↑ acidosis.

HHNK

Hyperglycemic hyperosmolar nonketotic syndrome (HHNK) occurs in people without history of diabetes or with mild type 2 diabetes, resulting in persistent hyperglycemia leading to osmotic diuresis. Fluid shifts from intracellular to extracellular spaces to maintain osmotic equilibrium, but the increased glucosuria and dehydration results in hypernatremia and increased osmolarity. This condition is most common in those 50-70 years old and often is precipitated by an acute illness, such as a stroke, medications (thiazides), or dialysis treatments. HNNS differs from ketoacidosis because, while the insulin level is not adequate, it is high enough to prevent the breakdown of fat. Onset of symptoms often occurs over a few days. Glucose levels are often higher than those in DKA due to the gradual increase over time (often greater than 600), and the body living in a state of hyperglycemia, therefore the individual not symptomatic until the blood glucose level is at an extreme high.

Symptoms: Polyuria, dehydration, hypotension, tachycardia, changes in mental status, seizures, hemiparesis.

Diagnosis: ↑ glucose, Na, osmolality (urine and serum), BUN/Creatinine.

Treatment is similar to that for ketoacidosis:

- Insulin drip with frequent (hourly) blood sugar monitoring.
- Intravenous fluids and electrolytes.
- Correct blood glucose and other labs.

ACUTE HYPOGLYCEMIA

Acute hypoglycemia (hyperinsulinism) may result from pancreatic islet tumors or hyperplasia, increasing insulin production, or from the use of insulin to control diabetes mellitus. Hyperinsulinism can cause damage to the central nervous and cardiopulmonary systems, interfering with functioning of the brain and causing neurological impairment. Other causes may include: genetic defects (chromosome 11: short arm), severe infections, and toxic ingestion of alcohol or drugs (salicylates).

Symptoms include:

- Blood glucose <50-60 mg/dL.
- Central nervous system: seizures, altered consciousness, lethargy, and poor feeding with vomiting, myoclonus, respiratory distress, diaphoresis, hypothermia, and cyanosis.
- Adrenergic system: diaphoresis, tremor, tachycardia, palpitation, hunger, and anxiety.

Diagnosis: Blood work, patient history/presentation.

Treatment depends on underlying cause:

- Glucose/Glucagon administration to elevate blood glucose levels.
- Diazoxide (Hyperstat®) to inhibit release of insulin.
- Somatostatin (Sandostatin®) to suppress insulin production.
- Careful monitoring.

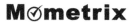

SIADH, Addison's Disease, and Thyroid Disorders

SIADH

Syndrome of inappropriate secretion of antidiuretic hormone (SIADH) is related to hypersecretion of the posterior pituitary gland. This causes the kidneys to reabsorb fluids, resulting in fluid retention, and triggers a decrease in sodium levels (dilutional hyponatremia), resulting in production of only concentrated urine. This syndrome may result from central nervous systems disorders, such as brain trauma, surgery, or tumors. It may also be triggered by other disorders, such as tumors of various organs, pneumothorax, acute pneumonia, and other lung disorders. Some medications (vincristine, phenothiazines, tricyclic antidepressants, and thiazide diuretics) may also trigger SIADH.

Symptoms: edema, dyspnea/crackles on auscultation, anorexia with nausea and vomiting, irritability, stomach cramps, alterations of personality, stupor and seizures (related to progressive sodium depletion)

Diagnosis: ↑ urine specific gravity, ↓ Na and serum osmolality.

Treatment includes: (treat underlying cause)

- Correct fluid volume excess and electrolytes
- Monitor urine output continuously: <0.5-1 mL/kg/hour is cause for concern.
- Seizure precautions
- With SIADH expect low serum sodium and serum osmolality with high urine osmolality.

ADRENAL INSUFFICIENCY (ADDISON'S DISEASE)

Adrenal/Adrenocortical insufficiency (Addison's disease) is caused by damage to the adrenal cortex, related to a variety of causes, such as autoimmune disease or genetic disorders, but it may relate to destructive lesions or neoplasms. Without treatment, the condition is life threatening.

Symptoms may be vague and the condition undiagnosed until 80-90% of the adrenal cortex has been destroyed:

- Chronic weakness and fatigue
- Abdominal distress with nausea and vomiting
- Salt or licorice craving, resulting from deficiency of aldosterone
- Pigmentary changes in skin and mucous membranes, hyperpigmentation
- Hypotension
- Hypoglycemia
- Recurrent seizures (more common in children)

Treatment includes hormone replacement therapy with glucocorticoids (cortisol) and mineralocorticoids (aldosterone) may be taken orally, by monthly parenteral injections or by subcutaneous implantation of desoxycorticosterone acetate every 9-12 months.

Note: During times of stress or illness, the demand for glucocorticoids may increase and dosages up to 3 times the normal dosage may be needed to prevent an acute crisis.

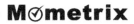

HYPERTHYROIDISM

Hyperthyroidism (thyrotoxicosis) usually results from excess production of thyroid hormones (Graves' disease) from immunoglobulins providing abnormal stimulation of the thyroid gland. Other causes include thyroiditis and excess thyroid medications.

Symptoms vary and may be non-specific, especially in the elderly:

- Hyperexcitability.
- Tachycardia (100-160) and atrial fibrillation.
- Increased systolic (but not diastolic) BP.
- Poor heat tolerance, skin flushed and diaphoretic.
- Dry skin and pruritis (especially in the elderly).
- Hand tremor, progressive muscular weakness.
- Exophthalmos (bulging eyes).
- Increased appetite and intake but weight loss.

Treatment includes:

- Radioactive iodine to destroy the thyroid gland. Propranolol may be used to prevent thyroid storm. Thyroid hormones are given for resultant hypothyroidism.
- Antithyroid medications, such as Propacil® or Tapazole® to block conversion of T4 to T3.
- Surgical removal of thyroid is used if patients cannot tolerate other treatments or in special circumstances, such as large goiter. Usually one-sixth of the thyroid is left in place and antithyroid medications are given before surgery.

HYPOTHYROIDISM

Hypothyroidism occurs when the thyroid produces inadequate levels of thyroid hormones. Conditions may range from mild to severe myxedema. There are a number of causes:

- Chronic lymphocytic thyroiditis (Hashimoto's thyroiditis).
- Excessive treatment for hyperthyroidism.
- Atrophy of thyroid.
- Medications, such as lithium, iodine compounds.
- Radiation to the area of the thyroid.
- Diseases that affect the thyroid, such as scleroderma.
- Iodine imbalances.

Symptoms may include chronic fatigue, menstrual disturbances, hoarseness, subnormal temperature, low pulse rate, weight gain, thinning hair, thickening skin. Some dementia may occur with advanced conditions. Clinical findings may include increased cholesterol with associated atherosclerosis and coronary artery disease. Myxedema may be characterized by changes in respiration with hypoventilation and CO_2 retention resulting in coma. Treatment involves hormone replacement with synthetic levothyroxine (Synthroid®) based on TSH levels, but this increases the oxygen demand of the body, so careful monitoring of cardiac status must be done during early treatment to avoid myocardial infarction while reaching euthyroid (normal) level.

Hematology

Hematologic Disorders

ANEMIA

Anemia occurs when there is an insufficient number of red blood cells to sufficiently oxygenate the body. As a result of the decreased level of oxygen being supplied to the organs, the body will attempt to compensate by increasing cardiac output and redistributing blood to the brain and heart. In return, the blood supply to the skin, abdominal organs and kidneys is decreased. Anemia can occur from blood loss, increased destruction of red blood cells (hemolytic anemia) or as a result of a decreased production in red blood cells.

Signs and symptoms: Pallor, fatigue, hypotension, weakness and mental status changes. As perfusion decreases and the body attempts to compensate for the lack of oxygenation, tachycardia, chest pain, and shortness of breath may occur. In hemolytic anemias, jaundice and splenomegaly may occur as the result of the breakdown of red blood cells and the excretion of bilirubin.

Diagnosis: A complete blood count, reticulocyte count and iron studies may be used to diagnose anemia.

Treatment: The treatment of anemia is focused on treating the underlying cause. Parenteral iron may be given for patients with iron deficiency anemias caused from chronic blood loss, or inadequate iron intake or absorption. Blood transfusions are used to treat patients with active bleeding as well as those patients who are displaying significant clinical symptoms.

Erythropoietin stimulating proteins may also be utilized to decrease the need for a transfusion.

DISSEMINATED INTRAVASCULAR COAGULATION

PATHOLOGY

Disseminated intravascular coagulation (DIC) (consumption coagulopathy) is a secondary disorder that is triggered by another, such as trauma, congenital heart disease, necrotizing enterocolitis, sepsis, and severe viral infections. DIC triggers both coagulation and hemorrhage through a complex series of events. Trauma causes tissue factor (transmembrane glycoprotein) to enter the circulation and bind with coagulation factors, triggering the coagulation cascade. This stimulates thrombin to convert fibrinogen to fibrin, causing aggregation and destruction of platelets and forming clots that can be disseminated throughout the intravascular system. These clots increase in size as platelets adhere to the clots, causing blockage of both the microvascular systems and larger vessels, and this can result in ischemia and necrosis. Clot formation triggers fibrinolysis and plasmin to breakdown fibrin and fibrinogen, causing destruction of clotting factors, resulting in hemorrhage. Both processes, clotting and hemorrhage, continue at the same time, placing the patient at high risk for death, even with treatment.

SYMPTOMS AND TREATMENT

The onset of **symptoms of DIC** may be very rapid or a slower chronic progression from a disease. Those who develop the chronic manifestation of the disease usually have fewer acute symptoms and may slowly develop ecchymosis or bleeding wounds.

95

Symptoms include:

- Bleeding from surgical or venous puncture sites.
- Evidence of GI bleeding with distention, bloody diarrhea.
- Hypotension and acute symptoms of shock.
- Petechiae and purpura with extensive bleeding into the tissues.
- Laboratory abnormalities:
    - Prolonged prothrombin and partial prothrombin times.
    - Decreased platelet counts and fragmented RBCs.
    - Decreased fibrinogen.

Treatment includes:

- Identifying and treating underlying cause.
- Massive blood transfusion protocol: Replacement of blood products, such as platelets and fresh frozen plasma.
- Anticoagulation therapy (heparin) to increase clotting time.
- Cryoprecipitate to increase fibrinogen levels.
- Coagulation inhibitors and coagulation factors.

ITP

The autoimmune disorder **idiopathic thrombocytopenic purpura (ITP)** causes an immune response to platelets, resulting in decreased platelet counts. ITP affects primarily children and young women although it can occur at any age. The acute form primarily occurs in children, but the chronic form affects primarily adults. Platelet counts are usually 150,000-400,000 per cu/mL. With ITP, platelet levels are less than 100,000. Maintaining a platelet count of at least 30,000 is necessary to prevent intracranial hemorrhage, the primary concern. The cause of ITP is unclear and may be precipitated by viral infection, sulfa drugs, and conditions, such as lupus erythematosus. ITP is usually not life threatening and can be controlled. **Symptoms** include:

- Bruising and petechiae with hematoma in some cases.
- Epistaxis.
- Increased menstrual flow in post-puberty females.

Treatment includes:

- Corticosteroids depress immune response and increase platelet count.
- Splenectomy may be indicated for chronic conditions.
- Platelet transfusions.
- Avoiding aspirin, ibuprofen or other NSAIDs.

HITTS

Heparin-induced thrombocytopenia and thrombosis syndrome (HITTS) occurs in patients receiving heparin for anticoagulation. There are two types:

- **Type I** is a transient condition occurring within a few days and causing depletion of platelets (<100,000 mm³), but heparin may be continued as the condition usually resolves without intervention.
- **Type II** is an autoimmune reaction to heparin that occurs in 3-5% of those receiving unfractionated heparin and also occurs with low-molecular weight heparin. It is characterized by low platelets (<50,000 mm³) that are ≥50% below baseline. Onset is 5-14 days but can occur within hours of heparinization. Death rates are <30%. Heparin-antibody complexes form and release platelet factor 4 (PF4), which attracts heparin molecules and adheres to platelets and endothelial lining, stimulating thrombin and platelet clumping. This puts the patient at risk for thrombosis and vessel occlusion rather than hemorrhage, causing stroke, myocardial infarction, and limb ischemia with symptoms associated with the site of thrombosis. Treatment includes:
  - Discontinuation of heparin.
  - Direct thrombin inhibitors (lepirudin, argatroban).
  - Monitor for s/s of thrombus/embolus.

REOPRO-INDUCED COAGULOPATHY

ReoPro® (abciximab) is used to prevent cardiac ischemia for those undergoing percutaneous cardiac intervention. It inhibits the aggregation of platelets. It is used with aspirin and/or weight-adjusted low dose heparin and potentiates the action of anticoagulants. However, its use with non-weight adjusted longer acting heparin can cause thrombocytopenia with increased risk of hemorrhage, especially with readministration of the drug, which can induce the formation of antibodies and an allergic reaction that is characterized by anaphylaxis and thrombocytopenia, referred to as **ReoPro-induced coagulopathy**. Because of the danger of hemorrhage, ReoPro® is contraindicated if there is active bleeding or a history of bleeding or CVA within the 2 years prior, history of a CVA, platelet count <100,000 mm³, or recent history of oral anticoagulation. Careful monitoring of platelet counts prior to administration and the use of weight-adjusted low dose heparin is important to prevent bleeding. Heparin should be discontinued after the PCI.

IMMUNE DEFICIENCIES

There are multiple disorders that fall into the category of **primary immunodeficiency diseases.** These disorders are genetic or inherited disorders in which the body's immune system does not function properly. These disorders may involve low levels of antibodies, defects in the antibodies, or defects in cells that make up the immune system (T-cells, B-cells). Common variable immune deficiency is a common immune deficiency diagnosed in adulthood. This disorder is characterized by low levels of serum immunoglobins and antibodies, which substantially increases the risk of infection.

Signs and symptoms: Recurrent infections are the hallmark sign of immune deficiency disorders. Recurrent infections most often involve the ears, sinuses, bronchi, and lungs. Lymphadenopathy may occur as well as splenomegaly. GI symptoms may include abdominal pain, nausea, vomiting, and diarrhea and weight loss. Some patients may experience polyarthritis. Granulomas are also common and may occur in the lungs, lymph nodes, liver and skin.

Diagnosis: A physical assessment and patient history are used to diagnose immune deficiency disorders. Since immune deficiency disorders are genetic or inherited, family history should also be evaluated. Lab tests such as serum antibodies, serum immunoglobin levels and a complete blood count may also be used to assist in the diagnosis of immune deficiency disorders.

Treatment: Patients with immune deficiency disorders often receive immunoglobulin replacement. Long term antibiotics may also be administered for recurrent infections. Educate patients to frequently wash hands, cook foods thoroughly, avoid large crowds, and other infection prevention techniques.

LEUKOPENIA

Leukopenia is defined as a decrease in white blood cells. Neutropenia is defined as a low number of neutrophils and is often used interchangeably with the term leukopenia. With a decrease in the number of circulating white blood cells, the patient is at an increased risk for the development of an infection. Leukopenia and neutropenia can occur from either a decrease in the production of white blood cells or an increase in their destruction. Infections, malignancy, autoimmune disorders, medications (including chemotherapy) and a history of radiation therapy may contribute to the development of leukopenia/neutropenia.

Signs and symptoms: Malaise, fever, chills, night sweats, and shortness of breath, headache, cough, abdominal pain, tachycardia and hypotension. The neutropenic/leukopenic patient is at risk for the development of infections including pneumonia, skin infections, urinary tract infections and gastrointestinal infections. In addition, the patient is at an increased risk for sepsis.

Diagnosis: Complete blood count including an absolute neutrophil count. In addition, a bone marrow biopsy may be performed to determine the cause of the decrease in neutrophils.

Treatment: Supportive therapy is used in the treatment of leukopenia including the aggressive treatment of infections that may develop. Precautions should be taken to protect the patient from additional infections including strict adherence to sterile technique and infection control procedures. Hematopoietic growth factors may also be given to stimulate the production of neutrophils.

THROMBOCYTOPENIA

Thrombocytopenia is a deficiency of circulating platelets in the blood. It can be caused by a decrease in the production of platelets from the bone marrow or an increase in destruction of platelets. Thrombocytopenia may also be caused from the use of heparin. Heparin induced thrombocytopenia can occur after heparin therapy (average 4-14 days post therapy) and is characterized by a decrease in platelet count to less than 50% of baseline or the occurrence of an unexplained thrombolytic event. A decreased production of platelets within the bone marrow can occur as a result of malignancy, bone marrow failure, infection, alcohol abuse, or a nutritional deficiency. An increase in the destruction of platelets may occur in disseminated intravascular coagulation, vasculitis, thrombotic thrombocytopenic purpura, sepsis or idiopathic thrombocytopenic purpura.

Signs and symptoms: Signs and symptoms may include petechiae, ecchymosis, bleeding from the mouth or gums, epistaxis, pallor, weakness, fatigue, splenomegaly, blood in the urine or stool and jaundice.

Diagnosis: Physical exam and lab studies including complete blood count, partial thromboplastin time and prothrombin time may be used to diagnosis thrombocytopenia. A bone marrow biopsy may be indicated to determine the cause of the decreased production of platelets.

Treatment: Treatment of thrombocytopenia involves identifying and treating the underlying cause. Medications that decrease the platelet count should be held. Platelet transfusions may be administered to patients with extremely low counts (less than 50,000) or if spontaneous bleeding occurs. Platelet transfusions are contraindicated in patients with thrombotic thrombocytopenia purpura.

TUMOR LYSIS SYNDROME

Tumor lysis syndrome occurs when intracellular contents are released from tumor cells, leading to electrolyte imbalances (hyperkalemia, hyperphosphatemia, hypocalcemia and hyperuricemia) when the kidneys are unable to excrete the large volume of metabolites. Tumor lysis syndrome is most common after treatment of hematologic malignancies but can occur due to any type of tumor that is sensitive to chemotherapy. The primary goals of therapy for tumor lysis syndrome are to increase urine production through IV hydration in order to prevent renal failure and to decrease uric acid concentration, usually with administration of allopurinol. The urine pH should be maintained at 7 or higher. Electrolyte levels should be closely monitored, as hyperkalemia is a risk. Patients at moderate risk (intermediate grade lymphomas, acute leukemias) should begin prophylactic allopurinol before chemotherapy; and those at higher risk (high grade lymphomas or acute leukemias with WBC count >50,000), rasburicase.

Assessment

RED BLOOD CELLS

Red blood cells (RBCs or erythrocytes) are biconcave disks that contain hemoglobin (95% of the cell's mass), which carries oxygen throughout the body. The heme portion of the cell contains iron, which binds to the oxygen. RBCs live about 120 days after which they are destroyed and their hemoglobin is recycled or excreted. Normal values of red blood cell count vary by gender:

- Males >18 years: 4.5-5.5 million per mm^3
- Females >18 years: 4.0-5.0 million per mm^3

The most common disorders of RBCs are those that interfere with production, leading to various types of anemia:

- Blood loss
- Hemolysis
- Bone marrow failure

The **morphology of RBCs** may vary depending upon the type of anemia:

- Size: Normocytes, microcytes, macrocytes
- Shape: Spherocytes (round), poikilocytes (irregular), drepanocytes (sickled)
- Color (reflecting concentration of hemoglobin): Normochromic, hypochromic

LABORATORY TESTS

Hemoglobin: Carries oxygen and is decreased in anemia and increased in polycythemia. Normal values:

- Males >18 years: 14.0-17.46 g/dl.
- Females >18 years: 12.0-16.0 g/dl.

Hematocrit: Indicates the proportion of RBCs in a liter of blood (usually about 3 times the hemoglobin number). Normal values:

- Males >18 years: 45-52%.
- Females >18 years: 36-48%

Mean corpuscular volume (MCV): Indicates the size of RBCs and can differentiate types of anemia. For adults, <80 is microcytic and >100 is macrocytic. Normal values:

- Males > 18 years: 84-96 μm^3.
- Females >18 years: 76-96 μm^3.

Reticulocyte count: Measures marrow production and should rise with anemia. Normal values:

- 0.5-1.5% of total RBCs.

C-reactive protein: Increases with inflammation in the body.

- Normal values: 2.6-7.6 µg/dL.

Erythrocyte sedimentation rate (sed rate): A non-specific test that decreases with inflammation. Values vary according to gender and age:

- <50: Males 0-15 mm/hr. Females 0-20 mm/hr.
- >50: Males 0-20 mm/hr. Females 0-30 mm/hr.

WBC COUNT AND DIFFERENTIAL

White blood cell (leukocyte) count is used as an indicator of bacterial and viral infection. WBC is reported as the total number of all white blood cells. Normal WBC for adults: 4,800-10,000. Acute infection will lead to a count > 10,000, while a WBC of 30,000+ indicates a severe infection. Viral infection results in a WBC of 4,000 and below. The **differential** provides the percentage of each different type of leukocyte. An increase in the white blood cell count is usually related to an increase in one type and often an increase in immature neutrophils, known as bands, referred to as a "shift to the left," an indication of an infectious process:

- **Immature neutrophils (bands):** 1-3%: Increase with infection.
- **Segmented neutrophils (segs):** 50-62%: Increase with acute, localized, or systemic bacterial infections.
- **Eosinophils:** 0-3%: Decrease with stress and acute infection.
- **Basophils:** 0-1%: Decrease during acute stage of infection.
- **Lymphocytes:** 25-40%: Increase in some viral and bacterial infections.
- **Monocytes:** 3-7%: Increase during recovery stage of acute infection.

COAGULATION PROFILE

The following are elements of the coagulation profile:

- **Prothrombin time (PT):**
  - *Normal = 10-14 seconds.*
  - Increases with anticoagulation therapy, vitamin K deficiency, ↓prothrombin, DIC, liver disease, and malignant neoplasm.

- **Partial thromboplastin time (PTT)**
  - *Normal = 30-45 seconds.*
  - Increases with hemophilia A & B, von Willebrand's, vitamin deficiency, lupus, DIC, and liver disease.

- **Activated partial thromboplastin time (aPTT)**
  - *Normal = 21-35 seconds*
  - Similar to PTT, but decreases in extensive cancer, early DIC and after acute hemorrhage. Monitors heparin dosage.

- **Thrombin clotting time (TCT) or Thrombin time (TT)**
  - *Normal = 7-12 seconds*
  - Used most often to determine dosage of heparin. Prolonged with multiple myeloma, abnormal fibrinogen, uremia, and liver disease.

- **Bleeding time**
  - *Normal = 2-9.5 minutes (Ivy method on the forearm).*
  - Increases with DIC, leukemia, renal failure, aplastic anemia, von Willebrand's, some drugs, and alcohol.

- **Platelet count**
  - *Normal = 150,000-400,000 per microliter.*
  - Increased bleeding risks when <50,000 and increased clotting risks when >750,000.

Review Video: The Coagulation Profile
Visit mometrix.com/academy and enter code: 423595

Procedures

TRANSFUSIONS

Blood components that are commonly used for transfusions include:

- **Packed red blood cells:** RBCs (250-300 mL per unit) should be warmed >30 °C (optimal 37 °C) before administration to prevent hypothermia and may be reconstituted in 50-100 mL of normal saline to facilitate administration. RBCs are necessary if blood loss is about 30% (1500-2000 mL) (Hgb ≤7). (Above 30% blood loss, whole blood may be more effective.) RBCs are most frequently used for transfusions.
- **Platelet concentrates:** Transfusions of platelets are used if the platelet count is <50,000 cells/mm³. One unit increases the platelet count by 5000-10,000 cells/mm³. Platelet concentrates pose a risk for sensitization reactions and infectious diseases. Platelet concentrate is stored at a higher temperature (20-24 °C) than RBCs. This contributes to bacterial growth, so it is more prone to bacterial contamination than other blood products and may cause sepsis. Temperature increase within 6 hours should be considered an indication of possible sepsis. ABO compatibility should be observed but is not required.
- **Fresh frozen plasma** (FFP) (obtained from a unit of whole blood frozen ≤6 hours after collection) includes all clotting factors and plasma proteins, so each unit administered increases clotting factors by 2-3%. FFP may be used for deficiencies of isolated factors, excess warfarin therapy, and liver-disease related coagulopathy. It may be used for patients who have received extensive blood transfusions but continue to hemorrhage. It is also helpful for those with antithrombin III deficiency. FFP should be warmed to 37 °C prior to administration to avoid hypothermia. ABO compatibility should be observed if possible, but it is not required. Some patients may become sensitized to plasma proteins.
- **Cryoprecipitate** is the precipitate that forms when FFP is thawed. It contains fibrinogen, factor VIII, von Willebrand, and factor XIII. This component may be used to treat hemophilia A and hypofibrinogenemia.

PRE-, INTRA-, AND POST-INTERVENTION MONITORING OF HEMATOLOGIC INTERVENTIONS
PLASMAPHERESIS

With **plasmapheresis,** whole blood is removed from the body, anticoagulant added, cellular components separated from the plasma (which is removed), and cellular components suspended in saline, albumin (most common) or other substitute for plasma. This is reinfused into the patient. The purpose is to remove harmful antibodies found in plasma. ACE inhibitors increase risk of hypotension and should be withheld for 24 hours before the procedure. Machine settings may vary. Typically, the patient's height and weight are entered into the automated system to aid in calculating the plasma volume. The patient must be carefully monitored during the procedure for signs of hypocalcemia (perioral/fingertip tingling, alterations in mental status, VT), which requires the administration of calcium; hypomagnesemia (confusion, headaches, dizziness, twitching), which requires administration of magnesium; and hypotension, which requires saline bolus. If the patient shows indications of transfusion reaction, the infusion must be discontinued and medications (diphenhydramine, corticosteroids) administered. The patient should be kept warm to avoid hypothermia. Post-procedure the patient may experience thrombocytopenia and hypofibrinogenemia, so the patient must be observed for signs of bleeding.

EXCHANGE TRANSFUSION

Exchange transfusions replace a person's blood with donor blood to remove sickled blood for sickle cell anemia or to remove toxins. Exchange may be complete or partial. An automated machine is generally used, and the time on the machine ranges from 1 to 4 hours. (If done manually, removal and replacement is done in cycles with blood first removed followed by replacement.) A catheter is inserted (usually in the arm) to drain the blood and another usually in the femoral area (under local or moderate sedation) to administer donor blood, plasma, or other substitute for plasma. During the exchange, the patient's VS must be carefully monitored. If the patient exhibits signs of hypocalcemia (perioral/finger tingling) then calcium is administered. Some may receive calcium routinely during administration. Blood may be taken from the femoral line for testing after the exchange. When the femoral catheter is removed, pressure must be applied to the area for at least 5 minutes and the patient instructed to lie flat for at least 30 minutes to prevent bleeding.

LEUKOCYTE DEPLETION

Red blood cell and platelet transfusions typically contain some leukocytes, which are recognized as foreign by the immune system of a patient receiving the transfusion, and this can lead to adverse reactions, especially in patients who are immunocompromised. **Leukocyte depletion** is carried out by various processes, including filtration. One disadvantage to leukodepletion of RBCs is that the process results in the loss of about 10% of the RBCs, and some hemolysis may occur. Leukocyte depleted RBCs are given in volumes of 200 to 250 mL within a 4-hour time period. The nurse should obtain the patient's transfusion history prior to the transfusion and must check the type and crossmatch and consent form and take baseline vital signs. A 22- to 24-gauge catheter is usually used for administration. The patient should be under direct observation for at least the first 15 minutes of the transfusion. Patient's vital signs should be monitored at 5 minutes, 15 minutes, and then at least every 30 minutes during the transfusion and one hour post-transfusion.

BLOOD CONSERVATION

Blood conservation includes methods to:

- **Minimize the loss of blood during surgical procedures**: May include regional anesthesia instead of general, positioning to reduce blood loss, cell salvage, autotransfusion, non-invasive monitoring (BP, pulse oximetry), limited blood draws, normovolemic hemodilution, and medications to reduce bleeding (vitamin K, tranexamic acid, desmopressin, somatostatin, vasopressin, recombinant factor VIIa).
- Lower the threshold for receiving transfusions: Transfusion threshold lowered from 10 to 7 g/dL.
- **Maintain the hematocrit at acceptable levels**: Administration of oral or parenteral iron therapy to increase tolerance for blood loss. Erythropoietin alpha may also be administered perioperatively to stimulate production of RBCs.
- **Ensure optimal oxygenation of tissue**: Hyperoxic ventilation during surgery, crystalloid/colloid volume replacement, and utilizing techniques to minimize consumption of oxygen.

Blood conservation includes a commitment to bloodless surgery as much as possible, especially through utilization of minimally-invasive procedures.

TRANSFUSION-RELATED COMPLICATIONS

There are a number of **transfusion-related complications**, which is the reason that transfusions are given only when necessary. Complications include:

- **Infection**: Bacterial contamination of blood, especially platelets, can result in severe sepsis. A number of infective agents (viral, bacterial, and parasitic) can be transmitted although increased testing of blood has decreased rates of infection markedly. Infective agents include HIV, hepatitis C and B, human T-cell lymphotropic virus, CMV, WNV, malaria, Chagas' disease and variant Creutzfeldt-Jacob disease (from contact with mad cow disease).
- **Transfusion-related acute lung injury** (TRALI): This respiratory distress syndrome occurs ≤6 hours after transfusion. The cause is believed to be antileukocytic or anti-HLA antibodies in the transfusion. It is characterized by non-cardiogenic pulmonary edema (high protein level) with severe dyspnea and arterial hypoxemia. Transfusion must be stopped immediately and the blood bank notified. TRALI may result in fatality but usually resolves in 12-48 hours with supportive care.
- **Graft vs. host disease:** Lymphocytes cause immune response in immunocompromised individuals. Lymphocytes may be inactivated by irradiation, as leukocyte filters are not reliable.
- **Post-transfusion purpura:** Platelet antibodies develop and destroy the patient's platelets, so the platelet count decreases about 1 week after transfusion.
- **Transfusion-related immunosuppression:** Cell-mediated immunity is suppressed, so the patient is at increased risk of infection and, in cancer patients, transfusions may correlate with tumor recurrence. This condition relates to transfusions that include leukocytes. RBCs cause a less pronounced immunosuppression, suggesting a causative agent is in the plasma. Leukoreduction is becoming more common to reduce transmission of leukocyte-related viruses.
- **Hypothermia**: This may occur if blood products are not heated. Oxygen utilization is halved for each 10 °C decrease in normal body temperature.

Gastrointestinal

Abdominal Trauma

SPLENIC INJURIES

The **spleen** is the most frequently injured solid organ in blunt trauma. Injuries to the spleen are the most common because it's not well protected by the rib cage and is very vascular. Symptoms may be very non-specific. Kehr sign (radiating pain in left shoulder) indicates intra-abdominal bleeding and Cullen sign (ecchymosis around umbilicus) indicates hemorrhage from ruptured spleen. Some may have right upper abdominal pain although diffuse abdominal pain often occurs with blood loss, associated with hypotension. Splenic injuries are **classified** according to the degree of injury:

- I: Tear in splenic capsules or hematoma.
- II: Laceration of parenchyma (<3 cm).
- III: Laceration of parenchyma (≥3cm).
- IV: Multiple lacerations of parenchyma or burst-type injury.

Treatment: Because removing the spleen increases the risk of life-threatening infections, every effort (bed rest, transfusion, reduced activity for at least 8 weeks) is done to avoid surgery (argon gas, fibrin "glue", or therapeutic ultrasound). Lab testing for the absence Howell-Jolly bodies indicates the spleen in functioning properly. If conservative efforts fail (usually occurs in first 72 hours), a splenectomy is performed. After surgery, the patient has an increased risk for infection and thrombosis. Lifetime anticoagulation therapy and vaccinations (combo of pneumonia/meningitis/influenza B vaccine) should be administered.

HEPATIC INJURIES

Hepatic injury is the most common cause of death from abdominal trauma. It is particularly danger as hematoma rupture can occur hours to 6 weeks after the time of injury. Because hepatic injury is often associated with multiple organ damage, symptoms may be non-specific and difficult to diagnose. Therefore, elevation in liver transaminase levels or elevation of right hemidiaphragm on Xray in trauma patients indicates damage that may require further examination. Liver injuries are classified according to the degree of injury:

- I: Tears in capsule with hematoma.
- II: Laceration(s) of parenchyma (<3 cm).
- III: Laceration(s) of parenchyma (≥3 cm).
- IV: Destruction of 25-75% of lobe from burst injury.
- V: Destruction of >75% of lobe from burst injury.
- VI: Avulsion [tearing away].

Hemodynamically stable patients are managed medically, but surgical repair may be necessary if the patient is unstable or bleeding. Hemorrhage is common complication of hepatic injury and may require ligation of hepatic arteries or veins. Treatment often includes intravenous fluids for fluid volume deficit as well as blood products (plasma, platelets) for coagulopathies. Surgical or angiographic embolization of the tear may be indicated in severe injury.

COMPARTMENT SYNDROME

Abdominal trauma with pronounced shock increases risk of **compartment syndrome**, in which the pressure in the abdomen increases to the point of acute ischemia and anoxia of the tissues. Causes include edema of the intestines (trauma/surgical manipulation), reduced expansion of abdominal cavity (burns), hemorrhage, and capillary leakage after excessive fluid resuscitation.

Signs/Symptoms: Increased airway pressures and acute respiratory distress syndrome, decreased U/O, and cerebral edema.

Diagnosis: Increased intra-abdominal pressure (>20 cmH$_2$O), measured by Foley catheter or NG tube with pressure transducer or water-column manometry; ↑ CVP and ICP, ↓ CO and GFR.

Treatment includes:

- Medications: Sudden release of pressure and reperfusion may cause acidosis, hyperkalemia, vasodilation, and cardiac arrest. The patient should be given crystalloid solutions before decompression. Treatment may also include milrinone, dopamine, and mannitol.
- Surgical decompression.

Prevention: If risk for compartment syndrome exists, the wound should not be closed, but left open and covered with a sterile dressing. Negative-pressure wound therapy may be used to decrease risk.

Peritonitis and Acute GI Bleed

PERITONITIS

Peritonitis (inflammation of the peritoneum) may be primary (from infection of blood or lymph) or, more commonly, secondary, related to perforation or trauma of the gastrointestinal tract. Common causes include perforated bowel, ruptured appendix, abdominal trauma, abdominal surgery, peritoneal dialysis or chemotherapy, or leakage of sterile fluids, such as blood, into the peritoneum.

Symptoms: Diffuse abdominal pain with rebound tenderness (Blumberg's sign), abdominal rigidity, paralytic ileus, fever (with infection), nausea and vomiting. sinus tachycardia

Diagnosis: Increased WBC (>15,000), abdominal Xray/CT, paracentesis, blood and peritoneal fluid culture.

Treatment includes:

- Intravenous fluids and electrolytes.
- Broad-spectrum antibiotics.
- Laparoscopy as indicated to determine cause of peritonitis and effect repair.

ACUTE GASTROINTESTINAL HEMORRHAGE

Gastrointestinal (GI) hemorrhage may occur in the upper or lower gastrointestinal track. The primary cause (50-70%) of GI hemorrhage is gastric and duodenal ulcers, generally caused by stress, NSAIDs or infection with *Helicobacter pylori*.

Symptoms: Abdominal pain and distention, coffee-ground emesis/ hematemesis, bloody or tarry stools, hypotension with tachycardia.

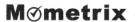

Diagnosis: Stool occult blood (Guaiac test), EGD, colonoscopy, GI Bleed scan.

Treatment includes:

- Medications: Fluid replacement with blood transfusions if necessary, antibiotic therapy for *Helicobacter pylori,* continuous pantoprazole IV to prevent further irritation.
- Endoscopic thermal therapy to cauterize or injection therapy (hypertonic saline, epinephrine, ethanol) to cause vasoconstriction.
- Arteriography with intraarterial infusion of vasopressin and/or embolizing agents, such as stainless-steel coils, platinum microcoils, or Gelfoam pledgets.
- Vagotomy and pyloroplasty if bleeding persists.

Prevention: Prophylactic medications (pantoprazole [Protonix] IV is common).

Bowel Obstructions, Infarctions, and Perforations

BOWEL OBSTRUCTIONS

Bowel obstruction occurs when there is a mechanical obstruction of the passage of intestinal contents because of constriction of the lumen, occlusion of the lumen, adhesion formation, or lack of muscular contractions (paralytic ileus). Symptoms include abdominal pain, rigidity, and distention, n/v, dehydration, constipation, and respiratory distress from the diaphragm pushing against the pleural cavity, sepsis and shock. Treatment includes strict NPO, insertion of naso/orogastric tube, IV fluids and careful monitoring; may correct spontaneously, severe obstruction requires surgery.

BOWEL INFARCTIONS

Bowel infarction is ischemia of the intestines related to severely restricted blood supply. It can be the result of a number of different conditions, such as strangulated bowel or occlusion of arteries of the mesentery, and may follow untreated bowel obstruction. People present with acute abdomen and shock, and mortality rates are very high even with resection of infarcted bowel. Treatment includes replacing volume, correcting the underlying issue, improving blood flow to the mesentery, insertion of NGT, and/or surgery.

INTESTINAL PERFORATION

Intestinal perforation is a partial or complete tear in the intestinal wall, leaking intestinal contents into the peritoneum. Causes include trauma, NSAIDs (elderly, patients with diverticulitis), acute appendicitis, PUD, iatrogenic (laparoscopy, endoscopy, colonoscopy, radiotherapy), bacterial infections, IBS, and ingestion of toxic substances (acids) or foreign bodies (toothpicks). The danger posed by infection after perforation varies depending upon the site. The stomach and proximal portions of the small intestine have little bacteria, but the distal portion of the small intestine contains aerobic bacteria, such as *E. coli,* as well as anaerobic bacteria.

Signs/Symptoms: (appear within 24-48 hours): Abdominal pain and distention and rigidity, fever, guarding and rebound tenderness, tachycardia, dyspnea, absent bowel sounds/paralytic ileus with nausea and vomiting; Sepsis and abscess or fistula formation can occur.

Diagnosis: Labs: ↑ WBC; lactic acid and pH change as late signs. Xray and CT will show free air in abdominal cavity.

Treatment includes:

- Prompt antibiotic therapy, and surgical repair with peritoneal lavage.
- The abdominal wound may be left open to heal by secondary intention and to prevent compartment syndrome

GERD

GASTROESOPHAGEAL REFLUX

Gastroesophageal reflux (GERD) occurs when the lower esophageal sphincter fails to remain closed, allowing the contents of the stomach to back into the esophagus. This reflux of the acid containing contents of the stomach may cause irritation of the lining of the esophagus. Over time, damage to the lining of the esophagus can occur. In some patients, this may lead to the formation of Barrett's esophagus. In Barrett's esophagus, the lining of the esophagus begins to resemble the tissue lining the intestine. Patients with Barrett's esophagus have an increased risk of developing esophageal adenocarcinoma.

Signs and symptoms: Heartburn, dysphagia, belching, water brash, sore throat, hoarseness, and chest pain.

Diagnosis: Clinical signs/symptoms, ambulatory esophageal reflux monitoring (this test uses a thin pH probe that is placed in the esophagus). Data is collected on the amount of acid entering the esophagus along with the presence of clinical symptoms. Endoscopy may be used in the diagnosis of GERD in patients with persistent or progressive symptoms.

Treatment: GERD is often treated with proton pump inhibitors (inhibit gastric acid secretion). Surgical therapy may be utilized if medical management is unsuccessful. Patients are taught to eliminate foods that trigger symptoms (chocolate, caffeine, alcohol, and highly acidic foods). In addition, patients with GERD should avoid meals 2-3 hours before bed and may find it helpful to sleep with the head of the bed elevated to alleviate symptoms.

Hepatic Failure/Coma

PORTAL HYPERTENSION

Portal hypertension occurs when obstructed blood flow increases blood pressure throughout the portal venous system, preventing the liver from filtering blood and causing the development of collateral blood vessels that return unfiltered blood to the systemic circulation. Increasing serum aldosterone levels cause sodium and fluid retention in the kidneys, resulting in hypervolemia, ascites and esophageal varices. Portal hypertension can be caused by any liver disease, especially cirrhosis and inherited or acquired coagulopathies that cause thrombosis of the portal vein.

Symptoms: Ascites with distended abdomen, esophageal varices with bleeding, dyspnea, abdominal discomfort, fluid/electrolyte imbalances.

Diagnosis: Labs (CBC, BMP, liver panel, Hep B &C), abdominal ultrasound or CT/ MRI, EGD, Hemodynamic measurement of the hepatic venous pressure gradient (HVPG)

Treatment includes:

- Restricted sodium intake & use diuretics as needed.
- Endoscopic treatment of obstruction.
- Portal vein shunting redirecting blood from the portal vein to the vena cava.
- Liver transplant in severe cases.
- These patients are at high risk for esophageal varices, which, if they rupture, can cause instantaneous hemorrhage and death.

COMPENSATED HEPATIC CIRRHOSIS

Cirrhosis is a chronic hepatic disease in which normal liver tissue is replaced the fibrotic tissue that impairs liver function. *Compensated cirrhosis* usually involves non-specific symptoms, such as intermittent fever, epistaxis, ankle edema, indigestion, abdominal pain, and palmar erythema. *Decompensated cirrhosis* occurs when the liver can no longer adequately synthesize proteins, clotting factors, and other substances so that portal hypertension occurs. **Types** include:

- **Alcoholic**: Caused by chronic alcoholism; most common, resulting in fibrosis around the portal areas. The necrotic liver cells are replaced by fibrotic tissue, with areas of normal tissue in between, giving the liver a *hobnail appearance.*
- **Post-necrotic:** broad bands of fibrotic tissue result from acute viral hepatitis.
- **Biliary,** the least common type is caused by chronic biliary obstruction and cholangitis, with resulting fibrotic tissue around the bile ducts.

Symptoms: Hepatomegaly, palmar erythema. Spider nevi, epistaxis, jaundice and ascites, esophageal varices, generalized edema, chronic gastritis, ↓dietary intake, alterations in mentation, Dupuytren's contracture (hand), atrophy of gonads.

Diagnosis: Thrombocytopenia, ↓ albumin, Vit A, C, K; ↑ ammonia, bilirubin, AST/ALT. Can see on ultrasound and abdominal CT; magnetic resonance elastography (MRE) shows hardening of the liver.

Treatment (supportive) includes:

- Dietary supplements and vitamins; restrict sodium and fluids.
- Diuretics (potassium sparing) to decrease ascites/edema.
- Colchicine to reduce fibrotic changes.
- Liver transplant – only curative treatment.

ESOPHAGEAL VARICES

Esophageal varices are torturous, dilated veins in the submucosa of the esophagus (usually the distal portion). They are a complication of cirrhosis of the liver, in which obstruction of the portal vein causes an increase in collateral vessels and resulting decrease in circulation to the liver, increasing the pressure in the collateral vessels. This causes the vessels to dilate. Because they tend to be fragile and inelastic, they tear easily, causing sudden, massive esophageal hemorrhage.

Signs/Symptoms: Usually asymptomatic until rupture; projectile vomiting bright red blood, dark stools, and shock.

Diagnosis: EGD, capsule endoscopy, CT, and MRI.

Treatment (rupture) includes:

- Emergent fluid and blood replacement.
- IV vasopressin, somatostatin, and octreotide to ↓ venous pressure and provide vasoconstriction/clotting.
- Endoscopic injection with sclerosing agents and band ligation.
- Esophagogastric balloon tamponade using Sengstaken-Blakemore and Minnesota tubes: Note – always inflate gastric balloon first, keep scissors nearby in case of balloon migration, do not use longer than 24 hrs, as there is increased risk of ulceration from pressure.
- Transjugular intrahepatic portosystemic shunting (TIPS) creates a channel between systemic and portal venous systems to reduce portal hypertension.

HEPATIC COMA

Hepatic coma or **hepatic encephalopathy** occurs when the liver's inability to remove ammonia and other toxins from the bloodstream causes a decrease in neurologic function. Hepatic encephalopathy often occurs in patients with severe liver disease, most commonly in patients diagnosed with cirrhosis of the liver. The fibrous tissue that forms in cirrhosis affects the liver structure and impedes the blood flow to the liver, ultimately causing the liver to fail. There are four stages of hepatic encephalopathy ranging from grade 0 to grade 4. Grade 4 encephalopathy is defined as hepatic coma. Neurologic alterations may progress slowly and if left untreated may result in irreversible neurologic damage.

Signs and symptoms: Altered mental status, personality or mood changes, poor judgment, and poor concentration. As symptoms progress, patients may experience agitation, disorientation, drowsiness, increasing confusion, lethargy, slurred speech, tremors, and seizures. In grade 4 encephalopathy, patients become unresponsive and ultimately comatose.

Diagnosis: Physical assessment, lab tests including a complete blood count, liver function tests, serum ammonia levels, BUN, creatinine and electrolyte levels, CT or MRI of the brain, and electroencephalogram may be used to diagnose hepatic encephalopathy.

Treatment: Address precipitating factors such as infection, gastrointestinal bleeding, dehydration, hypotension, or alcohol use. Other treatment options may include limiting protein intake, administration of lactulose to prevent the absorption of ammonia, and the administration of an antibiotic such as neomycin, rifaximin, or Flagyl to reduce the serum ammonia level.

FULMINANT HEPATITIS

Fulminant hepatitis or **acute liver failure** is a potentially fatal disease that occurs in patients with otherwise normal liver function and no previous liver disease. Patients develop severe liver injury with hepatic encephalopathy and coagulopathy within 8 weeks of the onset of symptoms. Causes of fulminant hepatitis include exposure to toxins, viral hepatitis (Hepatitis A or Hepatitis B, with B being a more common cause), drug induced (most commonly acetaminophen), other viral infections including cytomegalovirus and herpes simplex virus, Wilson's disease and mushroom poisoning. Other complications such as acute respiratory failure, cerebral edema, and acute renal failure may develop along with the failure of the liver.

Signs and symptoms: Jaundice, headache, asterixis, mental status changes, agitation, disorientation, drowsiness, increasing confusion, lethargy, slurred speech, tremors, and seizures (due to hepatic encephalopathy), hyperventilation, cerebral edema, coagulopathy, hypoglycemia, flu-like symptoms, fever and an enlarged liver.

Diagnosis: Labs (bilirubin, creatinine and BUN, coagulation studies, serum ammonia, complete metabolic panel, and liver function tests). In addition, physical assessment, radiologic studies such as ultrasound, MRI and CT scan and liver biopsy may be used.

Treatment: Fulminant hepatitis carries a very high mortality rate (>80% without transplant). Liver transplant is the only treatment option for patients with fulminant hepatitis.

BILIARY ATRESIA

Biliary atresia is a rare life-threatening condition that occurs in infancy of unknown cause. Bile ducts are tubes that transport bile from the liver to the gallbladder (where it is stored) and the small intestine (where it aids in digestion). Biliary atresia occurs when the bile ducts (either inside or outside of the liver) become inflamed, causing damage to the ducts and an impedance of bile flow. Without treatment, the trapped bile causes damage to the liver eventually causing it to fail. The life expectancy for infants with untreated biliary atresia is approximately 2 years.

Signs and symptoms: Early identification is key in successfully treating biliary atresia. Signs and symptoms include dark urine, gray or white stools, slow weight gain and delayed growth, jaundice, abdominal swelling and itching.

Diagnosis: Physical assessment, abdominal films, ultrasound, lab tests including bilirubin levels, and liver biopsy.

Treatment: The only treatment options for biliary atresia are liver transplant or the Kasai procedure. Named after the surgeon who invented it, the Kasai procedure involves using a loop of intestine to act as a new bile duct and the damaged ducts are removed. Flow of bile is then restored to the small intestine. The Kasai procedure is most successful when performed on younger infants (less than 3 months old).

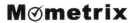

Malnutrition and Pancreatitis

MALNUTRITION AND MALABSORPTION IN CRITICALLY ILL PATIENTS

Malabsorption occurs when an abnormality or alteration in the gastrointestinal tract affects the absorption of nutrients through the small intestine. It can also occur with damage to the small intestine due to infection, trauma, surgery, or radiation therapy; patients in ICU's are at an increased risk due to multiple illnesses, intubation/prolonged NPO status, vasopressors decreasing blood flow to the bowel, and other factors that make receiving adequate nutrition difficult. Malabsorption often leads to **malnutrition**. Hospitalized malnourished patients are at a higher risk for infection, respiratory failure, heart failure, arrhythmias and delayed or decreased wound healing.

Signs and symptoms: Bloating, cramping, gas, chronic diarrhea, failure to thrive, muscle wasting, weight loss, steatorrhea, anemia, electrolyte imbalance and vitamin/mineral deficiencies.

Diagnosis: Serum electrolytes, complete blood count, ferritin, vitamin B12, folate, albumin, and protein. Stool fat testing may be performed to assess for the presence of fat in the stool that occurs in certain disorders that affect fat absorption. Endoscopy may be used to diagnose an abnormality in the mucosa lining of the bowel.

Treatment: Replacement of nutrients that have been lost as a result of malabsorption as well as treatment for the cause of the malabsorption. Supplemental treatment with enzymes found to be deficient may also be incorporated into the treatment plan.

Prevention: Ensure patients with prolonged "NPO" status have alternative means of nutrition (TPN, tube feeds, etc.).

ACUTE PANCREATITIS

Acute pancreatitis is related to chronic alcoholism or cholelithiasis in 90% of patients, but may have unknown etiology. It may also be triggered by a variety of drugs (tetracycline, thiazides, acetaminophen, and oral contraceptives). Complications may include shock, acute respiratory distress syndrome, and MODs.

Signs/Symptoms: acute pain (mid-epigastric, LUQ, or generalized), nausea and vomiting, abdominal distention.

Diagnosis: Serum lipase (>2x normal), amylase (less accurate), CT with contrast, abdominal U/S, MRI cholangiopancreatography, ERCP.

Treatment (supportive) includes:

- **Medications**: IV fluids, antiemetics, antibiotics (if necrosis is secondary to infection), analgesia; *NOTE: do not give morphine, can cause spasms in sphincter of Oddi, making pain worse.*
- **TPN, NPO, or restricted to clear liquids** may help manage vomiting, ileus, and aspiration.
- **Surgical**: may remove gallbladder and biliary duct obstructions if cause of recurrent pancreatitis.

Prevention: Avoid smoking and alcohol consumption; limit fat intake and increase fresh fruits/vegetables and water.

Nursing Actions

PHARMACOLOGICAL INTERVENTIONS FOR NAUSEA AND VOMITING

Medications for nausea/ vomiting include:

- **Metoclopramide** (Reglan®) is used to reduce nausea and vomiting from a wide range of causes. It is also a prokinetic drug that increases gastrointestinal contractions and promotes faster gastric emptying, so it is used for heartburn, GERD, and diabetic gastroparesis.
- **Ondansetron** (Zofran®) reduces vagal stimulation of medulla oblongata and is used for nausea related to chemotherapy.
- **Promethazine** (Phenergan®) is an antihistamine that works to prevent nausea and vomiting, especially in surgical patients. It has a sedative effect, so should be used with caution in patients with neurological or respiratory compromise. Promethazine is also extremely caustic to the tissues, causing necrosis if extravasated; it should be diluted before injection and administered through a central line intravenous piggyback when possible.

TROUBLE-SHOOTING PROBLEMS RELATED TO ENTERAL FEEDINGS

Feeding tubes are commonly found in the critical care setting, as many patients are intubated and unable to take oral nutrition or medication. General maintenance involves checking placement before flushing anything into tube (prevents aspiration), flushing the tubes with ≥30 cc water before and after use, and every 4 hours. Never crush enteric-coated medications, and keep the HOB ≥30° at all times during feeding to prevent aspiration. **Complications** include the following:

- **Vomiting / aspiration:** Placement, gastric emptying, formula intolerance.
  - o Confirm placement by checking pH (preferred to air bolus); Delay feeding one hour and check residual volume before resuming. Refrigerate formula, check expiration, use only for 24 hours.
- **Diarrhea:** Rapid feeding, antibiotics/medications, intolerance of formula or hypertonic formula, tube migration.
  - o ↓ rate of feeding, evaluate medications, avoid hanging feedings ≥8 hours, add fiber or decrease sodium in feed.
- **Displacement of Tube:**
  - o NG tube- replace using the other nostril, only if not surgically placed. G-tube/J-tube: cover site and notify physician. Prevention: secure all tubes with appropriate device, mark placement to identify migration.
- **Tube Occlusion:**
  - o Check for kinks/obvious problems. Aspirate fluid and instill warm water and aspirate to loosen occlusion. Physician may order enzyme or sodium bicarb solution.

TOTAL PARENTERAL NUTRITION

Total parenteral nutrition (TPN) is an intravenous hypertonic solution containing glucose, fat emulsion, protein, minerals, and vitamins. TPN is generally given through a central line (PICC if short-term), and used only when other methods of nutrition are not feasible. **Nursing considerations** include:

- **Infection prevention:** Use aseptic technique for feedings and dressing changes; change solution, filter, and tubing every 24 hours, discard cloudy solutions and monitor site for signs of infection.

- **Risk of embolus/contamination**: Use micropore filter (TPN without fat emulsion) or 1.2-micron filter (TPN with fat emulsion); can add heparin to solution. Never infuse any medication or product in same line as TPN; cannot draw blood from this line either. Label line as "TPN ONLY" to prevent these errors.
- **Malnutrition and electrolytes**: Check daily weight; BMP and CBC 3x a week until stable, then weekly. Check label and ingredients before administration; watch for signs of fluid overload. Cloudy blood specimen could indicate hyperlipidemia; also risk of hyper-ammonemia (Asterix, AMS) and azotemia (dehydration, ↑BUN).
- **Hyper/Hypoglycemia**: Initiate slowly, increasing rate over 24-48hrs. NEVER "catch-up" rate if there is a delay/pause in feeding; only administer with a pump and do not change rate without order. If bag runs out, hang a bag of D10W until new bag can be obtained. Monitor BG every 4-6 hours; may use sliding scale insulin.

BARRIERS TO NUTRITIONAL/FLUID ADEQUACY

CHEWING/SWALLOWING DIFFICULTIES

Dysphagia occurs in about 10% of noninstitutionalized older adults and even more in hospitalized patients. **Difficulty chewing and swallowing** is evident with solids (meat, bread) and thin liquids. There are a variety of causes:

- Stroke: About 30% have dysphagia.
- Neuromuscular diseases: Parkinson's disease, myasthenia gravis, multiple sclerosis, and ALS.
- Drugs: Phenothiazines.
- Dementia: Patients may not chew few adequately or may forget to swallow.
- Achalasia (failure of the esophagus to contract effectively and sphincter to relax).
- Esophageal stricture, diverticulum, or web (from iron deficiency) and cancer.
- Esophageal cancer.
- Dental problems.

Symptoms include chest tightness or pain, regurgitation, choking, esophageal reflux (especially when supine), and aspiration pneumonia. Weight loss and dehydration may result. **Diagnosis** is based on symptoms, barium swallow, and endoscopy. **Treatment** includes diagnosing and treating underlying causes and referring to therapist. Patient should sit upright to eat, avoid eating before lying down, chew foods carefully and sip water after swallowing, thicken thin liquids, use smaller utensils to limit bite-size, do strengthening exercises, and take medications to relax the esophagus (if indicated). In some cases, a feeding tube (PEG) may be necessary.

ALTERATIONS TO HUNGER AND THIRST AND INABILITY TO SELF-FEED

Barriers to nutritional/fluid adequacy include:

- **Hunger and thirst** are controlled by the hypothalamus, the blood glucose level, and the fullness of the stomach, intestines. Many different conditions (COPD, HIV, hepatitis, renal failure, hepatic failure, heart failure, pregnancy, metabolic disease) may result in loss of appetite. Additionally, many drugs (opioids, chemotherapeutic agents, antibiotics) may also cause loss of appetite or make foods taste bad. Loss of thirst may result from brain abnormalities, SIADH, hydrocephalus, and stroke. The underlying cause must be identified and treated if possible and the patient offered food and fluids frequently in small amounts. Some foods and fluids may be more palatable to patients than others.

- **Inability to self-feed** may result from weakness, paralysis, neurological disorders, psychiatric disorders, orthopedic disorders, or dementia. In some cases, patients may be able to manage food in different forms, such as finger foods or liquids in spill-proof cups with lids or mugs with double handles. If a patient must be fed or given liquids by a caregiver, then a schedule should be developed and food and liquids recorded and measured to ensure adequate nutrition and hydration.

LIVER FUNCTION STUDIES

Bilirubin: Shows the liver's ability to conjugate/excrete bilirubin

- Direct 0.0-0.3 mg/dL.
- Total 0.0-0.9 mg/dL.
- Urine bilirubin 0.

Total protein: Shows if the liver is producing normal protein levels

- Total Protein7.0-7.5 g/dL.
- Albumin: 4.0-5.5 g/dL.
- Globulin: 1.7=3.3 g/dL.
- Albumin/globulin (A/G) ratio: 1.5:1 to 2.5:1.

Alkaline phosphatase: Indicates biliary tract obstruction (in absence of bone disease)

- Alkaline phosphatase: 17-142 adults (varies with method).

AST (SGOT)/ ALT (SGPT): Increases with liver cell damage

- AST: 10-40 units.
- ALT 5-35 units.

Serum ammonia: Increases with liver failure

- Ammonia: 150-250 mg/dL

Will also see increase/abnormalities in lipids, cholesterol and clotting labs.

ABDOMINAL PRESSURE MONITORING

Abdominal pressure monitoring is indicated for ascites, abdominal trauma, major fluid resuscitation, and abdominal/retroperitoneal bleeding. Measurement of intra-abdominal pressure is by attaching a pressure transducer or water-column manometer to a Foley catheter in the bladder because bladder pressure correlates with abdominal pressure. The patient should be in supine flat position if possible. The bladder must be empty for accurate measurement. The catheter should be clamped and transducer zeroed at the iliac crest along the midaxillary line. Then, 2 to 25 mL (usually about 10 mL for critically ill) of fluid is injected into the bladder and left in place for 30 to 60 seconds before reading the pressure following a patient expiration. Compartment pressures should be <30 mmHg and the difference between diastolic BP and compartment pressure should be >30 mmHg. Intraabdominal pressure may also be checked with an indwelling NG tube. If risk for compartment syndrome exists, the wound should not be closed. Sudden release of pressure and reperfusion may cause acidosis, vasodilation, and cardiac arrest, so the patient should be given crystalloid solutions before decompression.

Procedures and Interventions

TYPES OF DRAINS

The following are different types of drains a patient may have, including pertinent nursing considerations:

- **Simple drains** are latex or vinyl tubes of varying sizes/length. They are usually placed through a stab wound near the area of involvement.
- **Penrose drains** are flat, soft rubber/latex tubes placed in surgical wounds to drain fluid by gravity and capillary action.
- **Sump drains** are double-lumen or tri-lumen tubes (with a third lumen for infusions). The multiple lumen produce venting when air enters the inflow lumen and forces drainage out of the large lumen.
- **Percutaneous drainage catheter** is inserted into wound to provide continuous drainage for infection/fluid collection. Irrigation of the catheter may be required to maintain patency. Skin barriers and pouching systems may also be necessary.
- **Closed drainage systems** use low-pressure suction to provide continuous gravity drainage of wounds. Drains are attached to collapsible suction reservoirs that provide negative pressure. The nurse must remember to always re-establish negative pressure after emptying these drains. There are two types in frequent use:
  - *Jackson-Pratt®* is a bulb-type drain that is about the size of a lemon. A thin plastic drain from the wound extends to a squeeze bulb that can hold about 100 mL of drainage.
  - *Hemovac®* is a round drain with coiled springs inside that are compressed after emptying to create suction. The device can hold up to 500 mL of drainage.

PEG TUBE

Percutaneous endoscopic gastrostomy (PEG), used for tube feedings, involves intubation of the esophagus with the endoscope and insertion of a sheathed needle with a guidewire through the abdomen and stomach wall so that a catheter can be fed down the esophagus, snared, and pulled out through the opening where the needle was inserted and secured. The PEG tube should not be secured to the abdomen until the PEG is fully healed, which usually takes 2 to 4 weeks, because tension caused by taping the tube against the abdomen may cause the tract to change shape and direction. The tract should be straight to facilitate insertion and removal of catheters. Once the tract has healed, the original PEG tube can generally be replaced with a balloon gastrostomy tube. External stabilizing devices can be applied to the skin to hold the tube in place but should be placed 1 to 2 cm above the skin surface to prevent excessive tension that may result in buried bumper syndrome (BBS) in which the internal fixation device becomes lodged in the mucosal lining of the gastric wall, resulting in ulceration.

GASTROINTESTINAL SURGERY

WHIPPLE

The **Whipple** (pancreaticoduodenectomy) procedure is used to surgically remove the head of the pancreas, the gallbladder, part of the bile duct, the duodenum, and sometimes the distal portion of the stomach. After excision, the remaining pancreas, bile duct, and intestinal stump are sutured to the intestine so that secretions empty into the intestine. The Whipple procedure may be done as an open procedure or laparoscopically. This procedure is used primarily for malignant or benign tumors of the head of the pancreas but can also be used for chronic pancreatitis, duodenal cancer, cancer of the ampulla, and cholangiocarcinoma. Whipple is recommended only if the cancer has not spread beyond the pancreas and has not invaded major vessels. Usually, the pancreas is still able to produce adequate insulin, but production of pancreatic enzymes may be impaired. A pylorus-preserving variation preserves the stomach and part of the pylorus to decrease nutritional deficiencies and weight loss associated with the standard Whipple.

Post-op treatment includes monitoring fluid/electrolyte balance and monitoring drains. These patients have a very high risk of developing numerous complications, including peritonitis, bowel obstruction, sepsis, acute abdomen, along with others.

ESOPHAGECTOMY AND ESOPHAGO-GASTRECTOMY

Esophageal cancer starts in the inner layer of the esophagus and spreads. It may develop after long-term reflux because of cell changes brought about by gastric acid. Symptoms include throat or epigastric discomfort, increasing dysphagia and inability to swallow solids, unexplained weight loss, hoarseness, hiccups, hematemesis, and the feeling of something in the throat. *Treatment* for esophageal cancer involves surgical removal of the affected portion of the esophagus. Two common procedures include:

- **Esophagectomy,** which is removal of all or part of the esophagus with the distal end resutured to the stomach or an intestinal graft used to replace the excised portion of the esophagus.
- **Esophago-gastrectomy** is removal of the distal portion of the esophagus, lymph nodes, and the upper portion of the stomach, after which the remaining esophagus and stomach are reattached.

POSTOPERATIVE MANAGEMENT FOR ESOPHAGECTOMY AND ESOPHAGO-GASTRECTOMY

Postoperative management for esophagectomy/gastrectomy includes the following:

- Monitor intubation and ventilation – at increased risk of acute respiratory distress syndrome; encourage pulmonary toilet; monitor chest tubes – notify physician of change in color or sudden increase in drainage (could indicate leak).
- Subcutaneous emphysema in chest / neck could indicate leak in the anastomosis and should be reported immediately.
- Manage pain, which is often severe; PCA or epidural may be used initially.
- Hemodynamics: IV fluids @ 100-200 mL/hr, bolus PRN – however, caution as increased risk of pulmonary edema.
- Monitor NG tube; *NEVER replace or irrigate the NG tube* – could damage anastomosis. Notify MD if complications arise.
- Maintain NPO for 5 to 7 days; nutrition per J-tube or TPN.
- Drains: Penrose, Jackson-Pratt, possible drainage collection bag at base of cervical incision for saliva if >250cc/8hr.
- NOTE: Patients often have HX of ETOH abuse – observe for signs of DTs/withdrawal.
- Prior to initiating oral intake, a fluoroscopic examination with water-soluble contrast will be done to check for leaks. If no leaks, patients begin with clear liquids and progress to 6 to 8 small meals per day.

ESOPHAGOGASTRODUODENOSCOPY

Esophagogastroduodenoscopy (EGD) uses a flexible fiberscope equipped with a lighted fiberoptic lens to allow direct inspection of the mucosa of the esophagus, stomach, and duodenum. The scope has a still or video camera attached to a monitor for viewing during the procedure. The scope may be used for biopsies or therapeutically to dilate strictures or treat gastric or esophageal bleeding. The patient is positioned on the left side (head supported) to allow saliva drainage. Conscious sedation (midazolam, propofol) is commonly used along with a topical anesthetic spray or gargle to facilitate placing the lubricated tube through the mouth into the esophagus. Atropine reduces secretions. A bite guard in the mouth prevents the patient from biting the scope. The airway must be carefully monitored through the procedure (which usually takes about 30 minutes), including oximeter to measure oxygen saturation. While perforation, bleeding, or infection may occur, most complications are cardiopulmonary in nature and relate to drugs (conscious sedation) used during the procedure, so reversal agents (flumazenil, naloxone) should be available.

BARIATRIC GASTROINTESTINAL SURGERY

Bariatric surgery is used to promote weight loss in the morbidly obese (100 pounds over normal weight or BMI of 35-40). Surgery is done to restrict intake and/or prevent absorption of calories. Procedures are open surgical or laparoscopic and include:

- **Banding** places a band around the upper portion of the stomach, creating a small pouch with a small distal opening to slow gastric emptying.
- **Sleeve gastrectomy** removes about 2/3 of stomach, and a distal part of the small intestine is attached, bypassing part of the small intestine, reducing absorption.
- **Roux-en-Y** uses staples and a vertical band to decrease the size of the stomach, creating a small pouch. Then a section of the small intestine is attached to the pouch, bypassing the first and second segments of the intestine to reduce absorption.
- **Gastric ballooning,** placing a balloon in the stomach and filling it with liquid to decrease stomach capacity is used primarily in Europe.

Nursing considerations: Use extreme caution with post-bariatric NG/PEG tubes – generally do not check placement/irrigate with normal amounts (risk of rupturing stomach); ensure patient maintains strict NPO. Increased risk of respiratory complications post-surgery.

Renal

Renal Disorders

INCONTINENCE

Urinary incontinence occurs more commonly in women than men and can range from an intermittent leaking of urine to a full loss of bladder control. Causes of urinary incontinence may include neurologic injury (including cerebral vascular accidents), infections, weakness of the muscles of the bladder and certain medications including diuretics, antihistamines and antidepressants. *Stress incontinence* is defined as an involuntary leakage of urine with sneezing, coughing, laughing, heavy lifting or exercise. *Urge incontinence* is defined as an uncontrollable need to urinate on a frequent basis. *Total incontinence* is the full loss of bladder control.

Signs and symptoms: Urinary frequency and urgency may accompany the inability to control urine. If urinary incontinence is severe, incontinence associated dermatitis may occur, predisposing the patient to skin breakdown and the development of pressure ulcers.

Diagnosis: Physical assessment and presence of symptoms. Ultrasound, urinalysis, urodynamic testing and cystoscopy may be used to determine the underlying cause.

Treatment: Treatment options are dependent on the type of urinary incontinence and the severity. Bladder training and pelvic muscle exercises may be utilized to strengthen muscles to control leakage of urine. In female patients with stress incontinence, a vaginal pessary may be inserted into the vagina to help support the bladder. Suburethral slings may also be surgically implanted to support the urethra. Anti-cholinergics, antispasmodics and tricyclic antidepressants may also be used in the treatment of urinary incontinence.

HYDRONEPHROSIS

Hydronephrosis is a symptom of a disease involving swelling of the kidney pelvises and calyces because of an obstruction that causes urine to be retained in the kidney. In chronic conditions, symptoms may be delayed until severe kidney damage has occurred. Over time, the kidney begins to atrophy. The primary conditions that predispose to hydronephrosis include:

- Vesicoureteral reflux.
- Obstruction at the ureteropelvic junction.
- Renal edema (non-obstructive).
- Any condition that impairs drainage of the ureters can cause backup of the urine.

Symptoms vary widely depending upon cause and whether the condition is acute or chronic.

- Acute episodes are usually characterized by flank pain, abnormal creatinine and electrolyte levels, and increased pH.
- The enlarged kidney may be palpable as a soft mass.

Treatment includes:

- Treatment requires identifying the cause of obstruction and correcting it to ensure adequate drainage.
- A nephrostomy tube, ureteral stent or pyeloplasty may be done surgically in some cases.
- A urinary catheter may be inserted if there is outflow obstruction from the bladder.

RENAL AND URETERAL CALCULI

Renal and urinary calculi occur frequently, more commonly in males, and can relate to diseases (hyperparathyroidism, renal tubular acidosis, gout) and lifestyle factors, such as sedentary work. Calculi can form at any age, most composed of calcium, and can range in size from very tiny to >6mm. Those <4mm can usually pass in the urine easily. *Diagnostic* studies include clinical findings, UA, pregnancy test to rule out ectopic pregnancy, BUN and creatinine if indicated, ultrasound (for pregnant women and children), IV urography. Helical CT (non-contrast) is diagnostic.

Symptoms occur with obstruction and are usually of sudden onset and acute:

- Severe flank pain radiating to abdomen and ipsilateral testicle or labium majus, abdominal or pelvic pain (young children).
- Nausea and vomiting.
- Diaphoresis.
- Hematuria.

Treatment includes:

- Instructions and equipment for straining urine.
- Antibiotics if concurrent infection.
- Extracorporeal shock-wave lithotripsy.
- Surgical removal: Percutaneous/standard nephrolithotomy.
- Analgesia: opiates and NSAIDs.

ACUTE TUBULAR NECROSIS

Acute tubular necrosis (ATN) occurs when a hypoxic condition causes renal ischemia that damages tubular cells of the glomeruli so they are unable to adequately filter the urine, leading to acute renal failure. Causes include hypotension, hyperbilirubinemia, sepsis, surgery (especially cardiac or vascular), and birth complications. ATN may result from nephrotoxic injury related to obstruction or drugs, such as chemotherapy, acyclovir, and antibiotics, such as sulfonamides and streptomycin. Symptoms may be non-specific initially and can include life-threatening complications.

Symptoms: Lethargy. Nausea and vomiting. Hypovolemia with low cardiac output and generalized vasodilation. Fluid and electrolyte imbalance leading to hypertension, CNS abnormalities, metabolic acidosis, arrhythmias, edema, and congestive heart failure. Uremia leading to destruction of platelets and bleeding, neurological deficits, and disseminated intravascular coagulopathy (DIC). Infections can include pericarditis and sepsis.

Treatment includes:

- Identifying and treating underlying cause, discontinuing nephrotoxic agents.
- Supportive care.
- Loop diuretics (in some cases), such as Lasix®.
- Antibiotics for infection (can include pericarditis and sepsis).
- Kidney dialysis.

ACUTE KIDNEY INJURY

Acute kidney injury (AKI), previously known as acute renal failure, is an acute disruption of kidney function that results in decreased renal perfusion, a decrease in glomerular filtration rate and a buildup of metabolic waste products (azotemia). Azotemia is the accumulation of urea, creatinine and other nitrogen containing end products into the bloodstream. The regulation of fluid volume, electrolyte balance and acid base balance is also affected. The causes of acute kidney injury are divided into pre-renal (caused by a decrease in perfusion), intrarenal or intrinsic (occurring within the kidney) and post-renal (caused by the inadequate drainage of urine). Acute kidney injury is common in hospitalized patients and even more commonly in critically ill patients, carrying a mortality rate of 50-80%. Risk factors for acute kidney injury include advanced age, the presence of co-morbid conditions, pre-existing kidney disease and a diagnosis of sepsis.

Signs and symptoms: Malaise, fatigue, lethargy, confusion, weakness, change in urine color, change in urine volume and flank pain.

Diagnosis: Urinalysis, serum BUN and creatinine levels, renal ultrasound, CT or MRI and renal biopsy.

Treatment: The treatment of acute kidney injury is based on the underlying cause. Treatment options may include fluid and electrolyte replacement, diuretic therapy, fluid restriction, renal diet, and low dose dopamine to increase renal perfusion. Hemodialysis may also be necessary in patients with acute kidney injury.

CHRONIC KIDNEY DISEASE

Chronic kidney disease (CKD) occurs when the kidneys are unable to filter and excrete wastes, concentrate urine, and maintain electrolyte balance because of hypoxic conditions, kidney disease, or obstruction in the urinary tract. It results first in azotemia (increase in nitrogenous waste in the blood) and then in uremia (nitrogenous wastes cause toxic symptoms.) When >50% of the functional renal capacity is destroyed, the kidneys can no longer carry out necessary functions and progressive deterioration begins over months or years. Symptoms are often non-specific in the beginning with loss of appetite and energy.

Symptoms and complications are as follows:

- Weight loss. Headaches, muscle cramping, general malaise.
- Increased bruising and dry or itching skin.
- Increased BUN and creatinine.
- Sodium and fluid retention with edema.
- Hyperkalemia. Metabolic acidosis. Calcium and phosphorus depletion, resulting in altered bone metabolism, pain, and retarded growth.
- Anemia with decreased production on RBCs. Increased risk of infection.
- Uremic syndrome.

Copyright © Mometrix Media. You have been licensed one copy of this document for personal use only. Any other reproduction or redistribution is strictly prohibited. All rights reserved.

Treatment includes:

- Supportive/symptomatic therapy.
- Dialysis and transplantation.
- Diet control: Low protein, salt, potassium, and phosphorus.
- Fluid limitations.
- Calcium and vitamin supplementation.
- Phosphate binders.

UREMIC SYNDROME

Uremic syndrome is a number of disorders that can occur with end-stage renal disease and renal failure, usually after multiple metabolic failures and decrease in creatinine clearance to <10 mL/min. There is compromise of all normal functions of the kidney: fluid balance, electrolyte balance, acid-base homeostasis, hormone production, and elimination of wastes. Metabolic abnormalities related to uremia include:

- **Decreased RBC production:** The kidney is unable to produce adequate erythropoietin in the peritubular cells, resulting in anemia, which is usually normocytic and normochromic. Parathyroid hormone levels may increase, causing calcification of the bone marrow, causing hypoproliferative anemia as RBC production is suppressed.
- **Platelet abnormalities:** Decreased platelet count, increased turnover, and reduced adhesion leads to bleeding disorders.
- **Metabolic acidosis:** The tubular cells are unable to regulate acid-base metabolism, and phosphate, sulfuric, hippuric, and lactic acids increase, leading to congestive heart failure and weakness.
- **Hyperkalemia:** The nephrons cannot excrete adequate amounts of potassium. Some drugs, such as diuretics that spare potassium may aggravate the condition.
- **Renal bone disease:** ↓ Calcium, ↑ phosphate, ↑ parathyroid hormone, ↓ utilization of vitamin D lead to demineralization. In some cases, calcium and phosphate are deposited in other tissues (metastatic calcification).
- **Multiple endocrine disorders:** Thyroid hormone production is decreased and reproductive hormones abnormalities may result in infertility/impotence. Males have ↓ testosterone but ↑ estrogen and LH. Females experience irregular cycles, lack of ovulation and menses. Insulin production may increase but with decreased clearance, resulting in episodes of hypoglycemia or decreased hyperglycemia in those who are diabetic.
- **Cardiovascular disorders:** Left ventricular hypertrophy is most common, but fluid retention may cause congestive heart failure and electrolyte imbalances, dysrhythmias. Pericarditis, exacerbation of valvular disorders, and pericardial effusions may occur.
- **Anorexia and malnutrition:** Nausea and poor appetite contribute to hypoalbuminemia, sometimes exacerbated by restrictive diets.

PYELONEPHRITIS

Pyelonephritis is a potentially organ-damaging bacterial infection of the parenchyma of the kidney. Pyelonephritis can result in abscess formation, sepsis, and kidney failure. Pyelonephritis is especially dangerous for those who are immunocompromised, pregnant, or diabetic. Most infections are caused by *Escherichia coli. Diagnostic* studies include urinalysis, blood and urine cultures. Patients may require hospitalization or careful follow-up.

Symptoms vary widely but can include:

- Dysuria and frequency, hematuria, flank and/or low back pain.
- Fever and chills.
- Costovertebral angle tenderness.
- Change in feeding habits (infants).
- Change in mental status (geriatric).
- Young women often exhibit symptoms more associated with lower urinary infection, so the condition may be overlooked.

Treatment includes:

- Analgesia.
- Antipyretics.
- Intravenous fluids
- Antibiotics: started but may be changed based on cultures.
  - IV ceftriaxone with fluoroquinolone orally for 14 days.
  - Monitor BUN. Normal 7-8 mg/dL (8-20 mg/dL >age 60). Increase indicates impaired renal function, as urea is end product of protein metabolism.

NEPHROTOXIC AGENTS

Medications are a common cause of renal damage, especially among older patients. The **nephrotoxic effects** may be reversible if the drug is discontinued before permanent damage occurs. Those at increased risk include patients who are older than 60, have a history of renal insufficiency, suffer from volume depletion, or have diabetes mellitus, sepsis, or heart failure. Initial signs may be quite subtle. Preventive measures include baseline renal function tests and monitoring of renal function and vital signs during treatment. The following are some common effects, and the drugs that may cause them:

- **Chronic interstitial nephritis**: Acetaminophen, lithium, carmustine, cisplatin, cyclosporine.
- **Acute interstitial nephritis**: NSAIDs, acyclovir, beta-lactams, rifampin, quinolones, sulfonamides, vancomycin, indinavir, loop/thiazide diuretics, lansoprazole, allopurinol, phenytoin, ranitidine.
- **Rhabdomyolysis**: Amitriptyline, diphenhydramine, doxylamine, benzodiazepines, haloperidol, lithium, ketamine, methadone, methamphetamine, statins.
- **Crystal nephropathy**: Acyclovir, foscarnet, ganciclovir, quinolones, sulfonamides, indinavir, methotrexate, triamterene.
- **Tubular cell toxicity**: Aminoglycosides, amphotericin B, pentamidine, adefovir, tenofovir, contrast dye, zoledronate.
- **Thrombotic microangiopathy**: Cyclosporine, clopidogrel, mitomycin-C, quinine.
- **Impaired intraglomerular hemodynamics**: NSAIDs, cyclosporine, tacrolimus, ACE inhibitors.
- **Glomerulonephritis**: NSAIDs, lithium, beta-lactams, interferon-alpha, gold therapy, pamidronate.

FLUID BALANCE/FLUID DEFICIT

Body fluid is primarily intracellular fluid (ICF) or extracellular space (ECF). By 3 years of age, the fluid balance has stabilized and remains throughout adulthood:

- ECF: 20-30% (intrastitial fluid, plasma, transcellular fluid).
- ICF: 40-50% (fluid within the cells).

The fluid compartments are separated by semipermeable membranes that allow fluid and solutes (electrolytes and other substances) to move by osmosis. Fluid also moves through diffusion, filtration, and active transport. In fluid volume deficit, fluid is out of balance and ECF is depleted; an overload occurs with increased concentration of sodium and retention of fluid. Signs of fluid deficit include:

- Thirsty, restless to lethargic.
- Increasing pulse rate, tachycardia.
- Fontanels depressed (infants).
- Decreased urinary output.
- Normal BP progressing hypotension.
- Dry mucous membranes.
- 3-10% decrease in body weight.

Free Water Deficit = (Weight [kg] x 0.6 [% of total body water which is about 60% in young males]) x ((Na/140)-1)

Electrolyte Imbalances

SODIUM

Sodium (Na) regulates fluid volume, osmolality, acid-base balance, and activity in the muscles, nerves and myocardium. It is the primary cation (positive ion) in ECF, necessary to maintain ECF levels that are needed for tissue perfusion:

- Normal value: 135-145 mEq/L.

HYPONATREMIA (<135)

May result from inadequate sodium intake or excess loss, through diarrhea, vomiting, NG suctioning. It can occur as the result of illness, such as severe burns, fever, SIADH, and ketoacidosis. **Symptoms vary:** Irritability to lethargy, alterations in consciousness. Cerebral edema with seizures and coma. Dyspnea to respiratory failure.

Treatment: Identify and treat underlying cause and provide Na replacement.

HYPERNATREMIA (>145)

May result from renal disease, diabetes insipidus, and fluid depletion. **Symptoms** include irritability to lethargy to confusion to coma, seizures, flushing, muscle weakness and spasms, and thirst. **Treatment** includes identifying and treating underlying cause, monitoring Na levels carefully, and IV fluid replacement.

POTASSIUM

Potassium (K) is the primary electrolyte in ICF with about 98% inside cells and only 2% in ECF, although this small amount is important for neuromuscular activity. K influences activity of the skeletal and cardiac muscles. K level is dependent upon adequate renal functioning because 80% is excreted through the kidneys and 20% through the bowels and sweat:

- Normal values: 3.5-5.5 mEq/L.
- Hypokalemia: <3.5 mEq/L. Critical value: <2.5 mEq/L.
- A healthy NPO patient will need about 40 mEq of K per day to maintain serum K levels. (Expect alterations in renal disease and other disease processes.)

HYPOKALEMIA

- Caused by loss of K through diarrhea, vomiting, gastric suction, and diuresis, alkalosis, decreased K intake with starvation, and nephritis. **Symptoms** include: Lethargy and weakness, nausea and vomiting, paresthesias and tetany, dysrhythmias with EKG changes: PVCs, flattened T waves, muscle cramps with hyporeflexia, hypotension.

Treatment: Identify and treat underlying cause and replace K. When possible, oral replacement is preferable to IV, as it allows slower adjustment of K levels. When given IV, K should be given no faster than 20 mEq/hour. *Note: K levels have a reciprocal relationship with serum pH.*

HYPERKALEMIA

Hyperkalemia (>5.5 mEq/L)

Critical value: >6.5 mEq/L

Caused by renal disease, adrenal insufficiency, metabolic acidosis, severe dehydration, burns, hemolysis, and trauma. It rarely occurs without renal disease but may be induced by treatment (such as NSAIDs and potassium-sparing diuretics). Untreated renal failure results in reduced excretion. Those with Addison's disease and deficient adrenal hormones suffer sodium loss that results in potassium retention.

- The **primary symptoms** relate to the effect on the cardiac muscle: Ventricular arrhythmias with increasing frequency that lead to cardiac and respiratory arrest. Weakness with ascending paralysis and hyperreflexia. Diarrhea. Increasing confusion.
- **Treatment** includes identifying underlying cause and discontinuing sources of increased K: Calcium gluconate to decrease cardiac effects. Sodium bicarbonate shifts K into the cells temporarily. Insulin and hypertonic dextrose shift K into the cells temporarily. Cation exchange resin (Kayexalate®) to decrease K (remember to never hold Kayexalate for diarrhea!), Peritoneal dialysis or hemodialysis.

Note: When a tourniquet is on, if a patient is opening and closing the hand, it can lead to falsely elevated K levels.

CALCIUM

More than 99% of **calcium (Ca)** is in the skeletal system with 1% in serum, but it is important for transmitting nerve impulses and regulating muscle contraction and relaxation, including the myocardium. Calcium activates enzymes that stimulate chemical reactions and has a role in coagulation of blood. Calcium levels should be interpreted with albumin levels. Ca^{++} is inversely proportional to pH of the blood. Normal values: 8.2 to 10.2 mg/dL.

Hypercalcemia (>10.2 mg/dL. Critical value: >12 mg/dL): May be caused by acidosis, kidney disease, hyperparathyroidism, prolonged immobilization, and malignancies. Crisis carries a 50% mortality rate.

- **Symptoms**: Increasing muscle weakness with hypotonicity. Anorexia, nausea and vomiting. Constipation. Bradycardia and cardiac arrest.
- **Treatment**: Treat underlying cause, diuretics, IV fluids, and phosphate.

Hypocalcemia: (<8.2. Critical value: <7 mg/dL). Hypocalcemia may be caused by hypoparathyroidism after thyroid and parathyroid surgery, pancreatitis, renal failure, inadequate vitamin D, alkalosis, magnesium deficiency and low serum albumin.

- **Symptoms**: Tetany, tingling, seizures, altered mental status, ventricular tachycardia, positive Trousseau's sign, positive Chvostek's sign, and hypotension.
- **Treatment**: Calcium replacement and vitamin D. It is preferable to give oral calcium, but if IV is given, carefully monitor EKG while giving 10% calcium gluconate 20 mL IV over 10 minutes.

PHOSPHORUS

Phosphorus, or phosphate, (PO_4) is necessary for neuromuscular and red blood cell function, the maintenance of acid-base balance, and provides structure for teeth and bones. About 85% is in the bones, 14% in soft tissue, and <1% in ECF. Normal values: 2.4 – 4.5 mEq/L

Hypophosphatemia (<2.4mEq/L)

Occurs with severe protein-calorie malnutrition, excess antacids with magnesium, calcium or albumin, hyperventilation, severe burns, and diabetic ketoacidosis.

- **Symptoms** include: Irritability, tremors, seizures to coma. Hemolytic anemia. Decreased myocardial function. Respiratory failure.
- **Treatment**: Identify and treat underlying cause and replace phosphorus.

Hyperphosphatemia (> 4.5 mEq/L)

Occurs with renal failure, hypoparathyroidism, excessive intake, and neoplastic disease, diabetic ketoacidosis, muscle necrosis, and chemotherapy.

- **Symptoms** include: Tachycardia. Muscle cramping, hyperreflexia, and tetany. Nausea and diarrhea.
- **Treatment**: Identify and treat underlying cause, correct hypocalcemia, and provide antacids and dialysis.

MAGNESIUM

Magnesium (Mg) is the second most common intracellular electrolyte (after potassium) and activates many intracellular enzyme systems. Mg is important for carbohydrate and protein metabolism, neuromuscular function, and cardiovascular function, producing vasodilation and directly affecting the peripheral arterial system. Normal values: 1.6 to 2.6 mEq/L.

Hypomagnesemia (Critical <1.2 mg/dL)

Occurs with chronic diarrhea, chronic renal disease, chronic pancreatitis, excess diuretic or laxative use, hyperthyroidism, hypoparathyroidism, severe burns, and diaphoresis.

- **Symptoms** include: Neuromuscular excitability/ tetany. Confusion, headaches and dizziness, seizure and coma. Tachycardia with ventricular arrhythmias. Respiratory depression.
- **Treatment**: Identify and treat underlying cause, provide magnesium replacement. IV magnesium is a vasodilator. Give at rate of 2 grams Magnesium IV over 60 mins.

Hypermagnesemia (Critical >4.9 mg/dL)

Occurs with renal failure or inadequate renal function, diabetic ketoacidosis, hypothyroidism, and Addison's disease.

- **Symptoms** include muscle weakness, seizures, and dysphagia with decreased gag reflex, tachycardia with hypotension.
- **Treatment**: Identify and treat underlying cause, IV hydration with calcium, and dialysis.

Medication Management

LOOP DIURETICS

Diuretics increase renal perfusion and filtration, thereby reducing preload and decreasing peripheral and pulmonary edema, hypertension, CHF, diabetes insipidus, and osteoporosis. There are different types of diuretics: Loop, thiazide, and potassium sparing.

Loop diuretics inhibit the reabsorption of sodium and chloride (primarily) in the ascending loop of Henle. They also cause increased secretion of other electrolytes, such as calcium, magnesium, and potassium, and this can result in imbalances that cause dysrhythmias. Other side effects include frequent urination, postural hypotension, and increased blood sugar and uric acid levels. They are short-acting so are less effective than other diuretics for control of hypertension:

- **Bumetanide** (Bumex®) is given intravenously after surgery to reduce preload or orally to treat heart failure.
- **Ethacrynic acid** (Edecrin®) is given intravenously after surgery to reduce preload.
- **Furosemide** (Lasix®) is used for the control of congestive heart failure as well as renal insufficiency. It is used after surgery to decrease preload and to reduce the inflammatory response caused by cardiopulmonary bypass (post-perfusion syndrome).

THIAZIDE DIURETICS

Thiazide diuretics inhibit the reabsorption of sodium and chloride primarily in the early distal tubules, forcing more sodium and water to be excreted. Thiazide diuretics increase secretion of potassium and bicarbonate, so they are often given with supplementary potassium or in combination with potassium-sparing diuretics. They have a long duration of action (12-72 hours, depending on the drug) so they are able to maintain control of hypertension better than short-acting drugs. They may be given daily or 3-5 days per week. There are numerous thiazide diuretics, including:

- Chlorothiazide (Diuril®)
- Bendroflumethiazide (Naturetin®)
- Chlorthalidone (Hygroton®)
- Trichlormethiazide (Naqua®)

Side effects include, dizziness, lightheadedness, postural hypotension, headache, blurred vision, and itching, especially during initial treatment. Thiazide diuretics cause sensitivity to sun exposure, so people should be counseled to use sunscreen.

POTASSIUM-SPARING DIURETICS

Potassium-sparing diuretics inhibit the reabsorption of sodium in the late distal tubule and collecting duct. They are weaker than thiazide or loop diuretics, but do not cause a reduction in potassium level; however, if used alone, they may cause an increase in potassium, which can cause weakness, irregular pulse, and cardiac arrest. Because potassium-sparing diuretics are less effective alone, they are often given in a combined form with a thiazide diuretic (usually chlorothiazide), which mitigates the potassium imbalance. Typical side effects include dehydration, blurred vision, nausea insomnia, and nasal congestion, especially in the first few days of treatment:

- **Spironolactone** (Aldactone®) is a synthetic steroid diuretic that increases the secretion of both water and sodium and is used to treat congestive heart failure. It may be given orally or intravenously.
- **Eplerenone** is an antimineralocorticoid similar to spironolactone but with fewer side effects.

Assessment and Diagnostics

URINALYSIS

The laboratory testing **urinalysis** consists of the following:

- **Color:** Pale yellow/ amber and darkens when urine is concentrated or other substances (such as blood or bile) or present.
- **Appearance:** Clear but may be slightly cloudy.
- **Odor:** Slight. Bacteria may give urine a foul smell, depending upon the organism. Some foods, such as asparagus, change odor.
- **Specific gravity:** 1.015 to 1.025. May increase if protein levels increase or if there is fever, vomiting, or dehydration.
- **pH:** Usually ranges from 4.5-8 with average of 5-6.
- **Sediment:** Red cell casts from acute infections, broad casts from kidney disorders, and white cell casts from pyelonephritis. Leukocytes >10/hpf are present with urinary tract infections.
- **Glucose, ketones, protein, blood, bilirubin, & nitrate:** Negative. Urine glucose may increase with infection (with normal blood glucose). Frank blood may be caused by some parasites and diseases but also by drugs, smoking, excessive exercise, and menstrual fluids. Increased red blood cells may result from lower urinary tract infections.
- **Urobilinogen:** 0.1-1.0 units.

RENAL FUNCTION STUDIES

Renal function studies include the following:

- **Specific gravity**:1.015-1.025: Determines kidney's ability to concentrate urinary solutes.
- **Osmolality (urine):** 350-900 mOsm/kg/24 hr: Shows early changes when kidney has difficulty concentrating urine.
- **Osmolality (serum):** 275-295 mOsm/kg: Gives a picture of the volume of solutes in the blood.
- **Uric acid:** 3.0-7.2 mg/dL: increases with renal failure.
- **Creatinine clearance (24-hour):** 75 to 125 mL/min.: Evaluates the amount of blood cleared of creatinine in 1 min. Approximates the GFR.
- **Serum creatinine:** 0.6-1.2mg/dL: Increase with decreased renal function, urinary tract obstruction, and nephritis.
- **Urine creatinine:** 11-26 mg/kg/24 hr: Product of muscle breakdown. Increase with decreased renal function.
- **Blood urea nitrogen (BUN):** 7-8 mg/dL (8-20 mg/dL >age 60): Increase indicates impaired renal function, as urea is end product of protein metabolism.
- **BUN/creatinine ratio:** 10:1: Increases with hypovolemia. With intrinsic kidney disease, the ratio is normal though increased BUN/Creatinine.

KIDNEY REGULATORY FUNCTIONS REGARDING FLUID BALANCE

Kidney regulatory functions include maintaining **fluid balance**. Fluid excretion balances intake with output so increased intake results in a large output and vice versa:

- **Osmolality** (the number of electrolytes and other molecules per kg/urine) measures the concentration or dilution. With dehydration, osmolality increases; with fluid retention, osmolality decreases. With kidney disease, urine is dilute and the osmolality is fixed.
- **Specific gravity** compares the weight of urine (weight of particles) to distilled water (1.000). Normal urine is 1.010-1.025 with normal intake. High intake lowers the specific gravity and low intake raises it. In kidney disease, it often does not vary.
- **Antidiuretic hormone** (ADH/vasopressin) regulates the excretion of water and urine concentration in the renal tubule by varying water reabsorption. When fluid intake decreases, blood osmolality rises and this stimulates release of ADH, which increases reabsorption of fluid to return osmolality to normal levels. ADH is suppressed with increased fluid intake, so less fluid is reabsorbed.

IVP

Intravenous pyelogram (IVP) is done to identify structural defects and tumors and to observe urinary structures. The patient is administered an IV contrast medium and may be administered antihistamine or corticosteroid before test to minimize allergic response. Serum creatinine and BUN are done prior to the IVP to ensure that the contrast medium can be excreted. During the procedure, radiographs are taken every minute x 5 and then after 15 minutes (giving the contrast medium time to pass into the bladder). A post-voiding radiograph shows how efficient the bladder is in emptying. Fluid intake should be increased post-procedure to flush contrast.

RADIO NUCLEOTIDE RENAL SCAN

Radionucleotide renal scan with dimercaptosuccinic acid (DMSA) requires IV administration of a radioactive element followed by a series of CT scans taken over 20 minutes to 4 hours. The scan is used to assess function and perfusion of the kidney and can detect lesions, atrophy and scars and differentiate among different causes for hydronephrosis. The patient must be well-hydrated and may need to be catheterized to measure output of urine.

RENAL BIOPSY

Renal biopsy to remove a small segment of cortical tissue helps to identify the extent of kidney disease with acute renal failure, transplant rejection, glomerulopathies, and persistent hematuria or proteinuria. Preoperative coagulation studies determine risk of bleeding. Biopsy is done percutaneously per needle biopsy (guided by fluoroscopy or ultrasound) or surgically through a small flank incision. A urine specimen must be obtained so it can be compared with a post-procedure specimen. Post-procedure:

- Maintain patient in supine position immediately after procedure for 4-6 hours and on bedrest overnight. Monitor urine for hematuria and compare with preop specimen.
- Monitor VS every 5 to 15 minutes for first hour and then less frequently. To minimize bleeding maintain BP<140/90.
- Note anorexia, vomiting, abdominal discomfort that suggest bleeding.
- Note pain: Severe colicky pain may indicate clot in the ureter.
- Monitor urinalysis and CBC post procedure.
- Maintain fluid intake at 3000 mL/day in absence of renal insufficiency.
- Provide blood component therapy and surgical repair if bleeding occurs.

RENAL ULTRASOUND

Renal ultrasound is a non-invasive method of viewing the urinary structures. Most patients that present with kidney disease of unknown origin should undergo renal ultrasound to assess for possible obstruction. Ultrasound uses ultrasonic sound waves transmitted by a transducer, which picks up reflected sound waves that a computer converts to electronic images. Ultrasound can show fluid accumulation, the movement of blood through the kidney, masses, malformations (congenital abnormalities), change in size of the kidney or other structures, and obstructions, such as renal calculi. Ultrasound is usually done before a renal biopsy, and may be done with a needle biopsy to guide placement of needle. Patient preparation includes drinking two 8-ounce glasses of water one hour before the examination to ensure that the bladder is full. The patient should be reminded not to urinate before the ultrasound. The patient usually remains in supine position throughout the procedure but may be asked to turn to the side. No special precautions are necessary post-procedure.

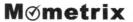

Interventions and Procedures

RENAL DIALYSIS

PERITONEAL DIALYSIS

Renal dialysis is used primarily for those who have progressed from renal insufficiency to uremia with end stage renal disease (ESRD). It may also be temporarily for acute conditions. People can be maintained on dialysis, but there are many complications associated with dialysis so many people are considered for renal transplantation. There are a number of different approaches to peritoneal dialysis:

- **Peritoneal dialysis:** An indwelling catheter is inserted surgically into the peritoneal cavity with a subcutaneous tunnel and a Dacron cuff to prevent infection. Sterile dialysate solution is slowly instilled through gravity, remains for a prescribed length of time, and is then drained and discarded.
- **Continuous ambulatory peritoneal dialysis:** A series of exchange cycles are repeated 24 hours a day.
- **Continuous cyclic peritoneal dialysis:** A prolonged period of retaining fluid occurs during the day with drainage at night.

Peritoneal dialysis may be used for those who want to be more independent, don't live near a dialysis center, or want fewer dietary restrictions.

HEMODIALYSIS

Hemodialysis, the most common type of dialysis, is used for both short-term dialysis and long-term for those with ESRD. Treatments are usually done 3 times weekly for 3-4 hours or daily dialysis with treatment either during the night or in short daily periods. Hemodialysis is often done for those who can't manage peritoneal dialysis or who live near a dialysis center, but it does interfere with work or school attendance and requires strict dietary and fluid restrictions between treatments. Short daily dialysis allows more independence, and increased costs may be offset by lower morbidity. A vascular access device, such as a catheter, fistula, or graft must be established for hemodialysis, and heparin is used to prevent clotting. With hemodialysis, blood is circulated outside of the body through a dialyzer (a synthetic semipermeable membrane), which filters the blood. There are many different types of dialyzers. High flux dialyzers use a highly permeable membrane that shortens the duration of treatment and decreases the need for heparin.

CONTINUOUS RENAL REPLACEMENT THERAPY

Continuous renal replacement therapy (CCRT) circulates the blood by hydrostatic pressure through a semipermeable membrane. It is used in critical care and can be instituted quickly:

- **Continuous arteriovenous hemofiltration** (CAVH) circulates blood from an artery (usually the femoral) to a hemofilter using only arterial pressure and not a blood pump. The filtered blood is then returned to the patient's venous system, often with added fluids to offset those lost. Only the fluid in filtered.
- **Continuous arteriovenous hemodialysis** (CAVHD) is similar to CAVH except that dialysate circulates on one side of the semipermeable membrane to increase clearance of urea.

- **Continuous venovenous hemofiltration** (CVVH) pumps blood through a double-lumen venous catheter to a hemofilter, which returns the blood to the patient in the same catheter. It provides continuous slow removal of fluid, is better tolerated with unstable patients, and doesn't require arterial access.
- **Continuous venovenous hemodialysis** is similar to CVVH but uses a dialysate to increase clearance of uremic toxins.

DIALYSIS COMPLICATIONS

There are many **complications** associated with dialysis, especially when used for long-term treatment:

- **Hemodialysis**: Long-term use promotes atherosclerosis and cardiovascular disease. Anemia and fatigue are common as are infections related to access devices or contamination of equipment. Some experience hypotension and muscle cramping during treatment. Dysrhythmias may occur. Some may exhibit dialysis disequilibrium from cerebral fluid shifts, causing headaches, nausea and vomiting, and alterations of consciousness.
- **Peritoneal dialysis:** Most complications are minor, but it can lead to peritonitis, which requires removal of the catheter if antibiotic therapy is not successful in clearing the infection within 4 days. There may be leakage of the dialysate around the catheter. Bleeding may occur, especially in females who are menstruating as blood is pulled from the uterus through the fallopian tubes. Abdominal hernias may occur with long use. Some may have anorexia from feeling of fullness or sweet taste in mouth from absorption of glucose.

RADICAL NEPHRECTOMY

Radical nephrectomy is done for adenocarcinoma of the kidney, which may be associated with paraneoplastic syndromes, and, because this type of cancer is associated with smoking, patients may have underlying coronary artery or respiratory disease. Some patients have erythrocytosis, but many are anemic and may require transfusions in preparation for surgery to increase hemoglobin to >10 g/dL. Surgery is done under endotracheal general anesthesia with an anterior subcostal, flank, or thoracoabdominal (preferred for large tumors) incision. The kidney and its adrenal gland with surrounding fat and fascia are removed together. Blood loss may be extensive because the tumors tend to be vascular and large, requiring multiple transfusions. However, controlled hypotension should be limited to brief periods because it may impair renal function. Mannitol is given prior to dissection. Continual direct arterial pressure monitoring and central venous cannulation must be done.

Nephron-sparing surgery (partial nephrectomy), often by laparoscopy, may be done if the renal cell carcinoma is <4 cm diameter. Postoperative analgesia and pulmonary hygiene are essential.

Integumentary

Integumentary Disorders and Complications

CELLULITIS

Cellulitis occurs when an area of the skin becomes infected, usually following injury or trauma to the skin. Cellulitis is most likely to be caused by staphylococcus or streptococcus bacteria. Patients with peripheral vascular disease, diabetes mellitus, and immunosuppression are at a higher risk for the development of cellulitis. Signs and symptoms include: pain, erythema, and warmth at the affected site that progresses rapidly. In addition, the patient may experience fever, chills, fatigue and malaise. Diagnosis is made by physical exam. Labs include complete blood count, culture of the involved area and blood. Treatment for cellulitis is the administration of antibiotics. Surgical irrigation and debridement may be indicated in severe cases.

SEPTIC ARTHRITIS

Septic arthritis is defined as an invasion of the joint space by bacteria, virus or fungi. Elderly patients, immunosuppressed patients, and those with prosthetic joints are at an increased risk for septic arthritis. The most commonly affected joints include the knee (#1), hip, shoulder, ankle and wrist. Signs and symptoms include joint pain, fever, impaired range of motion, chills, edema, erythema, warmth and the abnormal presence of fluid (effusion) surrounding the joint. Diagnosis is made by aspiration of the fluid with stain and culture, x-ray, and blood tests including CBC and cultures. Treatment is the administration of antibiotics. Surgical irrigation and debridement may also be indicated. The patient will likely undergo physical therapy as part of their recovery to improve and restore mobility and range of motion.

EXTRAVASATION

Extravasation occurs when an intravenously infused vesicant medication or fluid leaks from the vein and into the subcutaneous space. Vesicant medications are those that cause tissue injury if extravasated and that may ultimately lead to tissue necrosis. Extravasation and infiltration are similar in nature, with infiltration occurring when the infusate is a non-vesicant solution or medication. Extravasation occurs more commonly in peripheral IVs; however, it can also occur with central venous catheters. Common vesicant agents include several chemotherapeutic agents, vancomycin, electrolytes, dobutamine, norepinephrine, phenytoin, promethazine, propofol and vasopressin.

Signs and symptoms: Pain, burning, erythema and edema at the site of the extravasation. Often times, a blood return from the peripheral IV or central venous catheter is not present. Long term complications include complex regional pain syndrome, tissue necrosis, and nerve or tendon damage.

Diagnosis: physical assessment and review of patient symptoms and medications/infusions administered.

Treatment: Early recognition is key to the successful treatment of an extravasation. When an extravasation is suspected, the IV infusion should be immediately stopped and the infusion site assessed. For some medications, antidotes may be available to minimize the damage caused by the extravasation. Heat or cold therapy may also be utilized depending on the medication. In cases of severe damage, debridement, skin grafting and even amputation may result.

PRESSURE ULCERS

Pressure ulcers occur when pressure from the weight of the body causes a decrease in perfusion, affecting arterial and capillary blood flow and resulting ischemia. Ulcers may then develop from pressure, shearing and friction. Common pressure points include the occiput, scapula, sacrum, buttocks, ischium and heels. Patients with a decreased level of consciousness, brain/spinal cord injuries, peripheral neuropathies, malnutrition, dehydration, PVD, or impaired mobility are at a higher risk for pressure ulcers. Critically ill patients are at an increased risk due to prolonged immobility, sedation, and often incontinence of urine and stool. In addition, patients on vasopressors are at a higher risk due to the constriction of the peripheral circulation.

Signs and symptoms: Early stages – redness, tenderness and firmness at the site of the ulcer. Severe tissue injury – bone, muscle or tendons may be exposed, yellow or black wound base, pain and drainage at the site.

Diagnostics: Skin and wound assessment including staging of the ulcer.

Treatment: Wet-to-Dry dressings, Wound VAC® therapy, and hyperbaric oxygen may be used; a wound care consult is often advised. **Prevention**: begins with a risk assessment; the Braden scale is a commonly used scale. A score of 16 or below indicates that the patient is at risk. At-risk patients or patients with active ulcers should be placed on a turning and positioning schedule or specialty bed to relieve pressure. Moisture barriers and skin protectants may also be utilized.

NECROTIZING FASCIITIS

Necrotizing fasciitis is an infection that develops deep within the fascia, causing a rapidly developing tissue necrosis resulting in destruction and death of the soft tissue and nerves. Complications of necrotizing fasciitis may include the loss of the affected limb, sepsis and death. Group A Streptococcus, Klebsiella, Clostridium, Escherichia coli, Staphylococcus aureus and Aeromonas hydrophila are organisms that have the potential to cause necrotizing fasciitis.

Signs and symptoms: Edema, erythema and pain at the affected site. Nausea, vomiting, fatigue, malaise, fever and chills may also occur.

Diagnosis: Diagnosis is based on physical assessment and patient history. In addition, excisional deep skin biopsy and gram staining may be performed to determine the causative organism. CT/MRI may also be utilized to assess the extent of the infection.

Treatment: Treatment options for necrotizing fasciitis include antibiotics and fasciotomy with radical debridement. Hyperbaric oxygen therapy may also be utilized.

INFECTIOUS WOUNDS

All types of wounds have the potential to become infected. **Infectious wounds** are commonly health care acquired. Wound infections increase a patient's risk of sepsis, multisystem organ failure and death. Trauma patients are at an increased risk of developing an infected wound due to exposure to various contaminants that they may have encountered during their injury (e.g., dirt from a motor vehicle accident).

Signs and symptoms: Erythema, edema, induration, drainage, increasing pain and tenderness, fever, leukocytosis and lymphangitis.

Diagnosis: Wound infections are diagnosed by wound cultures (anaerobic and aerobic). Fluid or tissue biopsy may also be performed.

Treatment: Wound infections are treated with antibiotics and a wound care regimen that includes routine cleaning and dressing of the wound. Wound care treatment is based on the type and severity of the wound. Surgical irrigation and debridement may also be indicated. For deep, complex wounds, a wound-care consult is often indicated.

Surgical Wounds

Surgical wounds or incisions are made during a surgical procedure in a sterile, controlled environment. The American College of Surgeons has defined four classes of surgical wound types. This classification can help to predict how the wound will heal and the risk of infection.

- **Class I** is defined as clean (e.g., laparoscopic surgeries and biopsies).
- **Class II** is defined as clean contaminated (e.g., GI and GU surgeries).
- **Class III** is defined as contaminated (e.g., traumatic wounds such as a gunshot wound).
- **Class IV** is defined as dirty (e.g., traumatic wound from a dirty source).

Surgical wounds should be assessed for signs and symptoms of infection including erythema, edema, fever, increasing pain, and drainage. Surgical drains are commonly placed near the surgical incision to promote drainage – inspect drains for patency, amount and characteristics of drainage. Patients are often treated with antibiotics prophylactically to help prevent a surgical site infection. Wound vacuum assisted closure devices may also be utilized to remove blood or serous fluid from the surgical wound/incision site.

Traumatic Wounds

Traumatic wounds include cuts, punctures, lacerations, force trauma, gunshot wounds, bites, abrasions, crush injuries, degloving injuries and contusions. Trauma wounds can vary in severity and may be associated with serious underlying injuries. Once the patient is stabilized, wound management is initiated and should include thorough wound cleansing and debridement with removal of any foreign objects or materials. Irrigation and debridement are critical steps in minimizing the risk of infection. Signs and symptoms include bleeding, pain, erythema and edema. With severe traumatic injury patients may experience signs of hemorrhagic shock including heavy bleeding, loss of consciousness, tachypnea, tachycardia, hypotension, decreased urinary output and pallor.

Treatment of traumatic wounds is dependent on the location and severity of the wound. Treatment options may include irrigation and debridement, foreign body removal, wound closure including sutures, staples or fibrin glue, antibiotics, prophylactic tetanus injection, and fasciotomy.

Nursing Actions

Wound VACs

Wound vacuum-assisted closure (wound VAC) (AKA negative pressure wound therapy) uses subatmospheric (negative) pressure with a suction unit and a semi-occlusion vapor-permeable dressing. The suction reduces periwound and interstitial edema, decompressing vessels, improving circulation, stimulating production of new cells and decreasing colonization of bacteria. Wound VAC also increases the rate of granulation and re-epithelialization to hasten healing. The wound must be debrided of necrotic tissue prior to treatment. Wound VAC is used for a variety of difficult to heal wounds, especially those that show less than 30% healing in 4 weeks of post-debridement treatment or those with excessive exudate, including chronic stage II and IV pressure ulcers, skin

135

flaps, diabetic ulcer, acute wounds, burns, surgical wound and those with dehiscence, and nonresponsive arterial and venous ulcers. Contraindications include:

- Wound malignancy
- Untreated osteomyelitis
- Exposed blood vessels or organs
- Non-enteric, unexplored fistulas.

Nonadherent porous foam is cut to fit and cover the wound and is secured with occlusive transparent film with an opening cut to accommodate the drainage tube, which is attached to a suction cannister in a closed system. The pressure should be set between 75 and 125 psi and the dressing changed 2 to 3 times weekly.

PRESSURE REDUCTION SURFACES

Pressure reduction surfaces redistribute pressure to prevent pressure ulcers and reduce shear and friction. There are various types of support surfaces for beds, examining tables, operating tables, and chairs. Functions of pressure reduction surfaces include temperature control, moisture control, and friction/shear control. General use guidelines include:

- Pressure redistribution support surfaces should be used in beds, operating and examining tables for at-risk individuals.
- Patients with multiple ulcers, stage II or stage IV ulcers require support surfaces.
- Chairs should have gel or air support surfaces to redistribute pressure for chair bound patients, critically ill patients, or those who cannot move independently.
- Support surface material should provide at least an inch of support under areas to be protected when in use to prevent "bottoming out." (Check by placing hand palm-up under overlay below the pressure point.)
- Static support surfaces are appropriate for patients who can change position without increasing pressure to an ulcer.
- Dynamic support surfaces are needed for those who need assistance to move or when static pressure devices provide less than an inch of support.

INDWELLING FECAL MANAGEMENT SYSTEMS

Indwelling fecal management systems are used for incontinent clients with loose or watery stools in order to prevent skin breakdown, discomfort, odor, and contamination of wounds, and to control the spread of organisms, such as *Clostridium difficile,* in bedridden or immobile clients. A number of different devices, such as the Flexi-Seal® FMS, are available and work similarly. A typical management system includes:

- Silicone catheter, silicone retention balloon at end of catheter, a 45-mL syringe, and charcoal filter collection bags.

The application of the fecal management system is relatively simple: The catheter is inserted into the rectum and balloon inflated with water or saline (using the 45 mL syringe) to hold it in place and to block fecal leakage. Some systems, such as Flexi-Seal® FMS, have a pop-up button to indicate when the balloon is adequately filled for the size of the rectum. The catheter contains an irrigation port so that irrigating fluid can be instilled if necessary. The charcoal filter collection bag is attached to the end of the silicone catheter to contain fecal material.

Musculoskeletal

Nursing Role in Functional Issues

IMMOBILITY

Critical care patients are often **immobile** for extended periods of time, thereby increasing their risk of skin breakdown and the development of pressure ulcers, deep vein thrombosis, functional decline, decreased muscle mass, impaired coordination and gait, cardiovascular deconditioning, depression and constipation. Immobility leads to impaired physical functioning in which muscle mass is lost and weakness develops. Intensive care unit acquired weakness can develop during hospitalization and is associated with an increased hospital length of stay as well as an increased mortality rate. ICU acquired weakness may last years after discharge with residual effects often affecting the patient's quality of life. Progressive mobility is defined as the gradual progression of positioning and mobility techniques and should be utilized to improve muscle strength and provide the patient a greater ability to resume activities of daily living. Patients should be assessed daily for their readiness to progress in their mobility goals in order to prevent the adverse effects of immobility.

GAIT DISORDERS

Functional movement disorders are defined as an involuntary, abnormal movement of part of the body in which pathophysiology is not fully understood. Functional tremors are the most frequent type of functional movement disorder. Dystonia, myoclonus and Parkinsonism are other types of functional movement disorders. Functional gait disorders are another type of functional movement disorder and are common in the elderly. Gait disorders can manifest as a dragging gait, knee buckling, small slow steps or "walking on ice," swaying gait, fluctuating gait, hesitant gait, and hyperkinetic gait in which there is excessive movement of the arms, trunks and legs when ambulating. Patients with gait disorders are at an increased risk of falling. Gait disorders are diagnosed by a thorough clinical examination (including a neurologic assessment) and health history. Treatment for functional gait disorders includes strength and balance training. Assistive devices such as walkers and canes may also be utilized.

FALLS

Falls are the most commonly occurring adverse event in the hospital setting. Confusion and agitation are factors that contribute to an increased risk for falling. In addition, impaired balance or gait, orthostatic hypotension, altered mobility, a history of falling, advanced age and the use of certain medications are additional risk factors. Approximately 30% of patient falls result in injury, some of which can significantly contribute to an increase in morbidity and mortality including fractures and subdural hematomas. Both physical and environmental factors contribute to patient falls, some of which are preventable. Fall prevention strategies include utilization of a standardized fall risk assessment to determine the patient's level of risk and subsequent care planning and interventions individualized to the patient. Fall prevention should also be balanced with progressive mobility. Many falls are related to toileting needs and scheduled rounding to address those needs is a strategy that is often utilized.

Musculoskeletal Emergencies

COMPARTMENT SYNDROME

Compartment syndrome occurs when there is an increase in the amount of pressure within a grouping of muscles, nerves and blood vessels resulting in compromised blood flow to muscles and nerves. This is a medical emergency. If left untreated, tissue ischemia and eventual tissue death will occur. Compartment syndrome most often occurs after a fracture, particularly a long bone fracture, but can also occur with crushing syndrome and rhabdomyolysis. Risk factors include lower extremity trauma, massive tissue injury, venous obstruction, the use of certain medications (anticoagulants), burns and compressive dressings or casts. Compartment syndrome can affect the hand, forearm, upper arm, abdomen and lower extremities. It can be acute or chronic in nature with acute compartment syndrome requiring immediate intervention.

Signs and symptoms: intense pain, decreased sensation and paresthesia, firmness at the affected site, swelling and tightness at the affected site, pallor and pulselessness (late signs).

Diagnosis: physical assessment and the measurement of intra-compartmental pressures.

Treatment: The goal of treatment in compartment syndrome is decompression and the restoration of perfusion to the affected area. Surgical fasciotomy is often indicated to relieve pressure and prevent tissue death. Fasciotomy involves the opening of the skin and muscle fascia to release the pressure within the compartment and restore blood flow to the area.

Prevention: Leave large abdominal wounds open to drain, delay casting on affected extremities /use flexible casts. Watch circumferential burns closely, frequent neurovascular checks on those at risk.

OSTEOMYELITIS

Musculoskeletal infections encompass a variety of different disorders with differing pathologies. Osteomyelitis, cellulitis, and septic arthritis are examples of musculoskeletal infections that can be both serious and debilitating in nature.

Osteomyelitis is an infection of the bone that can occur from an open fracture or an infection that has occurred somewhere else in the body. In addition, wounds or soft tissue infections can progress and extend to the bone, also causing osteomyelitis to occur. Signs and symptoms of osteomyelitis include pain, swelling, erythema and possible drainage at the site. The patient may also experience fever and chills. Diagnosis includes lab work including a complete blood count, erythrocyte sedimentation rate (ESR), C-reactive protein (CRP), and blood cultures, as well as radiologic testing that may include CT, MRI, X-ray, bone scan or a bone biopsy. Treatment includes the administration of IV antibiotics. A needle aspiration may be performed to determine the organism and drain the area. Surgical irrigation and debridement may also be indicated.

RHABDOMYOLYSIS

Rhabdomyolysis occurs when damage of the cells of the skeletal muscles causes the release of toxins from injured cells into the bloodstream. Rhabdomyolysis may be caused by trauma, tissue ischemia, infection, certain medications (statins, selective serotonin reuptake inhibitors, lithium and antihistamines), sepsis, immobilization, extraordinary physical exertion, myopathies and cocaine or alcohol abuse. Additionally, rhabdomyolysis may occur with exposure to certain toxins such as snake/insect venoms or mushroom poisoning. In rare circumstances, the identifiable cause cannot be determined. The most serious complication of rhabdomyolysis is renal failure. Rhabdomyolysis may be life threatening. Early recognition and treatment are critical to avoid serious complications and for patients to make a full recovery.

Signs and symptoms: Electrolyte imbalance, muscle pain and weakness, fever, tachycardia, dehydration, fatigue, lethargy, hypotension and metabolic acidosis. Dark, reddish-brown urine may occur due to the presence of myoglobin released from the muscles and excreted into the urine.

Diagnosis: Laboratory studies such as creatinine kinase (CK) level, metabolic panel, urinalysis and blood gases.

Treatment: The treatment of rhabdomyolysis includes fluid administration to eliminate toxins and prevent renal failure. Bicarbonate may be administered to correct metabolic acidosis. Mannitol or dopamine may be administered to increase renal perfusion. Electrolyte replacement may also be indicated. In severe cases, emergency dialysis may be necessary.

Neurological

Delirium, Dementia, and Brain Death

DELIRIUM

Delirium is an *acute, sudden, and fluctuating change* in consciousness. Delirium occurs in 10-40% of hospitalized older adults and about 80% of patients who are terminally ill. Delirium may result from drugs, infections, hypoxia, trauma, dementia, depression, vision and hearing loss, surgery, alcoholism, untreated pain, fluid/electrolyte imbalance, and malnutrition. If left untreated, delirium greatly increases the risk of morbidity and death.

Signs/Symptoms: Reduced ability to focus/ sustain attention, language and memory disturbances, disorientation, confusion, audiovisual hallucinations, sleep disturbance, and psychomotor activity disorder

Diagnosis: Patient interview, history/chart/medication review, and possible blood tests to identify electrolyte imbalance/abnormalities.

Treatment includes:

- **Medications**: Trazodone, lorazepam, haloperidol – though these may make confusion worse in elderly patients
- **Procedures**: Provide a sitter to ensure safety, decreasing dosage of hypnotics and psychotropics, correct underlying cause.

Prevention: Reorient patient frequently, ensure adequate rest/nutrition, monitor response to medications, and treat infections and dehydration/malnutrition early.

AGITATION

Agitation is a common occurrence in the critically ill patient. Factors contributing to the development of agitation include drug or alcohol withdrawal, sleep deprivation, hypoxemia, electrolyte or metabolic imbalance, anxiety, pain and adverse drug reactions. Delirium, another common occurrence in the critically ill patient, may also include agitation as a manifestation. A high percentage of critically ill patients develop delirium.

Diagnosis: The physiologic effects of agitation may include increases in heart rate, respiratory rate, blood pressure, intracranial pressure and oxygen consumption. In addition, agitation can contribute to the self-removal of lines or tubes and combative behavior that may result in patient harm.

Treatment: Treatment of agitation involves the identification and correction of causative factors. The use of pharmacologic agents to manage pain, anxiety and agitation are often utilized. Non-pharmacologic interventions including verbal de-escalation (when possible), promoting of normal sleep patterns and relaxation techniques may also be effective. Early identification of signs and symptoms is also critical in the successful management of agitation.

DEMENTIA

Dementia is a chronic condition in which there is progressive and irreversible loss of memory and function. There are many types of dementia a nurse may encounter:

1. **Creutzfeldt-Jakob disease:** Rapidly progressive dementia with impaired memory, behavioral changes, and incoordination.
2. **Dementia with Lewy Bodies**: Similar to Alzheimer's, but symptoms may fluctuate frequently; may also include visual hallucinations, muscle rigidity, and tremors.
3. **Frontotemporal dementia:** Causes marked changes in personality and behavior; characterized by difficulty using and understanding language.
4. **Mixed dementia:** Combination of different types of dementia.
5. **Normal pressure hydrocephalus**: Characterized by ataxia, memory loss, and urinary incontinence.
6. **Parkinson's dementia**: Involves impaired decision making, and difficulty concentrating, learning new material, understanding complex language, and sequencing.
7. **Vascular dementia:** Memory loss may be less pronounced than that common to Alzheimer's, but symptoms are similar.

Nursing Considerations: Distraction is usually the best course of action to deter the patient with dementia. Re-orient frequently, but do not argue with patient. Avoid restraints or sedatives, which worsen confusion.

BRAIN DEATH

While each state has its own laws that describe the legal definition of **brain death,** most include some variation of this description:

- Brain death has occurred if the person has "sustained irreversible cessation of circulatory and respiratory functions; or has sustained irreversible cessation of all functions of the entire brain, including the brain stem."

Some states specify the number of physicians that must make the determination and others simply say the decision must be made in accordance with accepted medical practice. Criteria for determination of brain death include coma or lack of responsiveness, apnea (without ventilation), and absence of brainstem reflexes. In many states, findings must be confirmed by at least 2 physicians. **Tests used to confirm brain death** include:

- Cerebral angiograms: Delayed intracerebral filling or obstruction.
- EEG: Lack of response to auditory, visual, or somatic stimuli.
- Ultrasound (transcranial): Abnormal/lack of flow.
- Cerebral scintigrams: Static images at preset time intervals.
- Absence of oculocephalic reflex ("Doll's eyes"): patients eyes stay fixed when head is turned side to side
- Absence of oculovestibular reflex ("cold caloric"): When ice cold water is injected into the ear, the patient's eyes exhibit no response. The patient's HOB must be at least 20° for this test to be accurate.

Encephalopathy

HYPERTENSIVE ENCEPHALOPATHY AND CEREBRAL EDEMA

Hypertensive encephalopathy can occur as part of hypertensive crisis. With chronic hypertension, the brain adapts to higher pressures to regulate blood flow, but in a hypertensive crisis, autoregulation of the blood-brain barrier is overwhelmed and the capillaries leak fluid into the tissue and vasodilation takes place with resultant cerebral edema. Damage to arterioles occurs, causing increasing neurological deficits and papilledema. Hypertensive encephalopathy is relatively rare, but carries a high mortality rate and is most common in middle-aged males with long-standing hypertension. **Symptoms** usually develop over 1-2 days and include:

- Non-specific neurological deficits, such as weakness and visual abnormalities.
- Alterations in mental status, including confusion.
- Headache, often constant.
- Nausea and vomiting.
- Seizures.
- Coma.

TREATMENT FOR HYPERTENSIVE ENCEPHALOPATHY WITH CEREBRAL EDEMA

Hypertensive encephalopathy with cerebral edema requires prompt treatment in order to prevent neurological damage.

Treatment includes identifying and treating the underlying causes for the hypertensive crisis and taking steps to lower the blood pressure:

- **Nitroprusside sodium (Nitropress®)** is usually used initially to lower BP. However, caution must be used not to lower the blood pressure too quickly, as this can lead to cerebral ischemia.
- **Positioning** of patient to prevent obstruction of venous return from the head.
- **Monitoring blood gas** and maintaining $PaCO_2$ at 33-37 mmHg to facilitate vasoconstriction of cerebral arteries.
- **Preventing hyperthermia** with antipyretics and cooling devices.
- **BP monitoring** and maintenance.
- **Seizure control** with phenobarbital and/or phenytoin.
- **Lidocaine** through endotracheal tube or intravenously prior to nasotracheal suctioning.
- **Diuretics**, such as osmotic agents (mannitol) and loop diuretics (furosemide) to control fluid volume.
- **Controlling metabolic demand** by measures to increase pain control and reduce stimulation.
- **Barbiturates** (pentobarbital, thiopental) in high doses may be used if other treatments fail to decrease intracranial pressure.

CEREBRAL HYPOXIA

Cerebral hypoxia (hypoxic encephalopathy) occurs when the oxygen supply to the brain is decreased. If hypoxia is mild, the brain compensates by increasing cerebral blood flow, but it can only double in volume and cannot compensate for severe hypoxic conditions. Hypoxia may be the result of insufficient oxygen in the environment, inadequate exchange at the alveolar level of the lungs, or inadequate circulation to the brain. Brain cells may begin dying within 5 minutes if deprived of adequate oxygenation, so any condition or trauma that interferes with oxygenation can result in brain damage:

- Near-drowning.
- Asphyxia.
- Cardiac arrest.
- High altitude sickness.
- Carbon monoxide.
- Diseases that interfere with respiration, such as myasthenia gravis and amyotrophic lateral sclerosis.
- Anesthesia complications.

Symptoms include increasing neurological deficits, depending upon the degree and area of damage, with changes in mentation that range from confusion to coma. Prompt identification of the cause and increase in perfusion to the brain is critical for survival.

METABOLIC ENCEPHALOPATHY

Metabolic encephalopathy (hepatic encephalopathy) is damage to the brain resulting from a disturbance in metabolism, primarily hepatic failure to remove toxins from the blood. There may be impairment in cerebral blood flow, cerebral edema, or increased intracranial pressure. It can occur as the result of ingestion of drugs or toxins, which can have a direct toxic effect on neurons, but can also occur with liver disease, especially when stressed by co-morbidities, such as hemorrhage, hypoxemia, surgery, trauma, renal failure with dialysis, or electrolyte imbalances. **Symptoms** may vary:

- Irritability and agitation.
- Alterations in consciousness.
- Dysphonia.
- Lack of coordination, spasticity.
- Seizures are common and may be the presenting symptom.
- Disorientation progressing to coma.

Prompt diagnosis is important because the condition may be reversible if underlying causes are identified and treated before permanent neuronal damage occurs.

Treatment varies according to the underlying cause.

INFECTIOUS ENCEPHALOPATHY

Infectious encephalopathy is an encompassing term describing encephalopathies caused by a wide range of bacteria, viruses, or prions. Common to all infections are altered brain function that results in alterations in consciousness and personality, cognitive impairment, and lethargy. A wide range of neurological symptoms may occur: myoclonus, seizures, dysphagia, and dysphonia, neuromuscular impairment with muscle atrophy and tremors or spasticity. **Treatment** depends on the underlying cause and response to treatment. Prion infections are not treatable, but bacterial infections may respond to antibiotic therapy, and viral infections may be self-limiting. HIV-related encephalopathy results from opportunistic infections as immune responses decrease, usually indicated by CD4 counts <50. Aggressive antiretroviral treatment and treatment of the infection may reverse symptoms if permanent damage has not occurred for HIV-related encephalopathy. Treatment for other infectious encephalopathies varies according to the type of infection and underlying causes.

Aneurysms and AVMs

CEREBRAL ANEURYSMS

Cerebral aneurysms, weakening and dilation of a cerebral artery, are usually congenital (90%) while the remaining (10%) result from direct trauma or infection. Aneurysms usually range from 2-7 mm and occur in the Circle of Willis at the base of the brain. A rupturing aneurysm may decrease perfusion as well as increasing pressure on surrounding brain tissue. Cerebral aneurysms are classified as follows:

- **Berry/saccular:** The most common congenital type occurs at a bifurcation and grows from the base on a stem, usually at the Circle of Willis.
- **Fusiform**: Large and irregular (>2.5 cm) and rarely ruptures but causes increased intracranial pressure. Usually involves the internal carotid or vertebrobasilar artery.
- **Mycotic**: Rare type that occurs secondary to bacterial infection and aseptic emboli.
- **Dissecting**: Wall is torn apart and blood enters layers. This may occur during angiography or secondary to trauma or disease.
- **Traumatic Charcot-Bouchard (pseudoaneurysm):** Small lesion resulting from chronic hypertension.

ARTERIOVENOUS MALFORMATION

Arteriovenous malformation (AVM) is a congenital abnormality within the brain consisting of a tangle of dilated arteries and veins without a capillary bed. AVMs can occur anywhere in the brain and may cause no significant problems. Usually the AVM is "fed" by one or more cerebral arteries, which enlarge over time, shunting more blood through the AVM. The veins also enlarge in response to increased arterial blood flow because of the lack of a capillary bridge between the two. Because vein walls are thinner and lack the muscle layer of an artery, the veins tend to rupture as the AVM becomes larger, causing a subarachnoid hemorrhage. Chronic ischemia that may be related to the AVM can result in cerebral atrophy. Sometimes small leaks, usually accompanied by headache and nausea and vomiting, may occur before rupture. AVMs may cause a wide range of neurological symptoms, including changes in mentation, dizziness, sensory abnormalities, confusion, increasing ICP, and dementia.

Treatment includes:

- Supportive management of symptoms.
- Surgical repair or focused irradiation (definitive treatments).

Hemorrhage

INTRACRANIAL/INTRAVENTRICULAR HEMORRHAGE
EPIDURAL AND SUBDURAL

Epidural hemorrhage is bleeding between the dura and the skull, pushing the brain downward and inward. The hemorrhage is usually caused by arterial tears, so bleeding is often rapid, leading to severe neurological deficits and respiratory arrest.

Subdural hemorrhage is bleeding between the dura and the cerebrum, usually from tears in the cortical veins of the subdural space. It tends to develop more slowly than epidural hemorrhage and can result in a subdural hematoma. If the bleeding is acute and develops within minutes or hours of injury, the prognosis is poor. Subacute hematomas that develop more slowly cause varying degrees

144

of injury. Subdural hemorrhage is a common injury related to trauma but it can result from coagulopathies or aneurysms. Symptoms of acute injury may occur within 24-48 hours, but subacute bleeding may not be evident for up to 2 weeks after injury. Chronic hemorrhage occurs primarily in the elderly. Symptoms vary and may include bradycardia, tachycardia, hypertension, and alterations in consciousness. Older children and adults usually require surgical evacuation of the hematoma.

SUBARACHNOID

Subarachnoid hemorrhage (SAH) may occur after trauma but is common from rupture of a berry aneurysm or an arteriovenous malformation (AVM). However, there are a number of disorders that may be implicated: neoplasms, sickle cell disease, infection, hemophilia, and leukemia. The first presenting symptom may be complaints of severe headache, nausea and vomiting, nuchal rigidity, palsy related to cranial nerve compression, retinal hemorrhages, and papilledema. Late complications include hyponatremia and hydrocephalus. **Symptoms** worsen as intracranial pressure rises. SAH from aneurysm is classified as follows:

- **Grade I:** No symptoms or slight headache and nuchal rigidity.
- **Grade II:** Moderate to severe headache with nuchal rigidity and cranial nerve palsy.
- **Grade III:** Drowsy, progressing to confusion or mild focal deficits.
- **Grade IV:** Stupor, with hemiparesis (moderate to severe), early decerebrate rigidity, and vegetative disturbances.
- **Grade V:** Coma state with decerebrate rigidity.

Treatment includes:

- Identifying and treating underlying cause.
- Observing for re-bleeding.
- Anti-seizure medications (such as levetiracetam or phenytoin) to control seizures.
- Antihypertensives.
- Surgical repair if indicated.

CEREBRAL VASOSPASM

Cerebral vasospasm, a luminal narrowing of cerebral arteries, occurs in about 70% of patients after aneurysmal subarachnoid hemorrhage, resulting in ischemic stroke or death in about 15-20%. Onset is usually 4-12 days after initial rupture. The #1 sign of vasospasm is new onset lethargy, which requires a STAT transcranial doppler. If progressive neurological decline is noted, a STAT angiogram will be needed. The cause is unclear but may relate to narrowing caused by pressure of the clot on the arteries. The large arteries are usually affected, causing decreased perfusion to large cerebral areas. A number of therapies are under study, but 3 common approaches include:

- **Hypertensive hypervolemic hemodilution therapy** (HHH) involves using vasoactive drugs to ↑systolic BP to 150-160 while diluting the blood with intravenous fluids and volume expanders in order to improve perfusion. However, if done prior to clipping of the aneurysm, this poses a danger of rebleeding. Cerebral edema, increased intracranial pressure, cardiac failure, and electrolyte imbalance may also occur.
- **Nimodipine** every 4 hours for 21 days reduces/prevents vasospasm. IV magnesium and milrinone may also be used.
- **Cerebral angioplasty** may be done if medical approaches fail but poses a danger of perforation, thromboembolism, and stenosis.

Hydrocephalus

COMMUNICATING AND NONCOMMUNICATING

The ventricular system produces and circulates cerebrospinal fluid (CSF). The right and left lateral ventricles open into the third ventricle at the interventricular foramen (foramen of Monro). The aqueduct of Sylvius connects the third and fourth ventricles. The fourth ventricle, anterior to the cerebellum, supplies CSF to the subarachnoid space and the spinal cord (dorsal surface). The CSF circulates and then returns to the brain and is absorbed in the arachnoid villi. **Hydrocephalus** occurs when there is an imbalance between production and absorption of cerebrospinal fluid in the ventricles, resulting from impaired absorption or obstruction, which may be congenital or acquired. There are 2 common types of hydrocephalus:

- **Communicating:** CSF flows (communicates) between the ventricles but is not absorbed in the subarachnoid space (arachnoid villi).
- **Noncommunicating:** CSF is obstructed (non-communicating) between the ventricles with obstruction, often stenosis of the aqueduct of Sylvius but it can occur anywhere in the system.

SYMPTOMS

Symptoms of hydrocephalus depend on the age of onset. In *early infancy*, before closure of cranial sutures, head enlargement is the most common presentation, but in adults with less elasticity in the skull, neurological symptoms usually relate to increasing pressure on structures of the brain. Hydrocephalus may occur at any age, but the type that occurs in *young/middle-aged adults* is different than that common in children or those >50. Hydrocephalus in young and middle-aged adults may result from a congenital defect, hydrocephalus of infancy with shunt failure, or trauma and is characterized by:

- Headache relieved by vomiting, papilledema.
- Lack of bladder control.
- Strabismus and other visual disorders.
- Ataxia.
- Irritability.
- Lethargy.
- Confusion and impairment of cognitive abilities.

With **adult-onset normal pressure hydrocephalus** (>50) cerebrospinal fluid increases and dilates the ventricles, but frequently without increasing intracranial pressure. The cause is often unclear. Symptoms include gait disturbance, bladder control issues, and mild dementia. **Treatment** for all types of hydrocephalus involves shunting.

TREATMENT

Hydrocephalus is diagnosed through CT and MRI, which help to determine the cause. Treatment may vary somewhat depending upon the underlying disorder, which may require treatment. For example, if obstruction is caused by a tumor, surgical excision to directly remove the obstruction is required. Generally, however, most hydrocephalus is treated with shunts:

- **Ventricular-peritoneal shunt:** This procedure is the most common and consists of placement of a ventricular catheter directly into the ventricles (usually lateral) at one end with the other end in the peritoneal area to drain away excess CSF. There is a one-way valve near the proximal end that prevents backflow but opens when pressure rises to drain fluid. In some cases, the distal end drains into the right atrium.
- **Third ventriculostomy:** A small opening is made in the base of the third ventricle so CSF can bypass an obstruction. This procedure is not common and is done with a small endoscope.

Acute Spinal Cord Injury

Spinal cord injuries may result from blunt trauma (such as automobile accidents), falls from a height, sports injuries, and penetrating trauma (such as gunshot or knife wounds). Damage results from mechanical injury and secondary responses resulting from hemorrhage, edema, and ischemia. The type of symptoms relates to the area and degree of injury. About 50% of spinal cord injuries involve the cervical spine between C4 and C7 with a 20% mortality rate, and 50% of injuries result in quadriplegia. Neurogenic shock may occur with injury above T6, with bradycardia, hypotension, and autonomic instability. Patients may develop hypoxia because of respiratory dysfunction. With high injuries, up to 70% of patients will require a tracheostomy (especially at or above C3). Patients with paralysis are at high risk for pressure sores, urinary tract infections (from catheterization), and constipation and impaction. Management varies according to the level of injury but may include mobilization, mechanical ventilation, support surfaces, ROM, assisted mobility, rehabilitation therapy, analgesia, psychological counseling, bowel training, and skin care.

Neurologic Infectious Disease

BACTERIAL MENINGITIS

Bacterial meningitis may be caused by a wide range of bacteria, including *Streptococcus pneumoniae* and *Neisseria meningitidis*. Bacteria can enter the CNS from distant infection, surgical wounds, invasive devices, nasal colonization, or penetrating trauma. The infective process includes inflammation, exudates, WBC accumulation, and brain tissue damage with hyperemia and edema. Purulent exudate covers the brain and invades and blocks the ventricles, obstructing CSF and leading to increased intracranial pressure. **Symptoms** include abrupt onset, fever, chills, severe headache, nuchal rigidity, and alterations of consciousness with seizures, agitation, and irritability. Antibodies specific to bacteria don't cross the blood brain barrier, so immune response is poor. Some may have photophobia, hallucinations, and/or aggressive behavior or may become stuporous and lapse into coma. Nuchal rigidity may progress to opisthotonos. Reflexes are variable but Kernig and Brudzinski signs are often positive. Signs may relate to particular bacteria, such as rashes, sore joints, or draining ear. **Diagnosis** is usually based on lumbar puncture examination of cerebrospinal fluid and symptoms. **Treatment** includes IV antibiotics and supportive care: fluids, a dark and calm environment, measures to reduce ICP, etc.

FUNGAL MENINGITIS

Fungal meningitis is the least common cause of meningitis. It occurs when a fungal organism enters into the subarachnoid space, cerebral spinal fluid and meninges. Immune deficient patients such as those with HIV, cancer or immunodeficiency syndromes are most at risk for the development of fungal meningitis. The most common organisms causing fungal meningitis are candida albicans and Cryptococcus neoformans. Fungal meningitis caused by candida may occur in immunosuppressed patients, in those who have had a ventricular shunt placed, or in those that have had a lumbar puncture performed. Cryptococcus is a fungus found in soil throughout the world and does not usually affect people with a healthy immune system. Cryptococcal meningitis is most commonly seen in patients with HIV/AIDS and is one of the leading causes of death in HIV/AIDS patients in certain parts of Africa.

Signs and symptoms: Headache, fever, nausea and vomiting, stiff neck, photophobia and mental status changes.

Diagnosis: Lumbar puncture with subsequent culture of cerebral spinal fluid. In addition, blood cultures may be obtained as well as a CT of the head.

Treatment: The treatment of fungal meningitis involves a long course of anti-fungal medications, including Amphotericin B, flucytosine and fluconazole. Anticonvulsants may be administered for seizure control.

VIRAL INFECTIONS THAT CAN IMPACT THE NEUROLOGICAL SYSTEM

Many different types of **viral infections** can impact the neurological system either by direct infection transmitted through the bloodstream or by spreading along the nerve pathways (such as rabies). Common viral infections affecting the neurological system include:

- **Viral encephalitis**: Arboviral infections are transmitted from an animal host and an arthropod (typically a mosquito or tick), with humans typically dead-end hosts. Arboviral infections include western equine encephalitis, eastern equine encephalitis, St. Louis encephalitis, Powassan encephalitis, Colorado tick fever and La Crosse encephalitis. West Nile virus may also invade the CNS and cause encephalitis.
- **Viral meningitis**: Viral meningitis is usually self-limiting within 7 to 10 days and is less severe than bacterial meningitis.
- **Herpes virus**: Herpes simplex virus can invade the nervous system and cause herpes simplex encephalitis, which has a high mortality rate.
- **HIV**: Inflammation may affect the CNS and interfere with neuronal functions.

Neuromuscular Disorders

GUILLAIN-BARRÉ SYNDROME

Guillain-Barré syndrome (GBS) is an autoimmune disorder of the myelinated motor peripheral nervous system, causing ascending and descending paralysis. GBS is often triggered by a viral infection, but may be idiopathic in origin. Diagnosis is by history, clinical symptoms, and lumbar puncture, which often show increased protein with normal glucose and cell count although protein may not increase for a week or more.

> **Review Video: Guillain-Barre Syndrome**
> Visit mometrix.com/academy and enter code: 742900

Symptoms include:

- Numbness and tingling with increasing weakness of lower extremities that may become generalized, sometimes resulting in complete paralysis and inability to breathe without ventilatory support.
- Deep tendon reflexes are typically absent and some people experience facial weakness and ophthalmoplegia (paralysis of muscles controlling movement of eyes).

Treatment includes:

- Supportive: Fluids, physical therapy, antibiotics for infections.
- Patients should be hospitalized for observation and placed on ventilator support if forced vital capacity is reduced.
- While there is no definitive treatment, plasma exchange or IV immunoglobulin may shorten the duration of symptoms.

MUSCULAR DYSTROPHY

Muscular dystrophies are genetic disorders with gradual degeneration of muscle fibers and progressive weakness and atrophy of skeletal muscles and loss of mobility. Pseudohypertrophic (Duchenne) muscular dystrophy is the most common form and the most severe. It is an X-linked disorder in about 50% of the cases with the rest sporadic mutations, affecting males almost exclusively. Children typically have some delay in motor development, with difficulty walking and have evidence of muscle weakness by about age 3. Pseudohypertrophic refers to enlargement of muscles by fatty infiltration associated with muscular atrophy, which causes contractures and deformities of joints. Abnormal bone development results in spinal and other skeletal deformities. The disease progresses rapidly, and most children are wheelchair bound by about 12 years of age. As the disease progresses, it involves the muscles of the diaphragm and other muscles needed for respiration. Mild to frank mental deficiency is common. Facial, oropharyngeal, and respiratory muscles weaken late in the disease. Cardiomegaly commonly occurs. Death most often relates to respiratory infection or cardiac failure by age 25. Treatment is supportive.

CEREBRAL PALSY

Cerebral palsy (CP) is a non-progressive motor dysfunction related to CNS damage associated with congenital, hypoxic, or traumatic injury before, during, or ≤2 years after birth. It may include visual defects, speech impairment, seizures and mental retardation. There are 4 types of motor dysfunction:

- **Spastic**: Damage to the cerebral cortex or pyramidal tract. Constant hypertonia and rigidity lead to contractures and curvature of the spine.
- **Dyskinetic**: Damage to the extrapyramidal, basal ganglia. Tremors and twisting with exaggerated posturing and impairment of voluntary muscle control.
- **Ataxic**: Damage to the extrapyramidal cerebellum. Atonic muscles in infancy with lack of balance, instability of muscles and poor gait.
- **Mixed**: Combinations of all three types with multiple areas of damage.

Characteristics of CP include:

- Hypotonia or hypertonia with rigidity and spasticity.
- Athetosis (constant writhing motions).
- Ataxia.
- Hemiplegia (one-sided involvement, more severe in upper extremities).
- Diplegia (all extremities involved, but more severe in lower extremities).
- Quadriplegia (all extremities involved with arms flexed and legs extended).

MYASTHENIA GRAVIS

Myasthenia gravis is an autoimmune disorder that results in sporadic, progressive weakness of striated (skeletal) muscles because of impaired transmission of nerve impulses. Myasthenia gravis usually affects muscles controlled by the cranial nerves although any muscle group may be affected. Many patients also have thymomas. Signs and symptoms include weakness and fatigue that worsens throughout the day. Patients often exhibit ptosis and diplopia. They may have trouble chewing and swallowing and often appear to have masklike facies. If respiratory muscles are involved, patients may exhibit signs of respiratory failure. Myasthenic crisis occurs when patients can no longer breathe independently. Diagnosis includes tests include electromyography and the Tensilon test (IV injection of edrophonium or neostigmine, which improves function if patient has myasthenia gravis). CT or MRI to diagnose thymoma. Treatment includes anticholinesterase drugs (neostigmine, pyridostigmine) relieve some muscle weakness but lose effectiveness as the disease progresses. Corticosteroids may be used. Thymectomy is performed if thymoma present. Tracheotomy and mechanical ventilation may be needed for myasthenic crisis.

Seizure Disorders

EPILEPSY

Epilepsy is diagnosed based on a history of seizure activity as well as supporting EEG findings. Treatment is individualized. First line treatments include antiepileptic medications for partial and generalized tonic-clonic seizures. Usually treatment is started with one medication, but this may need to be changed, adjusted, or an additional medication added until the seizures are under control or to avoid adverse effects, which include allergic reactions, especially skin irritations, and acute or chronic toxicity. Milder reactions often subside with time or adjustment in doses. Toxic reactions may vary considerably, depending upon the medication and duration of use, so close monitoring is essential. Severe rash and hepatotoxicity are common toxic reactions that occur with many of the antiepileptic drugs. Dosages of drugs may need to be adjusted to avoid breakthrough seizures during times of stress, such as during illness or surgery. Alcohol/drug abuse and sleep deprivation may also cause breakthrough seizures. Most anticonvulsant drugs are teratogenic.

SEIZURE DISORDERS
PARTIAL SEIZURES

Partial seizures are caused by electrical discharges to a localized area of the cerebral cortex, such as the frontals, temporal, or parietal lobes with seizure characteristics related to area of involvement. They may begin in a focal area and become generalized, often preceded by an aura.

- **Simple partial:** Unilateral motor symptoms including somatosensory, psychic, and autonomic.
  - Aversive: Eyes and head turned away from focal side
  - Sylvan (usually during sleep): Tonic-clonic movements of the face, salivation, and arrested speech.
- **Special sensory:** Various sensations (numbness, tingling, prickling, or pain) spreading from one area. May include visual sensations, posturing or hypertonia.
- **Complex (Psychomotor):** No loss of consciousness, but altered consciousness and non-responsive with amnesia. May involve complex sensorium with bad tastes, auditory or visual hallucinations, feeling of déjà vu, strong fear. May carry out repetitive activities, such as walking, running, smacking lips, chewing, or drawling. Rarely aggressive. Seizure usually followed by prolonged drowsiness and confusion. Most common ages 3 through adolescence.

GENERALIZED SEIZURES

Generalized seizures lack a focal onset and appear to involve both hemispheres, usually presenting with loss of consciousness and no preceding aura.

- **Tonic-clonic (Grand Mal):** Occurs without warning.
  - Tonic period (10-30 seconds): Eyes roll upward with loss of consciousness, arms flexed; stiffen in symmetric tonic contraction of body, apneic with cyanosis and salivating.
  - Clonic period (10 seconds to 30 minutes, but usually 30 seconds). Violent rhythmic jerking with contraction and relaxation. May be incontinent of urine and feces. Contractions slow and then stop.

Following seizures, there may be confusion, disorientation, and impairment of motor activity, speech and vision for several hours. Headache, nausea, and vomiting may occur. Person often falls asleep and awakens conscious.

- **Absence (Petit Mal):** Onset between 4-12 and usually ends in puberty. Onset is abrupt with brief loss of consciousness for 5-10 seconds and slight loss of muscle tone but often appears to be daydreaming. Lip smacking or eye twitching may occur.

STATUS EPILEPTICUS

Status epilepticus (SE) is usually generalized tonic-clonic seizures that are characterized by a series of seizures with intervening time too short for regaining of consciousness. The constant assault and periods of apnea can lead to exhaustion, respiratory failure with hypoxemia and hypercapnia, cardiac failure, and death.

Causes: Uncontrolled epilepsy or non-compliance with anticonvulsants, infections, such as encephalitis, encephalopathy or stroke, drug toxicity (isoniazid), brain trauma, neoplasms, metabolic disorders.

Treatment includes:

- Anticonvulsants usually beginning with a fast-acting benzodiazepine (lorazepam), often in steps, with administration of medication every 5 minutes until seizures subside.
- If cause is undetermined, acyclovir and ceftriaxone may be administered.
- If there is no response to the first 2 doses of anticonvulsants (refractory SE), rapid sequence intubation (RSI), which involves sedation and paralytic anesthesia, may be done while therapy continues. Combining phenobarbital and benzodiazepine can cause apnea, so intubation may be necessary.
- Antiepileptic medications are added.

Brain Tumors

Any type of **brain tumor** can occur in adults. Brain tumors may be primary, arising within the brain, or secondary as a result of metastasis:

- **Astrocytoma**: This arises from astrocytes, which are glial cells. It is the most common type of tumor, occurring throughout the brain. There are many types of astrocytomas, and most are slow growing. Some are operable while others are not. Radiation may be given after removal. Astrocytomas include glioblastomas, aggressively malignant tumors occurring most often in adults 45-70.
- **Glioblastoma**: This is the most common and most malignant adult brain tumor/astrocytoma. Treatment includes a surgery, radiation, and chemotherapy, but survival rates are very low.
- **Brain stem glioma**: This may be fast or slow growing but is generally not operable because of location although it may be treated with radiation or chemotherapy.
- **Craniopharyngioma**: This is a congenital, slow-growing, recurrent (especially if >5 cm) and benign cystic tumor but difficult to resect, and treated with surgery and radiation.
- **Meningioma**: Slow growing recurrent tumors are usually benign and most often occur in women, ages 40 to 70; however, they can cause severe impairment/death, depending on size and location. Meningiomas are surgically removed if causing symptoms.
- **Ganglioglioma**: This can occur anywhere in the brain, usually slow growing and benign.
- **Medulloblastoma**: There are many types of medulloblastoma, most arising in the cerebellum, malignant, and fast growing. Surgical excision is done and often followed by radiation and chemotherapy although recent studies show using just chemotherapy controls recurrence with less neurological damage.
- **Oligodendroglioma**: This tumor most often occurs in the cerebrum, primarily the frontal or temporal lobes, involving the myelin sheath of the neurons. It is slow growing and most common in those age 40-60.
- **Optical nerve glioma**: This slow growing tumor of the optic nerve is usually a form of astrocytoma. It is often associated with neurofibromatosis type I (NF1), occurring in 15-40%. Despite surgical, chemotherapy or radiotherapy treatment, it is usually fatal.

Strokes

HEMORRHAGIC STROKES

Hemorrhagic strokes account for about 20% of all strokes and result from a ruptured cerebral artery, causing not only lack of oxygen and nutrients but also edema that causes widespread pressure and damage:

- **Intracerebral** is bleeding into the substance of the brain from an artery in the central lobes, basal ganglia, pons, or cerebellum. Intracerebral hemorrhage usually results from atherosclerotic degenerative changes, hypertension, brain tumors, anticoagulation therapy, or use of illicit drugs, such as cocaine.
- **Intracranial aneurysm** occurs with ballooning cerebral artery ruptures, most commonly at the Circle of Willis.
- **Arteriovenous malformation**. Rupture of AVMs is a cause of brain attack in young adults.
- **Subarachnoid hemorrhage** is bleeding in the space between the meninges and brain, resulting from aneurysm, AVM, or trauma. This type of hemorrhage compresses brain tissue.

Treatment includes: The patient may need airway protection/artificial ventilation if neurologic compromise is severe. Blood pressure is lowered to control rate of bleeding, but with caution to avoid hypotension and resulting cerebral ischemia (Goal – CPP >70). Sedation can lower ICP and blood pressure, and seizure prophylaxis will be indicated as blood irritates the cerebral cells. An intraventricular catheter may be used in ICP management; correct any clotting disorders if identified.

ISCHEMIA STROKES

Strokes (brain attacks, cerebrovascular accidents) result when there is interruption of the blood flow to an area of the brain. The two basic types are ischemic and hemorrhagic. About 80% are **ischemic**, resulting from blockage of an artery supplying the brain:

- **Thrombosis** in large artery, usually resulting from atherosclerosis, may block circulation to a large area of the brain. It is most common in the elderly and may occur suddenly or after episodes of transient ischemic attacks.
- **Lacunar infarct** (a penetrating thrombosis in small artery) is most common in those with diabetes mellitus and/or hypertension.
- **Embolism** travels through the arterial system and lodges in the brain, most commonly in the left middle cerebral artery. An embolism may be cardiogenic, resulting from cardiac arrhythmia or surgery. An embolism usually occurs rapidly with no warning signs.
- **Cryptogenic** has no identifiable cause.

Medical management of ischemic strokes with tissue plasminogen activator (tPA) (Activase®), the primary treatment, should be initiated within 3 hours (or up to 4.5 hours if inclusion criteria are met):

- **Thrombolytic,** such as tPA, which is produced by recombinant DNA and is used to dissolve fibrin clots. It is given intravenously (0.9 mg/kg up to 90 mg) with 10% injected as an initial bolus and the rest over the next hour.
- **Antihypertensives** if MAP >130 mmHg or systolic BP >220.
- **Cooling** to reduce hyperthermia.

- **Osmotic diuretics** (mannitol), hypertonic saline, loop diuretics (Lasix®), and/or corticosteroids (dexamethasone) to ↓ cerebral edema and intracranial pressure.
- **Aspirin/anticoagulation** may be used with embolism.
- Monitor and treat hyperglycemia.
- **Surgical Intervention:** Used when other treatment fails, may go in through artery and manually remove the clot.

Traumatic Brain Injury

BLUNT HEAD TRAUMA

Head trauma can occur as the result from intentional or unintentional blunt or penetrating trauma, such as from falls, automobile accidents, sports injuries, or violence. The degree of injury correlates with the impact force. The skull provides protection to the brain, but a severe blow can cause significant neurological damage. Blunt trauma can include:

- **Acceleration-deceleration injuries** are those in which a blow to the stationary head causes the elastic skull to change shape, pushing against the brain, which moves sharply backward in response, striking against the skull.
- **Bruising** can occur at the point of impact (*coup*) and the point where the brain hits the skull (*contrecoup*). So, a blow to the frontal area can cause damage to the occipital region.
- **Shear injuries,** where vessels are torn, results from sudden movement of the brain.
- **Severe compression** may force the brain through the tentorial opening, damaging the brainstem.

COMPLICATIONS OF HEAD TRAUMA
CEREBRAL EDEMA AND INCREASED ICP

Head injuries that occur at the time of trauma include fractures, contusions, hematomas, and diffuse cerebral and vascular injury. These injuries may result in hypoxia, **increased intracranial pressure,** and **cerebral edema**. Open injuries may result in infection. Patients often suffer initial hypertension, which increases intracranial pressure, decreasing perfusion. Often the primary problem with head trauma is a significant increase in swelling, which also interferes with perfusion, causing hypoxia and hypercapnia, which trigger increased blood flow. This increased volume at a time when injury impairs auto-regulation increases cerebral edema, which, in turn, increases intracranial pressure and results in a further decrease in perfusion with resultant ischemia. If pressure continues to rise, the brain may herniate. Concomitant hypotension may result in hypoventilation, further complicating treatment. **Treatments** include:

- Monitoring ICP and CCP.
- Providing oxygen.
- Elevating head of bed and maintaining proper body alignment.
- Giving medications: Analgesics, anticonvulsants, and anesthetics.
- Providing blood/fluids to stabilize hemodynamics.
- Managing airway, providing mechanical ventilation if needed.
- Providing osmotic agents, such as mannitol and hypertonic saline solution, to reduce cerebral edema.

CONCUSSIONS, CONTUSIONS, AND LACERATIONS

A variety of different injuries can occur as a result of **head trauma**:

- **Concussions** are diffuse areas of bleeding in the brain, one of the most common injuries and are usually relatively transient, causing no permanent neurological damage. They may result in confusion, disorientation, and mild amnesia, which last only minutes or hours.
- **Contusions/lacerations** are bruising and tears of cerebral tissue. There may be petechial areas at the impact site (coup) or larger bruising. Contrecoup injuries are less common in children than in adults. Areas most impacted by contusions and lacerations are the occipital, frontal, and temporal lobes. The degree of injury relates to the amount of vascular damage, but initial symptoms are similar to concussion; however, symptoms persist and may progress, depending upon the degree of injury. Lacerations are often caused by fractures.

FRACTURES

Fractures are a common cause of penetrating wounds causing cerebral lacerations. Open fractures are those in which the dura is torn, and closed is when the dura remain intact. While fractures by themselves do not cause neurological damage, force is needed to fracture the skull, often causing damage to underlying structures. Meningeal arteries lie in groves on the underside of the skull, and a fracture can cause an arterial tear and hemorrhage. Skull fractures include:

- **Basilar:** Occurs in bones at the base of the brain and can cause severe brainstem damage. May see bruising around the ear ("Battles sign") and leaking of CSF from nose and ears ("Halo sign"—bloody fluid will develop a ring of clear fluid when placed on gauze or linens).
- **Comminuted:** Skull fractures into small pieces.
- **Compound:** Surface laceration extends to include a skull fracture.
- **Depressed:** Pieces of the skull are depressed inward on the brain tissue, often producing dural tears.
- **Linear/hairline:** Skull fracture forms a thin line without any splintering.

TRAUMATIC BRAIN INJURY

Traumatic brain injury (TBI) occurs when an external force damages the brain, thereby causing an alteration in its function. TBIs can be classified as mild, moderate or severe. Common causes of traumatic brain injury include falls, motor vehicle accidents, and assaults. Traumatic brain injuries are more common in males than females.

Signs and symptoms: Signs and symptoms of a traumatic brain injury may not be immediately present, depending on the severity of the injury. Symptoms may be subtle initially and then worsen. Symptoms include: loss of consciousness, headache, blurred vision, confusion, nausea, vomiting, fatigue, somnolence, dizziness, loss of balance or coordination, seizures, tinnitus, slurred speech and photosensitivity.

Diagnosis: X-rays of the spine, CT and MRI of the head and angiography if penetrating injury occurred. The Glasgow coma scale is most commonly used to assess neurologic status in the TBI patient.

Treatment: Treatment of TBI includes frequent monitoring of vital signs, fluid balance and neurologic status. Intracranial pressure may also be monitored. Mannitol and hypertonic saline may be administered to decrease intracranial pressure and cerebral edema. Antiepileptic medications may be utilized to prevent or minimize seizure activity. In cases of severe injury, decompressive craniotomy and initiation of a hypothermia protocol may be used to reduce intracranial pressure, cerebral edema and cell death.

Neurologic Medication Management

HYPERTONIC SALINE SOLUTION

Hypertonic saline solution (HSS) has a sodium concentration higher than 0.9% (NS) and is used to reduce intracranial pressure/cerebral edema and treat traumatic brain injury. Concentrations usually range from 2% to 23.4%. The hypertonic solution draws fluid from the tissue through osmosis. As edema decreases, circulation improves. HSS also expands plasma, increasing CPP, and counteracts hyponatremia that occurs in the brain after injury. **Administration**:

- Peripheral lines: HSS <3% only.
- Central lines: HSS ≥3%

HSS can be administered continuously at rates varying from 30 mL to 150 mL/hr. Rate must be carefully controlled. Fluid status must be monitored to prevent hypovolemia, which increases risk of renal failure. Boluses (typically 30 mL of 23.4%) may be administered over 15 minutes for acute increased ICP or transtentorial herniation. **Laboratory monitoring** includes:

- Sodium (every 6 hours): Maintain at 145 to 155 mmol/L. Higher levels can cause heart/respiratory/renal failure.
- Serum osmolality (every 12 hours): Maintain at 320 mOsm/L. Higher levels can cause renal failure.

MANNITOL

Mannitol is an osmotic diuretic that increases excretion of both sodium and water and reduces intracranial pressure and brain mass, especially after traumatic brain injury. Mannitol may also be used to shrink the cells of the blood-brain barrier in order to help other medications breach this barrier. Mannitol is administered per intravenous infusion:

- 2 g/kg in a 15% to 25% solution over one-half to one hour.

Cerebral spinal fluid pressure should show decrease within 15 minutes. Fluid and electrolyte balances must be carefully monitored as well as I&O's and body weight. Concentrations of 20% to 25% require a filter. Crystals may form if the mannitol solution is too cold and the mannitol container may require heating (in 80 °C water) and shaking to dissolve crystals, but solution should be cooled to below body temperature prior to administration. Mannitol cannot be administered in polyvinylchloride bags as precipitates form. Side effects include fluid and electrolyte imbalance, nausea, vomiting, hypotension, tachycardia, fever, and urticaria.

NEUROMUSCULAR BLOCKADE

Neuromuscular blockade relaxes muscles for surgical procedures, aids in intubation, reduces extreme agitation and skeletal muscle activity, facilitates mechanical ventilation, and prevents increased ICP with intracranial hypertension. Sedatives/analgesics should be given prior to and during neuromuscular blockade to prevent awareness of paralysis and pain, an extremely traumatic experience. Neuromuscular blocking agents (NMBA) may cause muscle weakness, myopathy, and bronchoconstriction from release of histamine. Apnea and airway obstruction may occur:

- **Depolarizing agents** (agonists), such as succinylcholine, bind directly to acetylcholine receptors, blocking access and activating the receptor to depolarize. Some drugs potentiate effects: Numerous antibiotics (streptomycin, tetracycline, and clindamycin), antiarrhythmics (quinidine, CCBs), lithium carbonate, and magnesium sulfate. Side effects include myalgia, malignant hyperthermia, and severe anaphylactic/anaphylactoid reactions.
- **Non-depolarizing agents** (antagonists) bind directly to acetylcholine receptors, blocking access, but do not activate the receptors, so depolarization does not occur. Non-depolarizing agents are further classified by duration of action: short acting (mivacurium, rapacuronium), intermediate acting (rocuronium, vecuronium, atracurium, cisatracurium), and long acting (pancuronium, doxacurium, pipecuronium). Non-depolarizing NMBAs have slower onset and longer duration than succinylcholine.

ANTICONVULSANTS

Carbamazepine (Tegretol®) Use: Partial, tonic-clonic, and absence seizures. Analgesia for trigeminal neuralgia. Side effects: Dizziness, drowsiness, nausea, and vomiting. Toxic reactions include severe skin rash, agranulocytosis, aplastic anemia, and hepatitis

Clonazepam (Klonopin®) Use: Akinetic, absence, and myoclonic seizures. Lennox-Gastaut syndrome Side effects: Behavioral changes, hirsutism or alopecia, headaches, and drowsiness. Toxic reactions include hepatotoxicity, thrombocytopenia, ataxia, and bone marrow failure.

Ethosuximide (Zarontin®) Use: Absence seizures. Side effects: Headaches and gastrointestinal disorders. Toxic reactions include skin rash, blood dyscrasias (sometimes fatal), hepatitis and lupus erythematosus.

Felbamate (Felbatol®) Use: Lennox-Gastaut syndrome. Side effects: Headache, fatigue, insomnia, and cognitive impairment. Toxic reactions include aplastic anemia and hepatic failure. It is recommended only if other medications have failed.

Fosphenytoin (Cerebyx®) Use: Status epilepticus. Prevention and treatment during neurosurgery. Side effects: CNS depression, hypotension, cardiovascular collapse, dizziness, nystagmus, pruritus.

Gabapentin (Neurontin®) Use: Partial seizures, diabetic neuropathy, post-herpetic neuralgia. Side effects: Dizziness, somnolence, drowsiness, ataxia, weight gain, and nausea. Toxic reactions include hepatotoxicity and leukopenia.

Lamotrigine (Lamictal®): Use: Partial and primary generalized tonic-clonic seizures. Lennox-Gastaut syndrome. Side effects: Tremor, ataxia, weight gain, dizziness, headache, and drowsiness. Toxic reactions include severe rash, which may require hospitalization.

Levetiracetam (Keppra®): Use: Partial onset, myoclonic, and generalized tonic-clonic seizures. Side effects: Idiopathic generalized epilepsy, dizziness, somnolence, irritability, alopecia, double vision, sore throat, and fatigue. Toxic reactions include bone marrow suppression and liver failure.

Oxcarbazepine (Trileptal®): Use: Partal seizures. Side effects- Double or abnormal vision, tremor, abnormal gait, GI disorders, dizziness, and fatigue. A toxic reaction is hepatotoxicity.

Phenobarbital (Luminal®): Use: Tonic-clonic and cortical local seizures. Acute convulsive episodes. Hypnotic for insomnia. Side effects: Sedation, double vision, agitation, and ataxia. Toxic reactions include anemia and skin rash.

Phenytoin (Dilantin®): Use: Tonic-clonic and complex partial seizures. Side effects: Nystagmus, vision disorders, gingival hyperplasia, hirsutism, dysrhythmias, and dysarthria. Toxic reactions include collapse of cardiovascular system and CNS depression.

Primidone (Mysoline®): Use: Grand mal, psychomotor, and focal seizures. Side Effects: double vision, ataxia, impotence, lethargy, and irritability. Toxic reactions include skin rash.

Tiagabine (Gabitril®): Use: Partial seizures. Side Effects: Concentration problems, weak knees, dysarthria, abdominal pain, tremor, dizziness, fatigue, and agitation.

Topiramate (Topamax®): Use: Partial and tonic-clonic seizures, migraines. Side Effects: anorexia, weight loss, somnolence, ataxia, and confusion. Toxic reactions include kidney stones.

Valproate/Valproic acid (Depakote®, Depakene®): Use: Complex partial, simple, and complex absence seizures. Bipolar disorder. Side Effects: weight gain, alopecia, tremor, menstrual disorders, nausea, and vomiting. Toxic reactions include hepatotoxicity, severe pancreatitis, rash, blood dyscrasias, and nephritis.

Zonisamide (Zonegran®): Use: Partial seizures. Side Effects: Anorexia, nausea, agitation, rash, headache, dizziness, and somnolence. Toxic reactions include leukopenia and hepatotoxicity.

THROMBOLYTICS

Thrombolytics are drugs used to dissolve clots in myocardial infarction, ischemic stroke, DVT, and pulmonary embolism. Thrombolytics may be given in combination with heparin or low-weight heparin to increase anticoagulation effect. Thrombolytics should be administered within 90 minutes but may be given up to 6 hours after an event. They may increase the danger of hemorrhage and are contraindicated with hemorrhagic strokes, recent surgery, or bleeding. Thrombolytics include:

- **Alteplase tissue-type plasminogen activator** (t-PA) (Activase®) is an enzyme that converts plasminogen to plasmin, which is a fibrinolytic enzyme. T-PA is used for ischemic stroke, MI, and pulmonary embolism and must be given IV within 3-4.5 hours or by catheter directly to the site of occlusion within 6 hours.
- **Anistreplase** (Eminase®) is used for treatment of acute MI and is given intravenously in a 30-unit dose over 2-5 minutes.
- **Reteplase** (Retavase®) is a plasminogen activator used after MI to prevent CHF (contraindicated for ischemic strokes). It is given in 2 doses, a 10-unit bolus over 2 minutes and then repeated in 30 minutes.
- **Streptokinase** (Streptase®) is used for pulmonary emboli, acute MI, intracoronary thrombi, DVT, and arterial thromboembolism. It should be given within 4 hours but can be given up to 24 hours. Intravenous infusion is usually 1,500,000 units in 60 minutes. Intracoronary infusion is done with an initial 20,000-unit bolus and then 2000 units per minute for 60 minutes.
- **Tenecteplase** (TNKase®) is used to treat acute MI with large ST elevation. It is administered in a one-time bolus over 5 seconds and should be administered within 30 minutes of event.

Contraindications to thrombolytic therapy include:

- Evidence of cerebral or subarachnoid hemorrhage or other internal bleeding or history of intracranial hemorrhage, recent stroke, head trauma, or surgery. Ruled out by CT scan before administration for ischemic stroke.
- Uncontrolled hypertension, seizures.
- Intracranial AVM, neoplasm, or aneurysm.
- Current anticoagulation therapy.
- Low platelet count (<100,000 mm^3).

Assessment

GLASGOW COMA SCALE

The **Glasgow coma scale** (GCS) measures the depth and duration of coma or impaired level of consciousness and is used for post-operative assessment. The GCS measures three parameters: Best eye response, best verbal response, and best motor response, with scores ranging from 3 to 15:

- **Eye opening:**
  - 4: Spontaneous.
  - 3: To verbal stimuli.
  - 2: To pain (not of face).
  - 1: No response.
- **Verbal:**
  - 5: Oriented.
  - 4: Conversation confused, but can answer questions.
  - 3: Uses inappropriate words.
  - 2: Speech incomprehensible.
  - 1: No response.
- **Motor:**
  - 6: Moves on command.
  - 5: Moves purposefully respond pain.
  - 4: Withdraws in response to pain.
  - 3: Decorticate posturing (flexion) in response to pain.
  - 2: Decerebrate posturing (extension) in response to pain.
  - 1: No response.

Injuries/conditions are classified according to the total score: 3-8 Coma; ≤ 8 severe head injury; 9-12 moderate head injury; 13-15 mild head injury.

INTRACRANIAL PRESSURE MONITORING AND MONROE-KELLIE HYPOTHESIS

Increasing **intracranial pressure (ICP)** is a frequent complication of brain injuries, tumors, or other disorders affecting the brain, so monitoring the ICP is very important. Increased ICP can indicate cerebral edema, hemorrhage, and/or obstruction of cerebrospinal fluid. The **Monroe-Kellie hypothesis** states that in order to maintain a normal ICP, a change in volume in one compartment must be compensated by a reciprocal change in volume in another compartment. There are 3 compartments in the brain: brain tissue, cerebrospinal fluid (CSF), and blood. The CSF and blood can change more easily to accommodate changes in pressure than tissue, so medical intervention focuses on cerebral blood flow and drainage. Normal ICP is 0-15 mmHg on transducer or 80-180 mmH$_2$O on manometer. As intracranial pressure increases, symptoms include:

- Headache.
- Alterations in level of consciousness.
- Restlessness.
- Slowly reacting or nonreacting dilated or pinpoint pupils.
- Seizures.
- Motor weakness.
- Cushing's triad (late sign):
  o Increased systolic pressure with widened pulse pressure.
  o Bradycardia in response to increased pressure.
  o Decreased respirations.

ICP MONITORING DEVICES

The **intracranial pressure (ICP) monitoring device** may be placed during surgery or a ventriculostomy performed in which a burr hole is drilled into the frontal area of the scalp and an **intraventricular catheter** threaded into the lateral ventricle. The intraventricular catheter may be used to monitor ICP and to drain excess CSF. Other monitoring devices include:

- **Intracranial pressure monitor bolt** (subarachnoid bolt) is applied through a burr hole with the distal end of the monitor probe resting in the subarachnoid space.
- **Epidural monitors** are placed into the epidural space.
- **Fiberoptic monitors** may be placed inside the brain.

The intraventricular catheter is the most accurate. CSF may be drained continuously or intermittently and must be monitored hourly for amount, color, and character. For ICP measurement, the patient's head must be elevated to 30 to 45° and the transducer leveled to the tragus of the ear or outer canthus of the eye, depending on facility policy. Normal ICP is 0-15 mmHg on transducer or 80-180 mmH$_2$O on manometer.

KERNIG'S SIGN, BRUDZINSKI SIGN, AND POSITIVE JOLT MANEUVER

Patients with bacterial meningitis may exhibit **signs** to help support the diagnosis. While the following are not universally present, they are specific to meningitis and are rarely positive with other disorders:

- **Kernig's sign:** Flex each hip and then try to straighten the knee while the hip is flexed. Spasm of the hamstrings makes this painful and difficult with meningitis.
- **Brudzinski sign:** With the patient lying supine, flex the neck by pulling head toward chest. The neck stiffness causes the hips and knees to pull up into a flexed position with meningitis.
- **Jolt accentuation maneuver:** (Used if nuchal rigidity is not present.) Ask patient to rapidly move his/her head from side to side horizontally. Increase in headache is positive for meningitis.

MEAN ARTERIAL PRESSURE

Mean arterial pressure (MAP) can be calculated as diastolic BP (DBP) + 1/3 pulse pressure. MAP has a direct effect on cerebral blood flow:

- Normal: 50 to 150 mmHg.
- <50 mmHg: Cerebral flow decreases, resulting in ischemia.
- >60 mmHg: Needed to perfuse coronary arteries.
- 70 to 90 mmHg: Needed to perfuse brains and other organs.
- 90 to 110 mmHg needed to increase cerebral perfusion after neurosurgical procedures.
- >150 mmHg: Cerebral blood vessels become maximally constricted and the brain barrier is disrupted, resulting in cerebral edema and increased ICP.

CEREBRAL PERFUSION PRESSURE

Cerebral perfusion pressure (CPP) is the pressure required to maintain adequate blood flow to the brain. CPP is based on mean arterial pressure (MAP), intracranial pressure (ICP), and jugular venous pressure (JVP). CPP is calculated as MAP – ICP (when ICP >JVP) OR MAP – JVP (when JVP > ICP):

- Normal: 60 to 100 mmHg.
- <100 mmHg: Hyperperfusion occurs with increased ICP.
- <60 mmHg: Hypoperfusion occurs with ischemia.
- <30 mmHg: Hypoperfusion is marked and incompatible with life.

SWALLOW EVALUATION TO ASSESS DYSPHAGIA

The purpose of a **swallow evaluation** to assess dysphagia is to determine which patients need further assessment or intervention. Indications may include stroke, oropharyngeal changes (tumor, surgery), tracheostomy, recurrent pneumonia, and unexplained loss of weight. The evaluation begins by questioning the patient about problems swallowing and the types of foods or substances that trigger these problems as well as the onset, the frequency, and the severity of the swallowing difficulties. During the evaluation, the patient should be sitting upright and the ability of the patient to chew and swallow carefully observed as well as the movements of the lips and cheeks, and jaw and the coordination of breathing and swallowing. The patient is given a variety of substances, ranging from water to thickened liquids to pureed, soft, and solid foods. During the evaluation, the patient is asked to speak and make certain sounds (a wet or gurgling sound may indicate aspiration), smack lips, open mouth, stick out the jaw and tongue. If swallowing difficulties are found, then dietary modification may be made, and some patients may need further testing, such as modified barium swallow, endoscopic examination, and/or pharyngeal manometry.

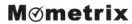

Procedures and Interventions

CLIPPING FOR TREATMENT OF ANEURYSM

Surgical clipping of a ruptured or large, unstable **aneurysm** is necessary because of the danger of rebleeding, 4% in the first 24 hours and 1-2% each day for the next month. Mortality rates with rebleeding are about 70%. Surgical repair is usually done within 48 hours. Clipping may be done prophylactically to prevent rupture. Clipping is done to secure the aneurysm without impairing circulation. Typically, a craniotomy is done and an incision is made into the brain to access the site of the aneurysm. When bleeding is controlled, a small spring-like clip (or sometimes multiple clips) is placed about the neck of the aneurysm. The bulging part of the aneurysm is drained with a needle to make sure that it does not refill and angiography may be done to ensure patency of the artery that feeds the aneurysm. It is possible during surgery for a clot to break away from the aneurysm with resultant extensive hemorrhage. Neurological damage may occur related to surgical manipulation, especially if access is difficult. Post-op monitoring includes frequent neurological checks – sometimes every hour, checking for s/s of stroke, hemorrhage or cerebral edema/ increased ICP. An angiogram may be performed after surgery to confirm placement of clips and ensure there are no leaks.

EMBOLIZATION FOR TREATMENT OF ANEURYSM OR AVM

Embolization is a minimally-invasive method that is an alternative to clipping for some aneurysms and is also used for AVMs. There are different types of embolization, but all use percutaneous transfemoral catheterization and fluoroscopy. The catheter is fed through the femoral and carotid artery to the area requiring repair:

- AVM repair introducing small silastic beads or glue into the feeder vessels, allowing blood flow to carry the material to the site. This may also be done prior to surgical repair.
- AVM or aneurysm repair placing one or more detachable balloons into the aneurysm or an AVM and inflating it with a liquid polymerizing agent that solidifies.
- Aneurysm repair with endovascular coiling involves feeding very small platinum coils through the catheter to fill the aneurysm.

Results of endovascular coiling have been very positive, with risk of death or disability at one year over 22% lower than those treated with clipping although distal ischemia related to emboli is a possible complication.

SURGICAL EXCISION OF AVM

Surgical excision of AVM is the definitive treatment for AVMs as both embolization and radiotherapy treatment pose the risk that the abnormal vessels will recur. Sometimes, 2-3 different surgeries may be required for large AVMs. Usually nonfunctioning brain tissue surrounds the AVM, so it's possible to remove the AVM without damaging brain tissue. However, reperfusion bleeding may occur as blood is diverted to surrounding arterials that had dilated because of chronic ischemia. The sudden increase in blood flow and pressure may cause leakage of blood from the vessels. There may be extensive blood loss during surgery, so constant monitoring of arterial pressure and multiple IV cannulas are important. Embolization may be done prior to surgery to reduce bleeding. Hyperventilation and mannitol are often used and β-blockers may be used to prevent hypertension and cerebral edema. Postoperatively, blood pressure is kept low to prevent reperfusion bleeding.

LUMBAR PUNCTURE

The **lumbar puncture** (spinal tap) is done between the 3rd and 4th or 4th and 5th lumbar vertebrae. Relieving intracranial pressure by withdrawing CSF may cause herniation of the brain, so lumbar puncture should be done with care in the presence of increased ICP. The patient is placed in the lateral recumbent position with knees drawn toward the chest during the procedure; however, it can be done with the patient sitting on the side of the bed. A local anesthetic is applied, and a needle is inserted into the subarachnoid space.

CSF analysis: Normal values: Clear and colorless; Protein: 15-45 mg/dL; Glucose: 60-80 mg/dL; Lactic acid: <25.2 mg/dL; Culture: Negative; RBCs: 0; WBCs: 0.5/mL

After the procedure the patient should remain in the prone position for at least 3 hours to reduce the chance of CSF leakage. If >20 mL of CSF is removed, then the patient should remain prone for 2 hours, side-lying (flat) for 2 or 3 hours and supine or prone for 6 additional hours. Spinal headache may occur; it may be treated with analgesics, fluids, and bed rest; however, if the headache is severe or persistent, the patient may have a CSF leak at the site. An **epidural blood patch** may be done, with venous blood withdrawn and then injected into the epidural space at the site of the puncture to seal the leaking opening.

EVACUATION OF HEMATOMAS

Evacuation of hematomas can be done in a number of different ways, including burr holes, needle aspiration, direct surgical craniotomy, or endoscopic craniotomy, but evacuation can pose considerable risks:

- **Epidural hematomas** are usually arterial but may be venous (20%) and are always medical emergencies and require craniotomy with evacuation before compression damage to the brain occurs. Prognosis is good if corrected early because underlying brain damage is rarely severe.
- **Subdural hematomas**, often from acceleration-deceleration accidents or abuse, involve damage to the brain tissue. Evacuation may be done if the hematoma is large and causing compression, but the brain tissue beneath hematomas is often extremely swollen. If the dura is opened, suddenly relieving the pressure may cause the brain to herniate through the opening, so aggressive therapy to reduce swelling preoperatively and careful surgical planning are necessary.

CRANIOTOMIES

Craniotomies for tumors or other surgical repair (AVMs, aneurysms) are increasingly done with micro-endoscopic equipment, but the surgical opening must be large enough to allow access and the use of necessary instruments. Procedures vary widely according to the reason for craniotomy, the type of tumor, and the age and condition of the patient. Direct craniotomies through the skull are needed in some instances, but newer approaches, including transnasal and transsphenoidal endoscopy are used when possible. Some areas of the brain are not accessible with craniotomy, but may be accessible through stereotactic radiosurgery with Gamma Knife® or CyberKnife®. Stereotactic radiosurgery is often used as a secondary treatment after primary removal of tumor for regrowth or residual tumor. Radiosurgery may be fractionated and given in a series of treatments. These non-invasive treatments are usually done while adults are awake.

POSTOPERATIVE CARE FOR CRANIOTOMY PATIENTS

In the post-operative period immediately following a **craniotomy**, the patient must be observed carefully for any **complications** or changes in condition:

- Intracranial pressure monitoring.
- Positioning: Head is usually positioned in midline, neutral position. The head of bed is elevated 30-45° for supratentorial surgery and is flat or only slightly elevated for infratentorial surgery.
- Fluid balance (intake and output).
- Wound care includes observation for swelling, drainage, and emptying and measuring any drainage devices (usually bulb drains) left in place.
- Oximetry and ABGs to ensure proper oxygenation.
- Analgesia and antiemetics are given routinely to maintain comfort and prevent stress/increased ICP from vomiting.
- Corticosteroids to reduce postoperative swelling.
- Anticoagulants (heparin) to prevent clotting.
- Monitor laboratory status:
  - Complete blood count to observe for blood loss/ infection.
  - Electrolyte levels, especially observing for hyponatremia and/or hyperkalemia.
  - Blood glucose level (may elevate with corticosteroids).
- Monitor thermoregulation and prevent hyperthermia.
- Anti-thromboembolism measures: Compression stockings or intermittent pneumatic compression.

NEUROSURGERY

Burr holes are small holes drilled through the skull, often as an emergent procedure to relieve increased intracranial pressure (such as from subdural, epidural hematoma, or hydrocephalus), to drain blood, or to remove foreign objects. Burr holes may also be used as access points for minimally-invasive surgeries on the brain, such as to remove a brain tumor. The burr holes are generally drilled with the patient under general anesthesia and the opening may be closed or left open with a drain in place. The patient must be monitored for indications of bleeding or other surgical complications. Perioperative complications may include increased intracranial pressure from cerebral edema, seizures, intracranial bleeding, and coma. The patient's vital signs and neurological signs should be closely monitored. If a drain is in place, the amount and character of the drainage should be monitored. The patient may receive prophylactic antibiotics to reduce the risk of infection.

VENTRICULAR DRAINS

Ventricular drains are inserted into one of the brain's lateral ventricles (usually on the right to prevent damage to the language center) to drain cerebrospinal fluid associated with hydrocephalus. The catheter is tunneled under the skin and sutured in place with an occlusive dressing covering the insertion site. The catheter drains into a collection chamber, which is separated from a drainage bag by a stopcock that can be opened or closed. A pressure scale (which should be leveled with zero at the tragus of the ear) is at the same level as the collection chamber. The target pressure should be determined by the neurosurgeon. The dressing should be changed only if soiled, and any indication of CSF leakage or blood in the CSF should be immediately reported. The CSF output should be measured and recorded hourly (after which the collection chamber is emptied into the drainage bag) and VS and neurological assessment at least every 4 hours. The catheter should be checked when the collection chamber is emptied to ensure it is patent and not kinked. During straining or activities that involve moving the patient, the drainage should be stopped, but for short periods only. Over drainage may result in headache.

LUMBAR DRAINS

A **lumbar drain** is inserted in the lumbar region (usually L3-L4 or L4-L5) into the arachnoid space in order to drain cerebrospinal fluid. Indications for a lumbar drain include shunt infection, increased intracranial pressure, hydrocephalus, thoracoabdominal aortic aneurysm repair, and dural fistula (traumatic/postoperative). The patient should be positioned with the head of bed elevated to 30 degrees and the transducer leveled to the phlebostatic axis or to the right atrium. The cerebrospinal fluid pressure should be monitored continuously and recorded at least every hour for the first 72 hours as well as the volume of drainage, which should be prescribed by the neurosurgeon. Over-drainage may cause a sudden decline in ICP and subarachnoid hemorrhage. Vital signs, neuromuscular and neurovascular checks should be carried out at least every hour for 24 hours. Systolic BP should be maintained ≥140 mmHg and fluid bolus administered for hypotension. After 24 hours, the patient may sit in a chair if stable, but CSF should not be drained while the patient is out of bed. Any sign of blood in CSF should be immediately reported to neurosurgeon. Hemoglobin should be maintained at >9mg/dL.

TRANSSPHENOIDAL HYPOPHYSECTOMY

The sella turcica is a depressed area that holds the pituitary gland (which extends down from the brain on a stalk) in the sphenoid bone at the base of the skull. Pituitary tumors < 10 mm diameter are removed in a **transsphenoidal hypophysectomy**. In addition to general anesthesia, supplemental infraorbital blocks may provide postoperative pain relief. Vasoconstrictors (such as epinephrine) with local anesthesia are usually administered intranasally to control bleeding. Microscopic surgery is done with an incision in the gingival mucosa beneath the upper lip then through the nasal septum and through the roof of the sphenoid cavity to access the base of the sella turcica and the pituitary tumor. Endoscopic surgery is done directly through the nares with removal of mucosa but no incision. After microscopic surgery, stents are placed in the nasal septum and the nose packed. With both procedures, nasal discharge must be observed for CSF leakage ("Halo sign") and the patient cautioned not to blow the nose.

NEURO-ENDOVASCULAR INTERVENTIONS

COILING

Coiling is a minimally-invasive procedure used to treat cerebral aneurysm. A catheter is inserted in the femoral area and advanced to the aneurysm. Then a microcatheter with coil attached is fed through the catheter into the aneurysm until the coil fills the aneurysm. The coil is separated with an electrical current and the catheter removed. In some cases, more than one coil may be needed. The coil is springlike and very thin. Blood enters the aneurysm about the coils and clots so that no further blood can enter, effectively sealing the aneurysm.

THROMBECTOMY

Thrombectomy is a procedure by which an endovascular clot is removed. Various techniques may be used, but a catheter is generally inserted into the femoral vein and advanced to the clot and then the clot may be suctioned, broken up mechanically and the pieces removed, or a helical thrombectomy device wrapped around the clot so that it can be removed. Thrombectomy is used as treatment for stroke to restore blood flow as well as for removal of clots in the arms or legs.

SPINAL IMMOBILIZATION

Spinal immobilization, once a standard for trauma patients, has been shown to have little effect and in some cases may cause harm. Because of these findings, spinal immobilization with backboard is now recommended only for patients with neurological complaints, such as numbness, tingling, weakness, paralysis, pain or tenderness in the spine, spinal deformity, blunt trauma associated with alterations of consciousness, and high energy injuries associated with drug/alcohol, inability of the patient to communicate, and/or distracting injury. Cervical collars for cervical spine immobilization are to be utilized for trauma based on the NEXUS criteria or Canadian C-spine rules (CCR). According to **NEXUS criteria**, a patient who exhibits all of the following does not require a cervical collar:

- Alert and stable.
- No intoxication.
- No midline tenderness of the spine.
- No distracting injury.
- No neurological deficit.

Spinal immobilization should be continued for the shortest time possible, so imaging, such as CT, should be carried out upon admission. Cervical collars are applied while the head is supported in neutral position, and the patient is logrolled onto a backboard and strapped in place.

Psychosocial

Psychosocial Disorders and Complications

VIOLENCE AND AGGRESSION

Violence and aggression are sometimes seen in critical care settings. The nurse must be aware of signs of impending violence or aggression in order to intervene and prevent injury to self or staff.

- **Violence** is a physical act perpetrated against an inanimate object, animal, or other person with the intent to cause harm. Violence often results from anger, frustration, or fear. It often occurs because the perpetrator believes that he is threatened in some way. Violence may occur suddenly without warning or following an escalating pattern of aggressive behavior.
- **Aggression** is the communication of a threat or intended act of violence that often occurs before the act of violence is carried out. This communication can occur verbally or nonverbally. Gestures, shouting, increasing volume of speech, invasion of personal space, and prolonged eye contact are all examples of aggression. The nurse should promptly recognize all forms of aggression and redirect or remove the patient from the situation to avoid an act of violence.

INJURIES CONSISTENT WITH DOMESTIC VIOLENCE

There are certain types of injuries that when found on a patient can indicate **domestic violence/abuse.** While obviously not any of these injuries exclusively is proof that abuse has occurred, the nurse should look at the entire clinical picture to determine whether abuse should be suspected. *A key factor in abuse is that the patient's story of how the injury occurred does not match with the pattern of the injury.*

Characteristic injuries include:

- Ruptured eardrum.
- Rectal/genital injury—burns, bites, trauma.
- Bruises in multiple stages of healing.
- Bites, rope and cigarette burns, welts in the outline of objects.

Patterns of injuries include:

- Bathing suit pattern— injuries on central parts of body usually covered with clothing.
- Head and neck injuries (50%).
- Bilateral arm/leg injury.

Defensive injuries include:

- Back of the body injury from being attacked while crouched on the floor, trying to protect face, or curled in the fetal position.
- Soles of the feet from kicking at perpetrator.
- Ulnar aspect of hand or palm from blocking blows.

167

SUICIDAL PATIENTS

Patients may attempt **suicide** for many reasons, including severe depression, social isolation, situational crisis, bereavement, or psychotic disorder.

Suicidal indications are as follows:

- Depression or dysphoria.
- Hostility to others.
- Problems with peer relationships, and lack of close friends.
- Post-crisis stress (divorce, death in family, graduation, college).
- Withdrawn personality; Quiet, lonely appearance, behavior.
- Change in behavior (dropping grades, unkempt appearance, change in sleeping patterns; A sudden increase in positive mood may indicate patient has a plan.)
- Co-morbid psychiatric problems (bipolar, schizophrenia); substance abuse.

The following are indicators of **high risk for repeated suicide attempt**:

- Violent suicide attempt (knives, gunshots).
- Suicide attempt with low chance of rescue.
- Ongoing psychosis or disordered thinking.
- Ongoing severe depression and feeling of helplessness.
- History of previous suicide attempts.
- Lack of social support system.

Nursing Considerations: Take all suicidal ideations seriously; do not minimize them. Suicidal patients should be watched continuously, given plastic utensils, break-away wall rails/shower heads, no cords/sharp instruments.

MEDICAL NON-ADHERENCE

Medical non-adherence is defined by the World Health Organization as "the extent to which a person's behavior corresponds with agreed upon recommendations from a health care provider." Recommendations may include medications, diet and other lifestyle modifications. Non-adherence with treatment regimens significantly contributes to hospital readmissions in patients with chronic diseases. It is also one of the most common causes of treatment failure.

There are many potential reasons why patient do not adhere to the recommendations of their health care provider. Factors may include the perception that the prescribed treatment is ineffective, the treatment has adverse or unpleasant side effects, or the cost of the treatment is too high. In addition, the patient may not fully understand the importance of the prescribed treatment or may forget to take medications as prescribed. The patient may encounter barriers that make it difficult to make necessary lifestyle modifications. Simplifying medication regimens and ensuring the patient has a thorough understanding of the prescribed treatment plan is critical in promoting adherence. Enlisting the support of family and friends and involving the patient and the family in the plan of care is also important. Discharge instructions should be written in terms that the patient understands and an assessment of the patient's level of understanding should be performed. Follow up phone calls may also be helpful in promoting adherence.

PTSD

Patients that experience a traumatic event may re-experience the trauma through distressing thoughts and recollections of the event. In addition, psychological effects of the trauma may include difficulty sleeping, emotional labiality and problems with memory and concentration. Patients may also wish to avoid places or activities that remind them of the trauma. These are all characteristics of **post-traumatic stress disorder (PTSD)** and may cause patients extreme distress and significantly impact their quality of life.

Signs and symptoms: Nightmares, flashbacks, insomnia, symptoms of hyperarousal including irritability and anxiety, avoidance, and negative thoughts and feelings about oneself and others.

Diagnosis: PTSD is diagnosed through psychological assessment and criteria defined in the Diagnostic and Statistical Manual of Mental Disorders, Fifth Edition (DSM-5).

Treatment: Pharmacologic therapy may be utilized to help control the symptoms of PTSD. Non-pharmacologic therapy options include group and individual/family therapy, cognitive behavioral therapy, and anxiety management / relaxation techniques. Hypnosis may also be utilized.

SCREENING FOR RISK-TAKING BEHAVIOR

The ability to assess outcomes and respond appropriately to risks are part of the decision-making process. Decision making can be impaired in patients with mental health disorders such as depression, anxiety, bipolar disorder, personality disorders, as well as in patients who have experienced a brain injury or have a dependence on drugs or alcohol. Health care providers should screen patients for the presence of high-risk behaviors. This may be accomplished through a self-administered questionnaire or through a patient interview with a trained clinician. Examples of **high-risk behaviors** include substance use/abuse, high risk sexual behaviors, high risk driving behaviors such as drinking and driving, speeding or riding with a drunk driver, and violence related behaviors. Patients with an increased response to risk taking may exhibit signs of impulsivity and sensation seeking. Conversely, other patients may exhibit abnormally cautious behavior.

INDICATORS OF SUBSTANCE ABUSE

Many people with **substance abuse** (alcohol or drugs) are reluctant to disclose this information, but there are a number of indicators that are suggestive of substance abuse:

Physical signs include:

- Burns on fingers or lips
- Pupils abnormally dilated or constricted, eyes watery
- Slurring of speech, slow speech
- Lack of coordination, instability of gait, tremors
- Sniffing repeatedly, nasal irritation, persistent cough
- Weight loss
- Dysrhythmias
- Pallor, puffiness of face
- Needle tracks on arms or legs

Behavioral signs include:

- Odor of alcohol/marijuana on clothing or breath
- Labile emotions, including mood swings, agitation, and anger
- Inappropriate, impulsive, and/or risky behavior, lying
- Missing appointments
- Difficulty concentrating/short term memory loss, blackouts
- Insomnia or excessive sleeping; disoriented/confused
- Lack of personal hygiene

ALCOHOL WITHDRAWAL

Chronic abuse of ethanol (alcoholism) can lead to physical dependency. Sudden cessation of drinking, which often happens in the inpatient setting, is associated with **alcohol withdrawal syndrome.** It may be precipitated by trauma or infection and has a high mortality rate, 5-15% with treatment and 35% without treatment.

Signs/Symptoms: Anxiety, tachycardia, headache, diaphoresis, progressing to severe agitation, hallucinations, auditory/tactile disturbances, and psychotic behavior (delirium tremens).

Diagnosis: Physical assessment, blood alcohol levels (on admission).

Treatment includes:

- Medication: IV benzodiazepines to manage symptoms; electrolyte and nutritional replacement, especially magnesium and thiamine.
- Use the CIWA scale to measure symptoms of withdrawal; treat as indicated.
- Provide an environment with minimal sensory stimulus (lower lights, close blinds) & implement fall and seizure precautions.
- Prevention: Screen all patients for alcohol/substance abuse, using CAGE or other assessment tool. Remember to express support and comfort to patient; wait until withdrawal symptoms are subsiding to educate about alcohol use and moderation.

DEVELOPMENTAL DELAYS AND INTELLECTUAL DISABILITY

Developmental delays occur when a patient does not progress mentally at the same rate as the general population. **Intellectual disability** is a condition in which individuals may have difficulty adapting to changing environments, need guidance in decision-making, and have self-care or communication deficits. Behaviors range from shy and passive to hyperactive or aggressive. Intellectual disability may be inherited (Tay-Sachs), toxin-related (maternal alcohol consumption), perinatal (hypoxia), environmental (lack of stimulation/neglect), or acquired (encephalitis, brain injury). Diagnosis involves performance results from standardized tests with behavior analysis. Intellectual disability classifications are based on IQ:

- 55 to 69 – Mild (85%): Educable to about 6th grade level. May not be diagnosed until adolescence. Usually able to learn skills and be self-supporting but may need assistance and supervision.
- 40 to 54 – Moderate (10%): Trainable and may be able to work and live in sheltered environments or with supervision.
- 25 to 39 – Severe (3-4%): Language usually delayed and can learn only basic academic skills and perform simple tasks.
- ≤25 – Profound (1-2%): Usually associated with neurological disorder with sensorimotor dysfunction. Require constant care and supervision.

Nursing Considerations: Always treat patients according to their developmental level, not their physical age. This is especially important when considering education and consent. People with developmental delays are at increased risk for injury and abuse.

ANXIETY AND DEPRESSION DUE TO INTENSIVE CARE STAYS

Anxiety and depression affect over half of patients who are treated in intensive care not only during the stay but also after discharge, especially if care is long-term or if their needs for moderate or high care continue. Additionally, studies have shown that those who suffer depression during and after ICU stays have increased risk of mortality over the next two years. Patients with anxiety may appear restless (thrashing about the bed), have difficulty concentrating, exhibit tachycardia and tachypnea, experience insomnia and feeling of dread, and complain of various ailments, such as stomach ache and headache. Symptoms of depression may overlap (and patients may have both anxiety and depression) and may also include fatigue, insomnia, withdrawal, appetite change, irritability, pessimistic outlooks, feelings of worthlessness, sadness, and suicidal ideation. Brief screening tools for anxiety and depression should be used with all ICU patients and interventions per psychological referral made as needed.

Nursing Actions

COGNITIVE ASSESSMENT

Individuals with evidence of dementia, delirium, or short-term memory loss should have cognition assessed. The mini-mental state exam (MMS) or the mini-cog test are both commonly used. These tests require the individual to carry out specified tasks, and are used as a baseline to determine change in mental status.

MMS:

- Remembering and later repeating the names of 3 common objects.
- Counting backward from 100 by 7s or spelling "world" backward.
- Naming items as the examiner points to them.
- Providing the location of the examiner's office, including city, state, and street address.
- Repeating common phrases.
- Copying a picture of interlocking shapes.
- Following simple 3-part instructions, such a picking up a piece of paper, folding it in half, and placing it on the floor.

A score of ≥24/30 is considered a normal functioning level.

Mini-cog:

- Remembering and later repeating the names of 3 common objects.
- Drawing the face of a clock, including all 12 numbers and the hands, and indicating the time specified by the examiner.

CONFUSION ASSESSMENT METHOD

The **Confusion Assessment Method** is an assessment tool intended to be used by those without psychiatric training in order to assess the progression of delirium in patients. The tool covers 9 factors, some factors have a range of possibilities, and others are rated only as to whether the characteristic is present, not present, uncertain, or not applicable. The tool also provides room to describe abnormal behavior. Factors indicative of delirium include:

1. **Onset**: Acute change in mental status.
2. **Attention**: Inattentive, stable or fluctuating.
3. **Thinking**: Disorganized, rambling conversation, switching topics, illogical.
4. **Level of consciousness:** Altered, ranging from alert to coma.
5. **Orientation**: Disoriented (person, place, and time).
6. **Memory**: Impaired.
7. **Perceptual disturbances:** Hallucinations, illusions.
8. **Psychomotor abnormalities:** Agitation (tapping, picking, moving) or retardation (staring, not moving).
9. **Sleep-wake cycle:** Awake at night and sleepy in the daytime.

*The tool indicates delirium if there is an acute onset, fluctuating inattention, and disorganized thinking OR altered level of consciousness.

ALCOHOL USE ASSESSMENT

The **Clinical Instrument for Withdrawal for Alcohol (CIWA)** is a tool used to assess the severity of alcohol withdraw. Each category is scored 0-7 points based on the severity of symptoms, except #10, which is scored 0-4. A score <5 indicates mild withdrawal without need for medications; for scores ranging 5-15, benzodiazepines are indicated to manage symptoms. A score >15 indicates severe withdrawal and the need for admission to the unit.

1. Nausea/Vomiting
2. Tremor
3. Paroxysmal Sweats
4. Anxiety
5. Agitation
6. Tactile Disturbances
7. Auditory Disturbances
8. Visual Disturbances
9. Headache
10. Disorientation or Clouding of Sensorium

The **CAGE** tool is used as a quick assessment to identify problem drinkers. Moderate drinking, (1-2 drinks daily or one drink a day for older adults) is usually not harmful to people in the absence of other medical conditions. However, drinking more can lead to serious psychosocial and physical problems. One drink is defined as 12 ounces of beer/wine cooler, 5 ounces of wine, or 1.5 ounces of liquor.

- **C** – *Cutting Down:* "Do you think about trying to cut down on drinking?"
- **A** – *Annoyed at Criticism:* Are people starting to criticize your drinking?
- **G** – *Guilty feeling:* "Do you feel guilty or try to hide your drinking?"
- **E** – *Eye opener*: "Do you increasingly need a drink earlier in the day?

"Yes" on one question suggests the possibility of a drinking problem. "Yes" on ≥2 indicates a drinking problem

COGNITIVE-BEHAVIORAL THERAPY

Cognitive-Behavioral Therapy (CBT) focuses on the impact that thoughts have on behavior and feelings, encouraging the individual to use the power of rational thought to alter perceptions. CBT centers on the concept of unlearning previous behaviors and learning new ones, questioning behaviors, and doing homework. This approach to counselling is usually short-term, about 12-20 sessions. The first sessions obtain a history, middle sessions focus on the problems, and the last sessions review and reinforce newly learned habits and thought patterns. Individuals are assigned "homework" during the sessions to practice new ways of thinking and to develop new coping strategies. The therapist helps the individual identify goals and then find ways to achieve those goals. CBT acknowledges that all problems cannot be resolved, but one can deal differently with problems. The therapist asks questions to determine the individual's areas of concern and encourages the individual to question his/her own motivations and needs. CBT is goal-centered, so each counselling session is structured toward a particular goal, such as coping techniques.

NONVIOLENT CRISIS INTERVENTION AND DE-ESCALATION TECHNIQUES

Nonviolent crisis intervention and de-escalation techniques begin with self-awareness because the normal response to aggression is a stress response (freezing, fight/flight, fear), and the nurse must control these responses in order to deal with the situation. The nurse should recognize signs of impending conflict (clenched fists, and sudden change in tone of voice or body stance, and change in eye contact). Steps include:

- Maintain social distance (≥12 feet) if possible and stay at the same level as the person (sitting or standing).
- Speak in a quiet calm tone of voice, limiting eye contact and avoiding changes in voice tone, facial expression, and gestures (especially avoid pointing or waving a finger at the person).
- Ask the person's name (if necessary) and use the name when addressing the person.
- Validate the person by acknowledging their issue, "I can see that you are angry about the changes in your treatment."
- Show empathy without being judgmental, "I'm sorry you are upset."
- Ignore questions that are challenging and avoid arguing.
- Practice active listening by paraphrasing and clarifying.
- Assist the person to explore options and the results of those options: "What is it that you would like to do?"

PHYSICAL RESTRAINTS

Restraints are used to restrict movement and activity when other methods of controlling patient behavior have failed and there is risk of harm to the patient/others. There are two primary types of restraints: violent (behavioral) and non-violent (clinical). Violent restraints are more commonly used in the psychiatric unit or when individuals exhibit aggressive behavior. More commonly, nonviolent restraints are used to ensure that the individual does not interfere with safe care. Non-violent restraints are commonly used in the confused elderly or intubated patient to prevent pulling out lines/removing equipment. The federal government and the Joint Commission have issued strict guidelines for temporary restraints or those not part of standard care (such as post-surgical restraint):

- Each facility must have a written policy & restraints are only used when ordered by a physician (usually require written/signed order every 24hrs and within 4 hours of restraint initiation).
- An assessment must be completed frequently, including circulation, toileting, and nutritional needs (generally every 1-2 hours).
- All alternative methods should be tried before applying a restraint & the least restrictive effective restraint should be used.
- A nurse must remove the restraint, assess, and document findings at least every 2 hours, every hour for violent restraints.

Key: Least restrictive option for the least amount of time.

CHEMICAL RESTRAINTS

Chemical restraints involve the use of pharmacological sedatives to manage an individual's behavior problems. This type of restraint is indicated only when severe agitation/violence put the patient at risk for injury to themselves or others. Chemical restraints inhibit the individuals' physical movements, making their behavior more manageable. It is important to realize that medication used on an ongoing basis as part of treatment is not legally considered a chemical restraint, even though the medications may be the same. There is little consensus about the use of chemical restraints, although benzodiazepines and antipsychotics are frequently used to control severe agitation (haloperidol, lorazepam, etc.). Oral medications should be tried first before injections, as oral medication is less coercive. It is important for the nurse to realize that chemical restraints are used as a last resort when other measures (such as de-escalation and environmental modification) have failed and there is an immediate risk of harm to the patient or others.

AGITATION

Identifying the underlying cause of **agitation** (impulsive/disruptive behavior, pacing, constant movement, excessive talking, outburst of anger) is essential for proper treatment as agitation may occur with drug/alcohol intoxication, psychiatric disorder (schizophrenia, bipolar disorder), delirium, dementia, hypothyroidism, neurological disease (brain injury, brain tumor), and various medications, and the underlying cause should be treated as well. Before medication, verbal attempts and de-escalation techniques to calm the patient should be made and observations made regarding what may have triggered the agitation so that it can be resolved. Medications used depend on the individual circumstances but may include benzodiazepine and first- or second-generation antipsychotics and should help to calm a patient so that diagnosis can be made or treatment carried out. The most commonly used first generation antipsychotics are haloperidol and droperidol. In acute settings, second-generation antipsychotics, such as olanzapine, aripiprazole, risperidone, quetiapine, and ziprasidone, are often the drugs of choice. Benzodiazepines, such as lorazepam and clonazepam, are often preferred when agitation results from drug/alcohol intoxication.

Multisystem

Acid-Base Imbalance

RESPIRATORY ACIDOSIS

Respiratory acidosis is precipitated by inadequate ventilation of alveoli, interfering with gaseous exchange so that carbon dioxide increases and oxygen decreases, causing excess carbonic acid (H_2CO_3) levels. The body maintains a normal pH by balancing bicarbonate (renal) with $PaCO_2$ (pulmonary) in a 20:1 ratio. If the pH alters, the system (renal or pulmonary) that is not causing the problem compensates. Respiratory acidosis is most common in acute respiratory disorders, such as pulmonary edema, pneumothorax, sleep apnea syndrome, atelectasis, aspiration of foreign objects, severe pneumonia, ARDS, administration of oxygen to treat chronic hypercapnia, or mechanical ventilation. Diseases with respiratory muscle impairment may also cause respiratory acidosis, such as muscular dystrophy, severe Guillain-Barre, and myasthenia gravis. Respiratory acidosis may be acute or chronic:

- **Acute**: Increased $PaCO_2$ with decreased pH caused by sudden decrease in ventilation.
- **Chronic**: Increased $PaCO_2$ with normal pH and serum bicarbonate (HCO_3^-) >30 mmHg with renal compensation.

ABG values in respiratory acidosis:

- pH <7.35.
- $PaCO_2$ >45 mmHg.
- Increased H_2CO_3.

SYMPTOMS AND TREATMENT

Acute Respiratory Acidosis

Symptoms include:

- Increased heart rate.
- Tachypnea. Hypertension.
- Confusion related to cerebrovascular vasodilation, especially if $PaCO_2$ >60 mmHg.
- Increased intracranial pressure with papilledema.
- Ventricular fibrillation.
- Hyperkalemia.

Chronic Respiratory Acidosis

Symptoms may be subtler with chronic respiratory acidosis because of the compensatory mechanisms. If the $PaCO_2$ remains >50 mmHg for long periods, the respiratory center becomes increasingly insensitive to CO_2 as a respiratory stimulus, replaced by hypoxemia, so supplemental oxygen administration should be monitored carefully to ensure that respirations are not depressed.

Treatment includes:

- Improving ventilation. Mechanical ventilation may be used with care.
- Medications as indicated (depending on cause): bronchodilators, anticoagulation therapy, diuretics, and antibiotics.
- Pulmonary hygiene.

RESPIRATORY ALKALOSIS

Respiratory alkalosis results from hyperventilation, during which extra CO_2 is excreted, causing a decrease in carbonic acid (H_2CO_3) concentration in the plasma. Respiratory alkalosis may be acute or chronic. Acute respiratory alkalosis is precipitated by anxiety attacks, hypoxemia, salicylate intoxication, pulmonary embolism, bacteremia (Gram-negative), and incorrect ventilator settings. Chronic respiratory alkalosis may result from chronic hepatic insufficiency, cerebral tumors, and chronic hypocapnia.

Characteristics: Decreased $PaCO_2$. Normal or decreased serum bicarbonate (HCO_3^-) as kidneys conserve hydrogen and excrete HCO_3^-. Increased pH.

Symptoms: Vasoconstriction with decreased cerebral blood flow resulting in lightheadedness, alterations in mentation, and/or unconsciousness, numbness and tingling, tinnitus, tachycardia and dysrhythmias.

Treatment: Identifying and treating underlying cause. If respiratory alkalosis is related to anxiety, breathing in a paper bag may increase CO_2 level. Some people may require sedation. ABG values in respiratory alkalosis:

- pH >7.45.
- $PaCO_2$ < 35 mmHg.
- Decreased H_2CO_3.

METABOLIC VS. RESPIRATORY ACIDOSIS

- **Pathophysiology**
  - *Metabolic:* Increase in fixed acid and inability to excrete acid or loss of base, with compensatory increased CO_2 excretion by lungs.
  - *Respiratory:* Hypoventilation and CO_2 retention, with renal compensatory retention of bicarbonate (HCO_3^-) and increased excretion of hydrogen.
- **Laboratory**
  - *Metabolic:* Decreased serum pH & PCO_2 normal if uncompensated. decreased if compensated. decreased HCO_3^-. Urine pH >6 if compensated.
  - *Respiratory:* Decreased serum pH and increased PCO_2. increased HCO_3^- if compensated and normal if uncompensated. Urine pH >6 if compensated.
- **Cause**
  - *Metabolic:* DKA, lactic acidosis, diarrhea, starvation, renal failure, shock, renal tubular acidosis, starvation:
  - *Respiratory:* COPD, overdose of sedative/barbiturate, obesity, pneumonia, muscle weakness, mech hypoventilation.

- **Symptoms**
  - *Metabolic:* Decreased LOC, confusion, HA, coma. decreased BP, N/V/D, arrhythmias, flushed skin, abd pain, deep inspired tachypnea.
  - *Respiratory:* Decreased LOC, dizziness, HA, coma, disorientation, seizures. Flushed skin, VF, Hypoventilation with hypoxia.

METABOLIC VS. RESPIRATORY ALKALOSIS

- **Pathophysiology**
  - *Metabolic:* Decreased strong acid or increased base, with compensatory CO_2 retention by lungs.
  - *Respiratory:* Hyperventilation and increased excretion of CO_2, with compensatory HCO_3^- excretion by kidneys.

- **Laboratory**
  - *Metabolic:* Increased serum pH. PCO_2 normal if uncompensated and increased if compensated. Increased HCO_3^- Urine pH >6 if compensated.
  - *Respiratory:* Increased serum pH. Decreased PCO_2. HCO_3^- normal if uncompensated and decreased if compensated. Urine pH >6 if compensated.

- **Causes**
  - *Metabolic:* Excessive vomiting, gastric suctioning, diuretics, potassium deficit, excessive mineralocorticoids and $NaHCO_3^-$ intake.
  - *Respiratory:* Encephalopathy, septicemia, brain injury, salicylate overdose, mechanical hyperventilation.

- **Symptoms**
  - *Metabolic:* dizziness, confusion, nervousness, anxiety, tremors, muscle cramps, tetany, seizures, n/v arrhythmias, anorexia, compensatory hypoventilation.
  - *Respiratory:* Light-headed, confused, and lethargic. Tachycardia and arrhythmias. Epigastric pain, nausea and vomiting. Hyperventilation.

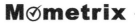

Comorbidities

BARIATRIC RELATED COMPLICATIONS IN CRITICALLY ILL PATIENTS

Obesity affects a large number of people worldwide and is directly and indirectly associated with a number of health-related problems. Obesity is defined as a body mass index of 30 or higher. Morbid obesity is defined as a progressive and often life-threatening disease caused by an excessive amount of fat storage and its associated co-morbidities. The bariatric critically ill patient is at risk for a number of complications including decreased oxygenation (due to excessive weight compressing the thoracic cavity and diaphragm, thereby impeding oxygenation), impaired immune function (due to protein-energy malnutrition) that may causes delayed healing and increase the risk of skin breakdown, increased metabolic demands and insulin resistance (potentially causing hyperglycemia and hyperlipidemia) and impaired cardiac function (caused by increased stroke volume, increased cardiac output and increased cardiac deconditioning.) Bariatric patients are also at an increased risk for psychosocial effects including negative body image and anxiety or depression.

CO-MORBIDITY IN PATIENTS WITH TRANSPLANT HISTORY

Patients requiring an **organ transplant** often present with additional clinical findings or **co-morbidities**. Depending on the type of transplant required, certain clinical conditions may preclude the patient from receiving a transplant. Common co-morbidities in patients who are pre-transplantation include cardiac disease, peripheral vascular disease, renal or hepatic disease, obesity and diabetes.

Post-transplantation, patients are at risk of developing additional co-morbidities. Potential complications of transplantation and/or side effects of the immunosuppressive regimen that patients are prescribed post-transplant may contribute to the development of additional medical issues. Typical immunosuppressive agents administered to post-transplant patients include corticosteroids, cyclosporine, monoclonal antibodies and antimetabolites. These agents often cause suppression of the bone marrow and the patient is at greater risk for the development of opportunistic infections. Potential complications of organ transplantation include bleeding, graft problems (including delayed function or graft failure), infections, graft versus host disease, renal disease, and acute or chronic rejection. Long term immunosuppression therapy may also increase the patient's risk for the development of certain types of cancers including lymphomas and Kaposi's sarcoma.

End of Life Care

NURSING ROLE IN END OF LIFE CARE

End of life care encompasses many dimensions. In the critical care setting, nursing staff caring for the dying patient must shift their priorities from life-saving interventions to providing comfort through the management of symptoms and addressing issues unique to the end of life. Nursing care of the dying patient includes providing supportive care and symptom management to ensure patient comfort and prevention of pain and suffering. Common symptoms occurring at the end of life include pain, dyspnea, anxiety and/or agitation, nausea and vomiting and depression. Additionally, the nurse serves as an advocate to the patient and family, providing education on end of life and supporting them in decision making. Emotional and spiritual support is another dimension of end of life care. The nurse serves to assess the emotional and spiritual needs of the patient and family and helps to coordinate resources to meet those needs. Goals of care are established with the patient and family and communicated to all members of the healthcare team.

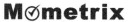

Healthcare Associated Infections

CLABSI

Intensive care patients routinely have central venous catheters placed for the administration of fluids, medications, parenteral nutrition and other supportive therapies. **Central line blood stream infections (CLABSI)** occur when a confirmed (by laboratory analysis) bloodstream infection occurs in a patient with a central line in place for greater than 2 calendar days on the date of the confirmed infection. Central line blood stream infections contribute to an increase in hospital length of stay, a marked increase in healthcare costs, and a higher mortality rate for those patients that acquire them. CLABSI is often a preventable occurrence and many evidence-based practices have been identified in their prevention. Strategies aimed at prevention of CLABSI include hand hygiene, strict aseptic technique in accessing and maintaining the catheter, thorough assessment of the catheter insertion site daily, and appropriate site care.

Signs and symptoms: Fever, chills, hypotension, tachycardia, erythema, edema and/or drainage at the catheter site, and pain/tenderness at the catheter site.

Diagnosis: CBC, blood cultures and culture of the catheter tip.

Treatment: Once the causative organism is identified, antimicrobial treatment will be initiated. The central venous catheter may also be removed.

CAUTI

Urinary tract infections that occur in the hospitalized patient are most often associated with the use of a urinary catheter. **Catheter associated urinary tract infections (CAUTIs)** occur when a urinary tract infection develops in a patient with an indwelling urinary catheter in place during the 48-hour period before the development of the infection. CAUTI is the most common healthcare associated infection. Like other health care associated infections, catheter associated urinary tract infections contribute to increased healthcare costs, increased length of stay and higher morbidity and mortality rates. Evidence based strategies aimed at prevention of CAUTI include using urinary catheters only when appropriately indicated, discontinuation of the urinary catheter as soon as possible, utilization of aseptic technique and sterile equipment during insertion, hand hygiene, utilization of a closed drainage system and securement of the urinary catheter.

Signs and symptoms: Fever, urinary urgency, urinary frequency, dysuria, pressure or pain in lower abdomen or back, flank pain, fatigue, nausea and vomiting, and mental status changes.

Diagnosis: Physical assessment, urinalysis and urine culture.

Treatment: Treatment of a catheter associated urinary treatment infection includes removal of the catheter, antibiotics and administration of fluids.

VAP/VAE

Ventilator associated events (VAE) include a broad range of complications that may occur in the ventilated patient. Aspiration is a potential complication of intubation and greatly increases the risk of developing ventilator associated pneumonia in the critical care patient. **Ventilator associated pneumonia (VAP)** is a healthcare associated infection that develops in a patient with an endotracheal tube or tracheostomy that has been mechanically ventilated for at least 48 hours when the infection is identified. Risk factors for the development of VAP include advanced age, immobility, post-operative patients and immunocompromised patients.

Signs and symptoms: Fever, purulent drainage/sputum, cough, hypoxemia.

Diagnosis: Physical assessment and chest x-ray to confirm the presence of infiltrates. Samples of respiratory secretions may also be obtained and sampled.

Treatment: Once the organism causing the pneumonia has been identified, treatment will include the administration of the appropriate antibiotic. Prevention includes keeping the HOB 30 degrees, frequent mouth care (usually every 2 hours), routine changing of in-line suction and tubing, and early mobility.

Hypotension

Hypotension is a frequent occurrence in the critically ill patient and is often an indication of deterioration. Causes of hypotension in the critically ill patient may include sepsis/septic shock, bleeding, acute heart failure, traumatic brain injury, hypovolemia, cardiogenic shock, anaphylaxis and the use of certain medications. Early recognition and treatment are critical in the management of hypotension as it may lead to multisystem organ failure and death.

Signs and symptoms: Hypotensive patients may experience oliguria and acute renal failure due to a decrease in renal perfusion. An altered level of consciousness may occur from the decreased perfusion to the brain. Acute coronary syndrome and myocardial ischemia may result from a decrease in cardiac perfusion.

Treatment: Treatment of hypotension should begin with the identification and treatment of the underlying cause. The goals of treatment are to increase blood pressure and cardiac output and decrease oxygen demand. Oxygenation and tissue perfusion must be maintained to prevent multisystem organ failure. Fluid resuscitation is often utilized as well as oxygen therapy and vasopressors (when fluid resuscitation is ineffective). Sedation and analgesia may be given to decrease oxygen demand; however, only with caution as these can lower blood pressure further. Supine positioning (not Trendelenburg, which is now contraindicated) is also a helpful but not long-lasting intervention.

Infectious Diseases

MRSA

Methicillin resistant staphylococcus aureus (MRSA) is a drug resistant form of staph aureus that accounts for 10-50% of all staph infections. It is associated with an increased risk of morbidity and mortality and can manifest as a skin infection, bloodstream infection, urinary tract, respiratory infection or wound infection. Risk factors for the development of MRSA are recent antibiotic therapy, recent or current hospitalization (risk increases with longer hospitalizations) and immunosuppression.

Signs and symptoms: Dependent on the site of infection—may include fever, chills, headache, fatigue, malaise, rash, shortness of breath, cough and delayed healing. Skin infection symptoms may include erythema, edema and drainage.

Diagnosis: The diagnosis of MRSA is made through a laboratory culture of the suspected site (i.e. wound, sputum, urine, blood).

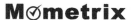

Treatment: MRSA is treated by antibiotic therapy. Laboratory cultures can assist in determining the sensitivity of the organism to antibiotics. Skin infections may require an irrigation and debridement.

MULTIDRUG RESISTANT VRE

Enterococcus bacteria may cause infections of the urinary tract, blood stream, endocardium and meninges. **Vancomycin resistant enterococcus (VRE)** is a drug resistant organism that is most likely to develop in hospitalized or immunosuppressed patients. Post-operative patients, patients who have been on long term antibiotic therapy and those with an indwelling intravenous or urinary catheter are also at an increased risk of developing VRE.

Signs and symptoms: Dependent on the site of infection—fever, chills, fatigue and malaise. Urinary tract infection symptoms may include back pain, urinary frequency and urgency and painful urination. Wound infection symptoms include erythema, edema, pain and drainage.

Diagnosis: The diagnosis of VRE is made through a laboratory culture of the suspected area.

Treatment: VRE is treated with antibiotic therapy. Laboratory cultures can assist in determining the sensitivity of the organism to antibiotics. These patients are placed in strict contact precautions.

CRE

Carbapenem resistant Enterobacteriaceae (CRE) are a family of resistant organisms that were formerly susceptible to the antibiotic class carbapenems. The majority of CRE infections are caused by the *Klebsiella pneumonia* organism. CRE infections are associated with an increased mortality rate and are more likely to occur in hospitalized patients who are mechanically ventilated, have an indwelling intravenous or urinary catheter or have received a long-term course of antibiotic therapy.

Signs and symptoms: Dependent on the site of infection—fever, chills, malaise and delayed wound healing. CRE infections may manifest as wound, urinary, respiratory or bloodstream infections.

Diagnosis: The diagnosis of CRE is made through a laboratory culture of the suspected area.

Treatment: CRE is treated with antibiotic therapy. Laboratory cultures can assist in determining the sensitivity of the organism to antibiotics. Hand hygiene, meticulous cleaning/sterilization of patient equipment and supplies and limited use of antibiotic therapy may be effective in decreasing the risk of healthcare acquired CRE infections. These patients are placed in strict contact precautions.

INFLUENZA-PANDEMIC AND EPIDEMIC

Pandemic influenza is defined as a global outbreak of the influenza virus that can occur when new strains of the virus or non-human strains of the virus, gain the ability to infect humans and spread rapidly. The rapid spread of the virus occurs when humans have little to no immunity. Symptoms are more severe in nature, causing more patients to become hospitalized. Fortunately, pandemic influenza outbreaks rarely occur. An influenza outbreak is defined as an **epidemic** when the total number of influenza related deaths exceed a certain percentage defined by the Center for Disease Control (CDC). An epidemic occurs when more cases of influenza are reported than expected in a given area or among a specific group of people over a particular period of time.

Signs and symptoms: Fever, chills, arthralgia, myalgia, upper respiratory symptoms (cough, sore throat, and rhinitis), headache, and fatigue. Nausea and vomiting may also be present.

Diagnosis: Diagnosis is made by physical assessment. Confirmation of influenza may be obtained by rapid influenza testing.

Treatment: Most commonly influenza is treated with fluids and rest. Anti-viral medications may be administered to decrease the duration of the illness. Pneumonia is common complication that may occur with influenza.

Multisystem Trauma

BURN INJURIES
SYSTEMIC COMPLICATIONS

Burn injuries begin with the skin but can affect all organs and body systems, especially with a major burn:

- **Cardiovascular**: Cardiac output may fall by 50% as capillary permeability increases with vasodilation and fluid leaks from the tissues.
- **Urinary**: Decreased blood flow causes kidneys to increase ADH, which increases oliguria. BUN and creatinine levels increase. Cell destruction may block tubules, and hematuria may result from hemolysis.
- **Pulmonary**: Injury may result from smoke inhalation or (rarely) aspiration of hot liquid. Pulmonary injury is a leading cause of death from burns and is classified according to degree of damage:
  - *First*: Singed eyebrows and nasal hairs with possible soot in airways and slight edema.
  - *Second*: (At 24 hours) Stridor, dyspnea, and tachypnea with edema and erythema of upper airway, including area of vocal cords and epiglottis.
  - *Third*: (At 72 hours) worsening symptoms if not intubated and if intubated, bronchorrhea and tachypnea with edematous, secreting tissue.
- **Neurological**: Encephalopathy may develop from lack of oxygen, decreased blood volume and sepsis. Hallucinations, alterations in consciousness, seizures and coma may result.
- **Gastrointestinal**: Ileus and ulcerations of mucosa often result from poor circulation. Ileus usually clears within 48-72 hours, but if it returns it is often indicative of sepsis.
- **Endocrine/Metabolic:** The sympathetic nervous system stimulates the adrenals to release epinephrine and norepinephrine to increase cardiac output and cortisol for wound healing. The metabolic rate increases markedly. Electrolyte loss occurs with fluid loss from exposed tissue, especially phosphorus, calcium and sodium, with an increase in potassium levels. Electrolyte imbalance can be life-threatening if burns cover >20% of BSA. Glycogen depletion occurs within 12-24 hours and protein breakdown and muscle wasting occurs without sufficient intake of protein.

MANAGEMENT

Management of burn injuries must include both wound care and systemic care to avoid complications that can be life threatening. Treatment includes:

- Establishment of airway and treatment for inhalation injury as indicated:
  - Supplemental oxygen, incentive spirometry, nasotracheal suctioning.
  - Humidification.
  - Bronchoscopy as needed to evaluate bronchospasm and edema.
  - β-Agonists for bronchospasm, followed by aminophylline if ineffective.
  - Intubation and ventilation if there are indications of respiratory failure. This should be done prior to failure. Tracheostomy may be done if ventilation >14 days.
- Intravenous fluids and electrolytes, based on weight and extent of burn. Parkland formula: Fluid replacement (mL) in first 24 hours = (mass in kg) × (body % burned) × 400.
- Enteral feedings, usually with small lumen feeding tube into the duodenum.
- NG tube for gastric decompression to prevent aspiration.
- Indwelling catheter to monitor urinary output. Urinary output should be 0.5-2 mL/kg/hr.
- Analgesia for reduction of pain and anxiety.
- Topical and systemic antibiotics.
- Wound care with removal of eschar and dressings as indicated.

TREATMENT PRIORITIZATION GUIDELINES FOR MULTISYSTEM TRAUMA

In order to give the trauma patient the best chance at survival, treatment must be appropriately **prioritized** and managed. Immediate priority should be given to maintaining the airway and ensuring adequate ventilation. Pre-hospital management should also include control of bleeding, prevention of shock, spine immobilization and neurological assessment. Upon arrival to the closest trauma center, the primary survey conducted by the healthcare trauma team is centered on determining which injuries are potentially life-threatening. Airway is the number one priority, followed by an assessment of hemodynamic status (assess for hypovolemia) and core body temperature (assess for hypothermia). Baseline data is also collected including laboratory studies, EKG, and radiologic testing. Treatment may include fluid resuscitation, the administration of blood products and surgical intervention (if indicated). Complications of multisystem trauma include disseminated intravascular coagulopathy, acute respiratory distress syndrome, renal failure, infection, compartment syndrome, dysrhythmias, and sepsis.

Pain

PAIN ASSESSMENT IN CRITICAL CARE PATIENTS

Pain is subjective and may be influenced by the individual's pain threshold (the smallest stimulus that produces the sensation of pain) and pain tolerance (the maximum degree of pain that a person can tolerate). The most common current pain assessment tool for adults and pre-teens/adolescents is the 1-10 scale:

- 0 = No pain.
- 1-2 = Mild pain.
- 3-5 = Moderate pain.
- 6-7 = Severe pain.
- 8-9 = Very severe pain.
- 10 = Excruciating pain.

However, there is more to pain assessment than a number on a scale. Assessment includes information about onset, duration, and intensity. Identifying what triggers pain and what relieves it can be very useful when developing a plan for pain management. Patients may show very different behavior when they are in pain: Some may cry and moan with minor pain, and others may exhibit little difference in behavior when truly suffering. Thus, judging pain by behavior can lead to the wrong conclusions.

ADVERSE SYSTEMIC EFFECTS OF PAIN

Acute pain causes **adverse systemic affects** that can negatively affect many body systems:

- **Cardiovascular**: Tachycardia and increased BP is a common response to pain, causing increased cardiac output and systemic vascular resistance. In those with pre-existing cardiovascular disease, such as compromised ventricular function, cardiac output may decrease. The increased myocardial need for oxygen may cause or worsen myocardial ischemia.
- **Respiratory**: Increased need for oxygen causes an increase in minute ventilation and splinting due to pain may compromise pulmonary function. If the chest wall movement is constrained, tidal volume falls, impairing the ability to cough and clear secretions. Bed rest further compromises ventilation.
- **Gastrointestinal**: Sphincter tone increases and motility decreases, sometimes resulting in ileus. There may be increased secretion of gastric acids, which irritate the gastric lining and can cause ulcerations. Nausea, vomiting, and constipation may occur. Reflux may result in aspiration pneumonia. Abdominal distention may occur.
- **Urinary**: Increased sphincter tone and decreased motility result in urinary retention.
- **Endocrine**: Hormone levels are affected by pain. Catabolic hormones, such as catecholamine, cortisol and glucagon increase and anabolic hormones, such as insulin and testosterone decrease. Lipolysis increases along with carbohydrate intolerance. Sodium retention can occur because of increased ADH, aldosterone, angiotensin, and cortisol. This in turn causes fluid retention and a shift to extracellular space.
- **Hematologic**: There may be reduced fibrinolysis, increased adhesiveness of platelets, and increased coagulation.
- **Immune**: Leukocytosis and lymphopenia may occur, increasing risk of infection.
- **Emotional**: Patients may become depressed, anxious, angry, depressed appetite, and sleep-deprived. This type of response is most common in those with chronic pain, who usually don't have typical systemic responses of those with acute pain.

184

PATIENT-CONTROLLED ANALGESIA

Patient-controlled analgesia (PCA) allows the patient to control administration of pain medication by pressing a button on an intravenous delivery system with a computerized pump. The device is filled with opioid (as prescribed) and must be programmed correctly and checked regularly to ensure that it is functioning properly and that controls are set. Current recommendations are that most patients that have an open (and some laparoscopic) surgical procedure use a PCA pump for pain control post operatively until they are tolerating fluids well orally. They may then be switched to oral pain medications. The most-commonly administered medications include morphine, meperidine, fentanyl, and hydromorphone. Most devices can be set to deliver continuous infusion of opioid as well as patient-controlled bolus. Each element must be set:

- **Bolus**: Determines the amount of medication received when the patient delivers a dose.
- **Lockout interval:** Time required between administrations of boluses.
- **Basal rate:** Rate at which continuous opioid is delivered per hour.
- **Limit** (usually set at 4 hours): Total amount of opioid that can be delivered in the preset time limit.

Important patient teaching includes instructing family members/others at bedside to never push the button for the patient (but can encourage when it is time). Also teach the patient that they cannot accidently overdose themselves to reduce fears and encourage use. Monitor for signs/symptoms of respiratory distress.

Sepsis and Shock

BACTEREMIA, SEPTICEMIA, AND SIRS

There are a number of terms used to refer to **severe infections** and often used interchangeably, but they are part of a continuum:

- **Bacteremia** is the presence of bacteria in the blood but without systemic infection.
- **Septicemia** is a systemic infection caused by pathogens (usually bacteria or fungi) present in the blood.
- **Systemic inflammatory response syndrome** (SIRS), a generalized inflammatory response affecting many organ systems, may be caused by infectious or non-infectious agents, such as trauma, burns, adrenal insufficiency, pulmonary embolism, and drug overdose. If an infectious agent is identified or suspected, SIRS is an aspect of sepsis. Infective agents include a wide range of bacteria and fungi, including *Streptococcus pneumoniae* and *Staphylococcus aureus*. SIRS includes 2 of the following:
  - Elevated (>38 °C) or subnormal rectal temperature (<36 °C).
  - Tachypnea or $PaCO_2$ <32 mmHg.
  - Tachycardia.
  - Leukocytosis (>12,000) or leukopenia (<4000).

SEPSIS, SEVERE SEPSIS, SEPTIC SHOCK, AND MODS

Infections can progress from bacteremia, septicemia, and SIRS to the following:

- **Sepsis** is presence of infection either locally or systemically in which there is a generalized life-threatening inflammatory response (SIRS). It includes all the indications for SIRS as well as one of the following:
  - Changes in mental status.
  - Hypoxemia without preexisting pulmonary disease.
  - Elevation in plasma lactate.
  - Decreased urinary output <5 mL/kg/hr for ≥1 hour.
- **Severe sepsis** includes both indications of SIRS and sepsis as well as indications of increasing organ dysfunction with inadequate perfusion and/or hypotension.
- **Septic shock** is a progression from severe sepsis in which refractory hypotension occurs despite treatment. There may be indications of lactic acidosis.

Multi-organ dysfunction syndrome (MODS) is the most common cause of sepsis-related death. Cardiac function becomes depressed, acute respiratory distress syndrome (ARDS) may develop, and renal failure may follow acute tubular necrosis or cortical necrosis. Thrombocytopenia appears in about 30% of those affected and may result in disseminated intravascular coagulation (DIC). Liver damage and bowel necrosis may occur.

SHOCK

There are a number of different types of **shock**, but there are general characteristics that they have in common. In all types of shock, there is a marked decrease in tissue perfusion related to hypotension, so that there is insufficient oxygen delivered to the tissues and, in turn, inadequate removal of cellular waste products, causing injury to tissue:

- Hypotension (systolic below 90 mmHg). This may be somewhat higher (110 mmHg) in those who are initially hypertensive.
- Decreased urinary output (<0.5 mL/kg/hr), especially marked in hypovolemic shock
- Metabolic acidosis.
- Peripheral/cutaneous vasoconstriction/vasodilation resulting in cool, clammy skin.
- Alterations in level of consciousness.

Types of shock are as follows:

- **Distributive:** Preload ↓, CO ↑, SVR ↓
- **Cardiogenic:** Preload ↑, CO ↓, SVR ↑
- **Hypovolemic:** Preload ↓, CO ↓, SVR ↑

SEPTIC SHOCK

Septic shock is caused by toxins produced by bacteria and cytokines that the body produces in response to severe infection, resulting in a complex syndrome of disorders. **Symptoms** are wide-ranging:

- Initial: Hyper- or hypothermia, increased temperature ($\uparrow$38 °C) with chills, tachycardia with increased pulse pressure, tachypnea, alterations in mental status (dullness), hypotension, hyperventilation with respiratory alkalosis ($PaCO_2$ ≤30 mmHg), increased lactic acid, and unstable BP, and dehydration with increased urinary output.
- Cardiovascular: Myocardial depression and dysrhythmias.
- Respiratory: Acute respiratory distress syndrome (ARDS).
- Renal: Acute kidney injury (AKI) with $\downarrow$ urinary output and $\uparrow$ BUN.
- Hepatic: Jaundice and liver dysfunction with $\uparrow$in transaminase, alkaline phosphatase and bilirubin.
- Hematologic: Mild or severe blood loss (from mucosal ulcerations), neutropenia or neutrophilia, decreased platelets, and DIC.
- Endocrine: Hyperglycemia, hypoglycemia (rare).
- Skin: Cellulitis, erysipelas, and fasciitis, acrocyanotic and necrotic peripheral lesions.

DIAGNOSIS AND TREATMENT

Septic shock is most common in newborns, those >50, and those who are immunocompromised. There is no specific test to confirm a diagnosis of septic shock, so diagnosis is based on clinical findings and tests that evaluate hematologic, infectious, and metabolic states: Lactic acid, CBC, DIC panel, electrolytes, liver function tests, BUN, creatinine, blood glucose, ABGs, urinalysis, ECG, radiographs, blood and urine cultures. **Treatment** must be aggressive and includes:

- Oxygen and endotracheal intubation as necessary.
- IV access with 2-large bore catheters and central venous line.
- Rapid fluid administration at 0.5L NS or isotonic crystalloid every 5-10 minutes as needed (to 4-6 L).
- Monitoring urinary output to optimal >30 mL/hr (>0.5-1 mL/kg/hr)
- Inotropic or vasoconstrictive agents (dopamine, dobutamine, norepinephrine) if no response to fluids or fluid overload.
- Empiric IV antibiotic therapy (usually with 2 broad spectrum antibiotics for both gram-positive and gram-negative bacteria) until cultures return and antibiotics may be changed.
- Hemodynamic and laboratory monitoring.
- Removing source of infection (abscess, catheter).

SHOCK STATES

DISTRIBUTIVE SHOCK

Distributive shock occurs with adequate blood volume but inadequate intravascular volume because of arterial/venous dilation that results in decreased vascular tone and hypoperfusion of internal organs. Cardiac output may be normal or blood may pool, decreasing cardiac output. Distributive shock may result from anaphylactic shock, septic shock, neurogenic shock, and drug ingestions.

Symptoms include:

- Hypotension (systolic <90 mmHg or <40 mmHg from normal), tachypnea, tachycardia (>90) (may be lower if patient receiving β-blockers); Hypoxemia.
- Skin initially warm, later hypoperfused.
- Hyper- or hypothermia (>38 °C or <36 °C).
- Alterations in mentation.
- Decreased urinary output.
- Symptoms related to underlying cause

Treatment includes:

- Treating underlying cause while stabilizing hemodynamics.
- Oxygen with endotracheal intubation if necessary.
- Rapid fluid administration at 0.25-0.5L NS or isotonic crystalloid every 5-10 minutes as needed to 2-3 L.
- Vasoconstrictive and inotropic agents (dopamine, dobutamine, norepinephrine) if necessary, for patients with profound hypotension.

NEUROGENIC SHOCK

Neurogenic shock is a type of distributive shock that occurs when injury to the CNS from trauma resulting in acute spinal cord injury (from both blunt and penetrating injuries), neurological diseases, drugs, or anesthesia, impairs the autonomic nervous system that controls the cardiovascular system. The degree of symptoms relates to the level of injury with injuries above T1 capable of causing disruption of the entire sympathetic nervous system and lower injuries causing various degrees of disruption. Even incomplete spinal cord injury can cause neurogenic shock.

Symptoms include:

- Hypotension and warm dry skin related to lack of vascular tone that results in hypothermia from loss of cutaneous heat.
- Bradycardia is a common but not universal symptom.

Treatment includes:

- ABCDE (airway, breathing, circulation, disability evaluation, exposure).
- Rapid fluid administration with crystalloid to keep mean arterial pressure at 85-90 mmHg.
- Placement of pulmonary artery catheter to monitor fluid overload.
- Inotropic agents (dopamine, dobutamine) if fluids don't correct hypotension.
- Atropine for persistent bradycardia.

ANAPHYLACTIC SHOCK

Anaphylactic reaction or **anaphylactic shock** may present with a few symptoms or a wide range of potentially lethal effects.

Symptoms:

Symptoms may recur after the initial treatment (biphasic anaphylaxis), so careful monitoring is essential:

- Sudden onset of weakness, dizziness, confusion.
- Severe generalized edema and angioedema. Lips and tongue may swell.
- Urticaria.
- Increased permeability of vascular system and loss of vascular tone – leading to severe hypotension & shock.
- Laryngospasm/bronchospasm with obstruction of airway causing dyspnea and wheezing.
- Nausea, vomiting, and diarrhea.
- Seizures, coma and death.

Treatments:

- Establish patent airway and intubate if necessary for ventilation.
- Provide oxygen at 100% high flow.
- Monitor VS.
- Administer epinephrine (Epi-pen® or solution).
- Albuterol per nebulizer for bronchospasm.
- Intravenous fluids to provide bolus of fluids for hypotension.
- Diphenhydramine if shock persists.
- Methylprednisolone if no response to other drugs.

HYPOVOLEMIC SHOCK/VOLUME DEFICIT

Hypovolemic shock occurs when there is inadequate intravascular fluid. The loss may be *absolute* because of an internal shifting of fluid, or an external loss of fluid, as occurs with massive hemorrhage, thermal injuries, severe vomiting or diarrhea, and internal injuries (such as ruptured spleen or dissecting arteries) that interfere with intravascular integrity. Hypovolemia may also be *relative* and related to vasodilation, increased capillary membrane permeability from sepsis or injuries, and decreased colloidal osmotic pressure that may occur with loss of sodium and some disorders, such as hypopituitarism and cirrhosis.

Hypovolemic shock is **classified** according to the degree of fluid loss:

- **Class I:** <750 mL or ≤15% of total circulating volume (TCV).
- **Class II:** 750-1500 mL or 15-30% of TCV.
- **Class III:** 1500-2000 mL or 30-40% of TCV.
- **Class IV:** >2000 mL or >40% of TCV.

SYMPTOMS AND TREATMENT

Hypovolemic shock occurs when the total circulating volume of fluid decreases, leading to a fall in venous return that in turn causes a decrease in ventricular filling and preload, indicated by ↓ in right atrial pressure (RAP) and pulmonary artery occlusion pressure (PAOP). This results in a decrease in stroke volume and cardiac output. This in turn causes generalized arterial vasoconstriction, increasing afterload (↑ systemic vascular resistance), causing decreased tissue perfusion.

Symptoms: Anxiety, pallor, cool and clammy skin, delayed capillary refill, cyanosis, hypotension, increasing respirations, weak, thready pulse.

Treatment is aimed at identifying and treating the cause:

- Administration of blood, blood products, autotransfusion, colloids (such as plasma protein fraction), and/or crystalloids (such as normal saline).
- Oxygen; intubation and ventilation may be necessary.
- Medications may include vasopressors, such as dopamine.
- *NOTE: Fluids must be given before starting vasopressors!

Sleep and Thermoregulation

SLEEP DISRUPTION

Sleep is an essential biological function. Patients admitted to the intensive care unit are at an increased risk for sleep disruption. Factors such as excessive noise levels, light, medications, frequent interventions by healthcare providers, and psychosocial stress may all contribute to sensory overload, thereby impacting a patient's ability to sleep or remain asleep. Patients may experience fragmented sleep due to frequent interruptions or they may have difficulty falling asleep. Often, patients experience a reduction in the amount of REM sleep. The physiologic impact of ineffective sleep may cause alterations in immune function, neurocognitive function, hormone regulation, respiratory and cardiac function and psychological well-being.

Signs and symptoms: Irritability, disorientation, lethargy, frequent yawning, depression and emotional lability.

Treatment: Creating a nocturnal environment for the critical care patient may help to promote a healthy sleeping pattern. Nursing interventions may include helping the patient to establish a normal sleep schedule (sleeping during night time hours and avoiding day time sleeping), managing the patient's pain, and decreasing stimulation (decreasing noise, modifying lighting, etc.) Patients may also benefit from relaxation techniques.

THERMOREGULATION IN CRITICALLY ILL PATIENTS

The hypothalamus, limbic system, lower brainstem, reticular formation, spinal cord and sympathetic ganglia all play a role in regulation of core temperature. The normal core body temperature of 35.5-37.5 degrees Celsius is a narrow range which is frequently disrupted in the critically ill patient. Impaired thermoregulation can occur in patients with sepsis, brain or spinal cord trauma, stroke, and tumors of the central nervous system. Mild hypothermia is common during deep sedation. Hypothermia (core temperature of <35 degrees Celsius) is associated with an increased risk of post-operative wound infections, blood loss and adverse cardiovascular events. Hypothermia may occur in trauma patients, patients with sepsis, post-operative patients and patients with severe burns. Hyperthermia (core temperature of >38 degrees Celsius) may occur in systemic inflammatory response syndrome, malignant hyperthermia, heat stroke, neuroleptic malignant syndrome, and serotonin syndrome. Hyperpyrexia occurs when the core temperature exceeds 40 degrees Celsius. Core temperatures exceeding 41.5 degrees Celsius may be life-threatening.

Toxic Ingestion/Inhalation

CARBON MONOXIDE POISONING

Carbon monoxide (CO) poisoning occurs with inhalation of fossil fuel exhausts from engines, emission of gas or coal heaters, indoor use of charcoal, and smoke and fumes. The CO binds with hemoglobin, preventing oxygen carriage and impairing oxygen delivery to tissue.

Diagnosis includes history, on-site oximetry reports, neurological examination, and CO neuropsychological screening battery (CONSB) done with patient breathing room air, CBC, electrolytes, ABGs, ECG, chest radiograph (for dyspnea); *pulse oximetry is not accurate in these patients.*

Symptoms: Cardiac: chest pain, palpitations, ↓ capillary refill, hypotension, cardiac arrest. CNS: malaise, nausea, vomiting, lethargy, stroke, coma, seizure. Secondary injuries: Rhabdomyolysis, AKI, non-cardiogenic pulmonary edema, multiple organ failure (MOF), DIC, and encephalopathy.

Treatment includes:

- Immediate support of airway, breathing, and circulation.
- Non-barometric oxygen (100%) by non-breathing mask with reservoir or ETT if necessary.
- Mild: Continue oxygen for 4 hours with reassessment.
- Severe: hyperbaric oxygen therapy (usually 3 treatments) to improve oxygen delivery.

CYANIDE POISONING

Cyanide poisoning, from hydrogen cyanide (HCN) or cyanide salts, can result from sodium nitroprusside infusions, inhalation of burning plastics, intentional or accidental ingestion or dermal exposure, occupation exposure, ingestion of some plant products, and the manufacture of PCP. Inhalation of HCN causes immediate symptoms; and ingestion of cyanide salts, within minutes.

Diagnosis is by history, clinical examination, normal PaO_2 and metabolic acidosis.

Symptoms: Increase in severity and alter with the amount of exposure: tachycardia, hypertension, leading to bradycardia, hypotension, and cardiac arrest. Pink or cherry-colored skin because of oxygen remaining in the blood. Headaches, lethargy, seizures, coma. dyspnea, tachypnea, and respiratory arrest.

Treatment includes:

- Supportive care as indicated.
- Removal of contaminated clothes.
- Gastric decontamination.
- Copious irrigation for topical exposure.
- Antidotes:
  - Amyl nitrate ampule cracked and inhaled 30 seconds.
  - Sodium nitrite (3%) 10 mL IV.
  - Sodium thiosulfate (25%) 50 mL IV.

GENERAL TREATMENT/REVERSAL AGENTS OF TOXIC INGESTIONS

Treatment for **toxic ingestions** is related to the type of toxin and whether or not it is identified:

- **Administration of reversal agent** if substance is known and an antidote exists. Antidotes for common toxins include:
  - Opiates: Naloxone (Narcan®).
  - Toxic alcohols: Ethanol infusion and/or dialysis.
  - Acetaminophen: N-acetylcysteine.
  - Calcium channel blockers, beta-blockers: Calcium chloride, Glucagon.
  - Tricyclic antidepressants: Sodium bicarbonate.
  - Ethylene glycol: Fomepizole.
  - Iron: Deferoxamine.
- **GI decontamination** at one time was standard procedures (Ipecac® and gastric lavage followed by activated charcoal). It is no longer advised for routine use although selective gastric lavage may be appropriate if done within 1 hour of ingestion.
- **Activated charcoal** (1 g/kg/wt) orally or per NG tube binds to many toxins if given within one hour of ingestion. It may also be used in multiple doses (q 4-6 hrs) to enhance elimination
- **Forced diuresis** with alkalinization of urine (>7.5) may prevent absorption of drugs that are weak bases or acids.

CAUSTIC INGESTIONS

Caustic ingestions of acids (pH <7) such as sulfuric, acetic, hydrochloric, and hydrofluoric found in many cleaning agents and alkalis (pH >7) such as sodium hydroxide, potassium hydroxide, sodium tripolyphosphate (in detergents) and sodium hypochlorite (bleach) can result in severe injury and death. Acids cause coagulation necrosis in the esophagus and stomach and may result in metabolic acidosis, hemolysis, and renal failure if systemically absorbed. Alkali injuries cause liquefaction necrosis, resulting in deeper ulcerations, often of the esophagus, but may involve perforation and abdominal necrosis with multi-organ damage.

Diagnosis is by detailed history, airway examination (oral intubation if possible), arterial blood gas, electrolytes, CBC, hepatic and coagulation tests, radiograph, and CT for perforations.

Symptoms: May vary but can include pain, dyspnea, oral burns, dysphonia, vomiting.

Treatment includes:

- Supportive and symptomatic therapy.
- <u>NO</u> ipecac, charcoal, neutralization, or dilution.
- NG tube for acids only to aspirate residual.
- Endoscopy in first few hours to evaluate injury/perforations.
- Sodium bicarbonate for pH <7.10.
- Prednisolone (alkali injuries).

Toxin/Drug Exposure

ALLERGIC REACTIONS

Exposure to certain toxins, medications, illegal substances and allergens can cause life threatening effects in some patients. The physiologic response of the patient is dependent on the agent and the degree of exposure. Tissue hypoperfusion and lactic acidosis often occur as a result of the exposure. This can lead to metabolic acidosis, shock, organ failure and death.

Signs and symptoms: In allergic type reactions, urticaria, pruritus, chest, back or abdominal pain, facial flushing, shortness of breath, wheezing and stridor may occur. Beta- and alpha-adrenergic responses may occur with exposure to amphetamines, cocaine, ephedrine, and pseudoephedrine. This response is manifested by diaphoresis, hypertension, tachycardia and mydriasis. Diarrhea, nausea and vomiting can occur with exposure to certain toxins.

Diagnosis: Physical assessment and testing to discover the toxin, drug or allergen the patient was exposed to. Labs—blood gases, BMP, complete blood count, toxicology screen, urinalysis, and allergy testing.

Treatment: Priority is to eliminate exposure to the drug/toxin/allergen. Antidotes (if available) may be administered in the case of toxin exposure. Activated charcoal may be administered in the case of medication/drug overdose. For allergic reactions, antihistamines and corticosteroids may be administered. Severe allergic reactions may need to be treated with epinephrine. Dialysis may be indicated in some patients. Sodium bicarbonate may be administered for the treatment of metabolic acidosis caused by many toxic reactions.

ACETAMINOPHEN TOXICITY

Acetaminophen toxicity from accidental or intentional overdose has high rates of morbidity and mortality unless promptly treated. *Diagnosis* is by history and acetaminophen level, which should be completed within 8 hours of ingestion if possible. Toxicity occurs with dosage >140 mg/kg in one dose or >7.5g in 24 hours.

Symptoms occur in stages:

1. (Initial) Minor gastrointestinal upset.
2. (Days 2-3) Hepatotoxicity with RUQ pain and increased AST, ALT, and bilirubin.
3. (Days 3-4) Hepatic failure with metabolic acidosis, coagulopathy, renal failure, encephalopathy, nausea, vomiting, and possible death.
4. (Days 5-12) Recovery period for survivors.

Treatment includes:

- GI decontamination with activated charcoal (orally or NG) <24 hours.
- Toxicity is plotted on the Rumack-Matthew nomogram with serum levels >150 requiring antidote. The antidote is most effective ≤8 hours of ingestion but decreases hepatotoxicity even >24 hours.
- Antidote: 72-hour N-acetylcysteine (NAC) protocol includes 140 mg/kg initially and 70 mg/kg every 4 hours for 17 more doses (orally or IV).
- Supportive therapy: Continuous dialysis, fluids, blood pressure medications.

AMPHETAMINE AND COCAINE TOXICITY

Amphetamine toxicity may be caused by IV, inhalation, or insufflation of various substances that include methamphetamine (MDA or "ecstasy"), methylphenidate (Ritalin®), methylenedioxymethamphetamine (MDMA), and ephedrine and phenylpropanolamine. *Cocaine* may be ingested orally, IV or by insufflation while crack cocaine may be smoked. Amphetamines and cocaine are CNS stimulants that can cause multi-system abnormalities.

Symptoms may include chest pain, dysrhythmias, myocardial ischemia, MI, seizures, intracranial infarctions, hypertension, dystonia, repetitive movements, unilateral blindness, lethargy, rhabdomyolysis with acute kidney failure, perforated nasal septum (cocaine) and paranoid psychosis (amphetamines). *Crack cocaine* may cause pulmonary hemorrhage, asthma, pulmonary edema, barotrauma, and pneumothorax. Swallowing packs of cocaine can cause intestinal ischemia, colitis, necrosis, and perforation. **Diagnosis** includes clinical findings, CBC, chemistry panel, toxicology screening, ECG, and radiography.

Treatment includes:

- Gastric emptying (<1 hour). Charcoal administration.
- IV access. Supplemental oxygen.
- Sedation for seizures: Lorazepam 2m, diazepam 5mg IV titrated in repeated doses. Agitation: Haloperidol.
- Hypertension: Nitroprusside/nicardipine, phentolamine IV.
- Cocaine quinidine-like effects: Sodium bicarbonate.

SALICYLATE TOXICITY

Salicylate toxicity may be acute or chronic and is caused by ingestion of OTC drugs containing salicylates, such as ASA, Pepto-Bismol®, and products used in hot inhalers.

Diagnosis is by ferric chloride or Ames Phenistix tests. Symptoms vary according to age and amount of ingestion. Co-ingestion of sedatives may alter symptoms.

Symptoms include:

- <150 mg/kg: Nausea and vomiting.
- 150-300 mg/kg: Vomiting, hyperpnea, diaphoresis, tinnitus, alterations in acid-base balance.
- >300 mg/kg (usually intentional overdose): Nausea, vomiting, diaphoresis, tinnitus, hyperventilation, respiratory alkalosis and metabolic acidosis.
- Chronic toxicity results in hyperventilation, tremor, and papilledema, alterations in mental status, pulmonary edema, seizures, and coma.

Treatment includes:

- Gastric decontamination with lavage (≤1 hour) and charcoal.
- Volume replacement (D5W).
- Sodium bicarbonate 1-2 mEq/kg.
- Monitoring of salicylate concentration, acid-base, and electrolytes every hour.
- Whole-bowel irrigation (sustained release tablets).

BENZODIAZEPINE TOXICITY

Benzodiazepine toxicity may result from accidental or intentional overdose with such drugs as Xanax®, Librium®, Valium®, Ativan®, Serax®, Versed®, and Restoril®. Mortality is usually the result of co-ingestion of other drugs.

Diagnosis is based on history and clinical exam, as benzodiazepine level does not correlate well with toxicity.

Symptoms: Non-specific neurological changes: Lethargy, dizziness, alterations in consciousness, ataxia. Respiratory depression and hypotension are rare complications. Coma and severe central nervous depression are usually caused by co-ingestions.

Treatment includes:

- Gastric emptying (<1 hour).
- Charcoal.
- Concentrated dextrose, thiamine and naloxone if co-ingestions suspected, especially with altered mental status.
- Monitoring for CNS/respiratory depression.
- Supportive care.
- Flumazenil (antagonist) 0.2 mg each minute to total 3 mg may be used in some cases but not routinely advised because of complications related to benzodiazepine dependency or co-ingestion of cyclic antidepressants. Flumazenil is contraindicated in patients with increased ICP.

ETHANOL OVERDOSE

Ethanol overdose affects the central nervous system as well as other organs in the body. Ethanol is absorbed through the mucosa of the mouth, stomach, and intestines, with concentrations peaking about 30-60 minutes after ingestion. If people are easily aroused, they can usually safely sleep off the effects of ingesting too much alcohol, but if the person is semi-conscious or unconscious, emergency medical treatment should be initiated.

Symptoms include:

- Altered mental status with slurred speech and stupor.
- Nausea and vomiting.
- Hypotension.
- Bradycardia with arrhythmias
- Respiratory depression and hypoxia.
- Cold, clammy skin or flushed skin (from vasodilation).
- Acute pancreatitis with abdominal pain.
- Lack of consciousness
- Circulatory collapse

Treatment includes:

- Careful monitoring of arterial blood gases and oxygen saturation.
- Ensure patent airway with intubation and ventilation if necessary.
- Intravenous fluids.
- Dextrose to correct hypoglycemia if indicated.
- Maintain body temperature (warming blanket).
- Dialysis may be necessary in severe cases.

ALCOHOL OVERDOSE

Alcohol is an inhibitory neurotransmitter that depresses the central nervous system. In most states, the legal intoxication blood alcohol level is defined as 100mg/dl. Blood alcohol levels of **500mg/dl or greater** are associated with a high mortality rate. The central nervous system depressant effect is further enhanced when alcohol is mixed with other agents.

Signs and symptoms: Acute mental status changes (confusion, disorientation, lethargy, coma), vomiting, seizures, hypothermia, bradypnea, loss of gag reflex, slurred speech, ataxia and incontinence.

Diagnosis: Physical exam and blood alcohol level. A CT of the head may be conducted to rule out other diagnoses that may mimic alcohol overdose. Other drug testing may be performed as well to assess for the presence of other substances.

Treatment: The treatment of alcohol overdose is dependent on the severity of the symptoms. Some patients may require intubation and mechanical ventilation if the central nervous system is significantly depressed. IV fluids are often administered along with Vitamin B to treat dehydration. Hemodialysis may also be necessary.

GASTRIC EMPTYING FOR TOXIC SUBSTANCE INGESTION

Gastric emptying for toxic substance ingestion should be done ≤60 minutes of ingestion for large life-threatening amounts of poison. The patient requires IV access, oximetry, and cardiac monitoring. Sedation (1-2 mg IV midazolam) or rapid sequence induction and endotracheal intubation may be necessary. Patients should be positioned in left lateral decubitus position with head down at 20° to prevent passage of stomach contents into duodenum although intubated patients may be lavaged in the supine position. With a bite block in place, an orogastric Y-tube (36-40 Fr. for adults) should be inserted after estimating length. Placement should be confirmed with injection of 50 mL of air confirmed under auscultation and aspiration of gastric contents, as well as abdominal Xray (pH may not be reliable depending on substance ingested). Irrigation is done by gravity instillation of about 200-300 mL warmed (45 °C) tap water or NS. The instillation side is clamped and drainage side opened. This is repeated until fluid returns clear. A slurry of charcoal is then instilled, and tube clamped and removed when procedures completed.

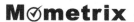

Life Threatening Maternal/Fetal Complications

ECLAMPSIA

Eclampsia is a progression of preeclampsia, which is a disorder that develops at around 20 weeks of gestation in approximately 5% of all pregnancies. Preeclampsia is characterized by hypertension associated (though not inconclusively) with proteinuria (300mg/24h) and edema (peripheral or generalized) or increase of ≥5 pounds of weight in one week after 20th week of gestation. Severe preeclampsia is BP ≥160/110. Symptoms include headache, abdominal pain, and visual disturbances. Initial treatment of pre-eclampsia is magnesium sulfate to prevent seizures in the mother. Severe cases may require the premature delivery of the infant to relieve the condition. If pre-eclampsia does not resolve and progresses to include tonic-clonic seizures, it is termed eclampsia, and this is life threatening. The seizure typically begins with facial twitching and then generalized seizures followed by loss of consciousness. If the patient arouses, she may be hyperventilating, confused, agitated, and combative. The patient may have multi-system derangements. Treatment for seizures is magnesium sulfate, but benzodiazepines or phenytoin may be used if magnesium sulfate is ineffective. Labetalol or hydralazine are given to lower BP. Immediate delivery of the fetus is imperative. Risk factors include teen pregnancy, primigravida, nulliparity, older mother, obesity, history of hypertension, gestational diabetes, SLE, and renal disease.

HELLP SYNDROME

HELLP syndrome occurs in 4 to 12% of those with pre-eclampsia, most often during weeks 27 to 37 but may develop within 24 hours post-partum, and is characterized by:

- **H**—hemolysis.
- **EL**—Elevated liver enzymes
- **LP**—low platelet count.

HELLP syndrome is most common in older multiparous mothers. Hypertension may be less pronounced than in others with preeclampsia. Pain in the right upper quadrant related to liver dysfunction may be misdiagnosed as gastrointestinal upset or gall bladder disease. Mothers often present with flu-like non-specific symptoms, including headache, nausea and vomiting and visual disturbances. Prompt diagnosis and treatment is necessary because of high mortality. Platelet transfusions are given if platelet count <20,000/mm³ or <50,000/mm³ with Caesarean. The primary treatment is immediate delivery of the fetus as the mother may develop hepatic hemorrhage or permanent liver damage. Both the mother and the fetus are at risk. Neonates are at increased risk and may require mechanical ventilation. Complications include abruptio placentae, DIC, and post-partum hemorrhage.

POSTPARTAL HEMORRHAGE

Postpartal hemorrhage may be early (≤24 hours) or late (≤6 weeks). Normal blood loss with vaginal delivery is about 500 mL and with Caesarean about 1000 mL. Blood loss is difficult to estimate because it is mixed with amniotic fluid and mucus, and hemorrhage may be internal and not obvious on examination. Usual indications of hemorrhage, such as increased pulse, decreased blood pressure, and decreased output of urine may be delayed until about 2 L of blood loss. A significant drop in hematocrit (10 points) is indicative of hemorrhage. Early hemorrhage poses more risk of mortality than late hemorrhage. When hemorrhage is suspected, such as with steady flow of lochia rubra, then the woman's vital signs should be checked every 5 to 15 minutes and perineal pads weighed (1 mL blood weighs about 1 g). A soft boggy uterus should be massaged frequently to maintain firmness, with clots expressed. IV access should be maintained. Urinary

197

output < 30 mL/hr. should be reported to physician. Risk factors include uterine atony, genital lacerations, hematomas, uterine inversion, uterine rupture, abnormal placental implantation, fetal macrosomia, grand multipara, primipara, weight gain/BMI, and coagulopathies.

AMNIOTIC EMBOLISM

Amniotic embolism (AKA amniotic fluid embolism) is a maternal complication that occurs during labor or immediately postpartum characterized by sudden hypotension, hypoxia, and coagulopathy, which can lead to massive hemorrhage, although presentation varies widely and some patients may exhibit only one primary symptom. Risk factors include older age, placental abnormalities, preeclampsia, medically-induced labor, polyhydramnios, and operative deliveries. Amniotic embolism occurs when amniotic fluid enters the circulatory system. In some patients, this triggers a number of life-threatening physiological reactions, which may include hypotension, fetal distress, pulmonary edema/ARDS, dyspnea, cyanosis, seizure, and cardiopulmonary arrest. Pulmonary constriction results in impaired flood flow to the heart and circulatory collapse. Both the patient and fetus are at risk of death. If the fetus has not been delivered, emergent Caesarean may be done to save the child. If the patient survives cardiovascular collapse, the patient should receive circulatory support, replacement blood products, oxygen, and supportive care. Survivors often suffer neurological impairment.

Post-Intensive Care Syndrome

Post-intensive care syndrome (PICS) refers to the disabilities that occur as the result of treatment in intensive care for critical illness, such as coronavirus patients with induced coma and weeks of mechanical ventilation. Impairments include:

- **Cognitive:** Difficulty speaking, impaired memory, difficulty concentrating, impaired executive function.
- **Psychological:** Depression, anxiety, PTSD, delirium, lack of motivation. PICS can affect family members and caregivers as well because of the emotional stress they encounter, primarily exhibited with psychological problems (grief, anxiety, depression, insomnia, PTSD).
- **Physical**: Generalized weakness, dyspnea, insomnia, lethargy, fatigue, difficulty walking.

These impairments may result from the critical illness or the interventions (medications, sedation, ventilation) that were included as part of treatment. Management includes early mobilization, orienting and interacting with patient, minimizing medications and sedation, avoiding hypoxemia and hypoglycemia, assessing for delirium, and treating depression. Patients may need physical therapy to regain strength, respiratory and/or cardiac therapy, and psychological counseling. Some impairments may remain chronic.

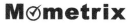

Malignant Hyperthermia

Malignant hyperthermia is a life-threatening condition triggered by genetic susceptibility to inhalational anesthetics (except nitrous oxide and succinylcholine). Signs may occur within 10-20 minutes of induction or delayed >24 hours. Risk factors include large, strong muscles and a history of unexplained fevers or family history of death after surgery. Effects include:

- Increased cytoplasmic calcium, causing muscle contractions, including Masseter spasm (jaw clamps shut).
- Hypermetabolism with increasing temperature.
- Cell leakage of potassium, myoglobin, and creatinine phosphokinase damages cells.

Sympathetic nervous system compensation:

- Vasodilation and increased perspiration to combat rising temperature, increased circulating catecholamines cause tachycardia and subsequent vasoconstriction and increases vascular resistance.
- Increased Cardiac output outpaces oxygen demand with decreased mixed venous O_2 and arterial oxygen, and development of lactic acidosis, hypotension, increased ventilation.

High temperature may be a late sign. Once temperature begins to increase, it may rise 1-2 °C every 5 minutes. Systemic manifestations may include cardiac dysrhythmias (ventricular), hemorrhage and/or DIC, increased ICP, kidney failure with oliguria, and cardiac arrest. Treatment includes stopping triggering agent, supportive treatment, and administration of dantrolene 1 mg/kg every five minutes until stabilized. Forced diuresis may be done to protect against renal failure. Internal and external cooling methods are used to reduce temperature.

Nursing Actions

TARGETED TEMPERATURE MANAGEMENT

Targeted temperature management (previously referred to as therapeutic hypothermia) is used to reduce ischemic tissue damage associated with cardiac arrest, ischemic stroke, traumatic brain/spinal cord injury, neurogenic fever, and subsequent coma (3 on Glasgow scale). Reducing the body's temperature to below normal range has a neuroprotective effect by making cell membranes less permeable, thus reducing neurologic edema and damage. Hypothermia should be initiated immediately after an ischemic event if possible but some benefit remains up to 6 hours. Hypothermia to 33 °C may be induced by cooled saline through a femoral catheter, reducing temperature 1.5-2 °C/hr, with by an electronic control unit. Hypothermic water blankets covering ≥80% of body the body surface can also lower body temperature. In some cases, both a femoral cooling catheter and water blanket are used for rapid reduction of temperature. Rectal probes are used to measure core temperature, but Foley temperature catheters are more common. Desflurane or meperidine is given to reduce the shivering response. Hypothermia increases risk of bleeding (decreased clotting time), infection (due to impairing leukocyte function and introducing catheters), arrhythmias, hyperglycemia, and DVT. Rewarming is done slowly at 0.5-1 °C/hr. through warmed intravenous fluids, warm humidified air, and/or warming blanket. The warming process is a critical time as it causes potassium to be moved from extracellular to intracellular spaces and the patient's electrolyte levels must be monitored regularly.

CONTINUOUS TEMPERATURE MONITORING

Continuous temperature monitoring may be carried out through a pulmonary artery catheter (most accurate but generally not recommended because of invasiveness and potential for complications), through rectal or Foley temperature probes, through probes fastened to the skin, or through wearable Bluetooth monitors (patch applied to the skin), which transmit information to an external monitor or the patient's electronic health record. For external temperature monitoring, the device must be applied properly and for the correct duration of time. (For example, the TempTraQ® wearable patch is applied in the underarm area and measures temperature for 72 hours.) Indications for continuous temperature monitoring include skin flaps to assess perfusion, patients with brain injuries to assess thermoregulation, immunocompromised patients to assess signs of infection, patients undergoing therapeutic hypothermia (such as post cardiac surgery or cardiac arrest), patients who are critically ill (and at risk for temperature dysregulation), and patients with malignant hyperthermia.

MINIMAL SEDATION

Minimal sedation includes local/topical anesthesia, peripheral nerve blocks, administration of <50% nitrogen oxide in oxygen by itself, or administration one sedative or analgesic medication in a dosage that does not typically require supervision. The patient should be fully aware and able to respond appropriately to verbal and tactile stimulation and to maintain an airway independently as these medications should not have cardiovascular or respiratory effects. The purpose of minimal sedation is to decrease perception of pain, relax the patient, and reduce fear. The patient's level of consciousness, sedation, and pain should be monitored throughout the procedure to ensure the dosage is adequate and the patient is not excessively sedated. Medications may include benzodiazepines (diazepam, lorazepam), and opioids (fentanyl, morphine, meperidine). Reversal agents (flumazenil, naloxone) should be available. Minimal sedation is often used during labor and delivery and for minor procedures, such as skin biopsies and removal of skin lesions.

CONTINUOUS VS. INTERMITTENT SEDATION

Sedation for critically ill patients may include:

- **Intermittent sedation** is that administered through IV push, so the expected duration is relatively short. Typical agents include benzodiazepines and opioids. Intermittent sedation is most often used for endoscopic procedures but is also sometimes used for patients who are on mechanical ventilation, especially if they have regular trials of weaning. Also, intermittent sedation is less likely to result in over sedation.
- **Continuous sedation** is that administered through a steady intravenous infusion to ensure longer-lasting sedation. Typical agents include opioids, midazolam, and propofol. Continuous sedation is more commonly used for patients on mechanical ventilation because it requires less intervention and maintains a steady blood level. Daily interruptions of continuous sedation may be carried out as a trial for weaning patients on mechanical ventilation.

With both intermittent sedation and continuous sedation, the patient's vital signs, respiratory status, temperature, and oxygen saturation should be monitored. Arousal scales (Richmond or Riker Agitation/Sedation Scales) should be utilized to assess arousal and to adjust sedation dosages.

NEUROMUSCULAR BLOCKADE AGENTS

Neuromuscular blocker agents are used for induced paralysis of those who have not responded adequately to sedation, especially for intubation and mechanical ventilation. NMBAs do not produce unconsciousness, amnesia, or analgesia, therefore it is critical that they are administered <u>after</u> the client has been adequately sedated. NMBAs include:

- **Depolarizing agents**: Succinylcholine. Risk for severe hyperkalemia after denervation injury persists for 7-10 days. Post-operative myalgia is common, and succinylcholine may trigger malignant hyperthermia and severe anaphylactic/anaphylactoid reactions.
- **Non-depolarizing agents**: Short acting (mivacurium, rapacuronium), intermediate acting (rocuronium, vecuronium, atracurium, cisatracurium), and long acting (pancuronium, doxacurium, pipecuronium). Should be given for ≤2 days for those on ventilators because they may develop persistent quadriparesis. Most are not associated with malignant hyperthermia.

Eye lubricant should be applied every 2 hours and the eyes kept closed. Range of motion exercises should not extend beyond normal range because of potential to damage joints. The patient must be repositioned frequently while paralyzed and on adequate support surface. Pupil reactivity should be assessed every 1 to 4 hours to evaluate neurological status. Temperature should be monitored hourly if <36 °C or if placed under a cooling blanket because heat production is depressed. After cessation, patient should be closely monitored to ensure that muscle function has returned to normal.

MODERATE (CONSCIOUS) SEDATION

The ASA sedation guidelines (2018) are intended for **moderate (AKA conscious) sedation** used for procedures, such as colonoscopy. Steps include:

- **Pre-procedure evaluation**: Includes review of health records, physical examination and laboratory testing as indicated a few days or weeks prior to the procedure and re-evaluating the patient again before the procedure.
- **Patient preparation**: Consult with specialist if indicated, ensure patient has informed consent and has been compliant with pre-procedure fasting, insert intravenous line.
- **Patient monitoring**: LOC (every 5 minutes), oxygenation/ventilation (capnography, pulse oximetry), and hemodynamic with designated person responsible for monitoring and recording.
- **Supplemental oxygen:** Use unless contraindicated by condition.
- **Emergency interventions**: Resuscitative equipment and reversal agents for opioids (naloxone) and benzodiazepines (Romazicon) must be present with person trained in assessment and use available.
- **Sedatives**: Combinations of drugs as appropriate may be used (benzodiazepines and dexmedetomidine) and analgesics (opioids).
- **Sedative (propofol, ketamine, etomidate) and analgesics (local anesthetics, NSAIDs, and opioids) intended for general anesthesia**: Care must be consistent with that of general anesthesia and IV medications administered incrementally.
- **Recovery care**: Monitor oxygenation, ventilation, and circulation every 5 to 15 minutes.

SEDATION USING PROPOFOL

Sedation used for drug-induced coma often includes **propofol**. Propofol is an IV non-opioid hypnotic anesthetic, the most common used for induction. It is also used for maintenance and postoperative sedation. Onset of action is rapid because of high lipid solubility, and propofol has a short distribution half-life and rapid clearance, so recovery is also fast. Propofol is metabolized by the liver as well as through the lungs. Propofol decreases cerebral blood flow, metabolic rate of oxygen consumption and ICP. Propofol causes vasodilation with resultant hypotension, but with bradycardia rather than tachycardia. Propofol is a respiratory depressant, resulting in apnea after induction and decreased tidal volume, respiratory rate, and hypoxic drive during maintenance. Propofol has antiemetic properties as well but does not produce analgesia.

DELAYED EMERGENCE

Delayed emergence (failure to emerge for 30-60 minutes after anesthesia ends) is more common in the elderly because of slowed metabolism of anesthetic agents but may have a variety of causes, such as drug overdose during surgery, overdose related to preinduction use of drugs or alcohol that potentiates intraoperative drugs. In this case, naloxone or flumazenil may be indicated if opioids or benzodiazepines are implicated. Physostigmine may also be used to reverse effects of some anesthetic agents. Hypothermia may also cause delay in emergence, especially core temperatures <33 °C, and may require forced-air warming blankets to increase the temperature. Other metabolic conditions, such as hypoglycemia or hyperglycemia may also affect emergence. Patients suffering from delayed emergence must be evaluated for perioperative stroke, especially after neurological, cardiovascular, or cerebrovascular surgery. Metabolic disturbance may also delay emergence.

POST-ANESTHETIC RESPIRATORY COMPLICATIONS

Post-operative respiratory complications are most common in the postanesthesia period, so monitoring of oxygen levels is critical to preventing hypoxemia:

- **Airway obstruction** may be partial or total. Partial obstruction is indicated by sonorous or wheezing respirations, and total by absence of breath sounds. Treatment includes supplemental oxygen, airway insertion, repositioning (jaw thrust), or succinylcholine and positive-pressure ventilation for laryngospasm. If edema of the glottis is causing obstruction, IV corticosteroids may be used.
- **Hypoventilation** ($PaCO_2$ >45 mmHg) is often mild but may cause respiratory acidosis. It is usually related to depression caused by anesthetic agents. A number of factors may slow emergence (hypothermia, overdose, metabolism) and cause hypoventilation. It may also be related to splinting because of pain, requiring additional pain management.
- **Hypoxemia** (mild is PaO_2 500-60 mmHg) is usually related to hypoventilation and/or increased right to left shunting and is usually treated with supplementary oxygen (30-60%) with or without positive airway pressure.

POST-ANESTHETIC CARDIOVASCULAR COMPLICATIONS

Cardiovascular complications after surgery are sometimes related to respiratory complications, which may need to be addressed as well. Complications include:

- **Hypotension** is most often mild and requires no specific treatment. It is most commonly caused by hypovolemia and is significant if BP falls 20-30% below normal baseline. A bolus (100-250 mL IV colloid) is used to confirm hypovolemia. If severe, then medications, such as vasopressors, may be indicated. Hypotension may occur with pneumothorax so careful respiratory assessment must be done.
- **Hypertension** usually occurs ≤ 30 minutes after surgery and is common in those with history of hypertension. It may be secondary to hypoxemia or metabolic acidosis. Mild increases usually don't require treatment but medications may be used for moderate (β-adrenergic blockers) or severe (nitroprusside).
- **Arrhythmias** usually relate to respiratory complications or effects of anesthetic agents. Bradycardia may relate to cholinesterase inhibitors, opioids, or propranolol. Tachycardia may relate to anticholinergics, β-agonists, and vagolytic drugs. Hypokalemia and hypomagnesemia may cause premature atrial and ventricular beats.

Professional Caring and Ethical Practice

Advocacy/Moral Agency

ACCN SYNERGY MODEL

The **ACCN Synergy model** of nursing practice, developed by the ACCN for nursing certification, places the needs of the patient as a central focus and defines the relationship between 8 patient characteristics and 8 nurse competencies. These competencies and characteristics are evaluated on a scale (1-5). **Patient characteristics** include resiliency, vulnerability, stability, complexity, resource availability, participation in care, participation in decision-making, and predictability. **Nurse competencies** include clinical judgment, advocacy, caring practices, collaboration, systems thinking, response to diversity, clinical inquiry, and facilitation of learning. The **system or healthcare environment** is the third element of the model. It provides support for the needs of the patients and empowers and nurtures the practice of nursing, caring, and ethical practice. All three of these systems are essential for Synergy. The needs of the patient are the driving force for nurse competencies and both are dependent on the healthcare system. When the needs, competencies, and system complement each other, Synergy is achieved, and outcomes for the nurse, the patient, and the system are optimized.

THREE LEVELS OF OUTCOMES

The **ACCN Synergy model** is based on three levels of quality outcomes (patient, nurse, and system). Six general indicators of quality outcomes include:

- Satisfaction of patient and family.
- Adverse incidents rates.
- Rate of complications.
- Adherence to discharge plans.
- Mortality rate.
- Length of stay in hospital.

These general outcomes are based on outcomes derived from the patient, the nurse, and the system:

- **Patient outcomes** include functional change, behavioral change, trust, ratings, satisfaction, comfort, and quality of life.
- **Nurse outcomes** include physiological changes, presence or absence of complications, extent to which care of treatment objectives were attained.
- **System outcomes** include recidivism, costs, and resource utilization.

ADVOCACY/MORAL AGENCY

Nurse competencies under the ACCN Synergy model include **advocacy/moral agency**:

- **Advocacy** is working for the best interests of the patient despite personal values in conflict and assisting patients to have access to appropriate resources.
- **Agency** is openness and recognition of issues and a willingness to act.
- **Moral agency** is the ability to recognize needs and take action to influence the outcome of a conflict or decision.

203

The **levels of advocacy/moral agency** include:

- **Level 1:** This nurse works on behalf of the patient, assesses personal values, has awareness of patient's rights and ethical conflicts, and advocates for the patient when consistent with the nurse's personal values.
- **Level 3:** This nurse advocates for the patient/family, incorporates their values into the care plan even when they differ from the nurse's, and can utilize internal resources to assist patient/family with complex decisions.
- **Level 5:** This nurse advocates for patient/family despite differences in values and is able to utilize both internal and external resources to help to empower patient/family to make decisions.

COMPLEMENTARY THERAPIES

Complementary therapies are used as well as conventional medical treatment and should be included if this is what the patient/family wants, empowering the family to take some control. Complementary therapies vary widely and most can easily be incorporated into the plan of care The National Center for Complementary and Alternative Medicine recognizes the following:

- Whole medical systems include medical systems, such as homeopathic, naturopathic medicine, acupuncture, and Chinese herbal medications.
- Mind-body medicine can include support groups, medication, music, art, or dance therapy.
- Biologically-based practices include the use of food, vitamins, or nutrition for healing.
- Manipulative/body-based programs include massage or other types of manipulation, such as chiropractic treatment.
- Energy therapies may be biofield therapies intended to affect the aura (energy field) that some believe surrounds all living things. These therapies include therapeutic touch and Reiki. Bioelectromagnetic-based therapies use a variety of magnetic fields.

ETHICAL ASSESSMENT

While the terms *ethics* and *morals* are sometimes used interchangeably, ethics is a study of morals and encompasses concepts of right and wrong. When making **ethical assessments,** one must consider not only what people should do but also what they actually do, as these two things are sometimes at odds. Ethical issues can be difficult to assess because of personal bias, and that is one of the reasons that sharing concerns with other internal sources and reaching consensus is so valuable. Issues of concern might include options for care, refusal of care, rights to privacy, adequate relief of suffering, and the right to self-determination. Internal sources might include the ethics committee, whose role is to make decisions regarding ethical issues. Risk management can provide guidance related to personal and institutional liability. External agencies might include government agencies, such as the public health department.

BENEFICENCE AND NONMALEFICENCE

Beneficence is an ethical principle that involves performing actions that are for the purpose of benefitting another person. In the care of a patient, any procedure or treatment should be done with the ultimate goal of benefitting the patient, and any actions that are not beneficial should be reconsidered. As conditions change, procedures need to be continually reevaluated to determine if they are still of benefit.

Nonmaleficence is an ethical principle that means healthcare workers should provide care in a manner that does not cause direct intentional harm to the patient:

- The actual act must be good or morally neutral.
- The intent must be only for a good effect.
- A bad effect cannot serve as the means to get to a good effect.
- A good effect must have more benefit than a bad effect has harm.

AUTONOMY AND JUSTICE

Autonomy is the ethical principle that the individual has the right to make decisions about his/her own care. In the case of children or patients with dementia who cannot make autonomous decisions, parents or family members may serve as the legal decision maker. The nurse must keep the patient and/or family fully informed so that they can exercise their autonomy in informed decision-making.

Justice is the ethical principle that relates to the distribution of the limited resources of healthcare benefits to the members of society. These resources must be distributed fairly. This issue may arise if there is only one bed left and two sick patients. Justice comes into play in deciding which patient should stay and which should be transported or otherwise cared for. The decision should be made according to what is best or most just for the patients and not colored by personal bias.

BIOETHICS

Bioethics is a branch of ethics that involves making sure that the medical treatment given is the most morally correct choice given the different options that might be available and the differences inherent in the varied levels of treatment. In the acute/critical care unit, if the patients, family members, and the staff are in agreement when it comes to values and decision-making, then no ethical dilemma exists; however, when there is a difference in value beliefs between the patients/family members and the staff, there is a bioethical dilemma that must be resolved. Sometimes, discussion and explanation can resolve differences, but at times the institution's ethics committee must be brought in to resolve the conflict. The primary goal of bioethics is to determine the most morally correct action using the set of circumstances given.

INFORMED CONSENT

Patients or guardians must provide **informed consent** for all treatment the patient receives. This includes a thorough explanation of all procedures and treatment and associated risks. Patients/guardians should be apprised of all options and allowed input on the type of treatments. Patients/guardians should be apprised of all reasonable risks and any complications that might be life threatening or increase morbidity. The American Medical Association has established guidelines for informed consent:

- Explanation of diagnosis.
- Nature and reason for treatment or procedure.
- Risks and benefits.
- Alternative options (regardless of cost or insurance coverage).
- Risks and benefits of alternative options.
- Risks and benefits of not having a treatment or procedure.
- Providing informed consent is a requirement of all states.

Note: A patient may waive their right to informed consent; if this is the case, the nurse should document the patient's refusal and proceed with the procedure. Also, informed consent is not necessary for procedures performed to save a life/limb in which the patient/family is unable to consent.

INCORPORATING PATIENT/FAMILY RIGHTS INTO PLAN OF CARE

In order for **patient/family rights** to be incorporated into the plan of care, the care plan needs to be designed as a collaborative effort that encourages participation of patients and family members. There are a number of different programs that can be useful, such as including patients and families on advisory committees. Additionally, assessment tools, such as surveys for patients/families, can be utilized to gain insight in the issues that are important to them. While infants and small children and sometimes the elderly cannot speak for themselves, "patient" is generally understood to include not only the immediate family but also other groups or communities who have an interest in the care of an individual or individuals. Because many hospital stays are now short-term, programs that include follow-up interviews and assessments are especially valuable in determining if the needs of the patient/family were addressed in the care plan.

CONFIDENTIALITY

Confidentiality is the obligation that is present in a professional-patient relationship. Nurses are under an obligation to protect the information they possess concerning the patient and family. Care should be taken to safeguard that information and provide the privacy that the family deserves. This is accomplished through the use of required passwords when family call for information about the patient and through the limitation of who is allowed to visit. There may be times when confidentiality must be broken to save the life of a patient, but those circumstances are rare. The nurse must make all efforts to safeguard patient records and identification. Computerized record keeping should be done in such a way that the screen is not visible to others, and paper records must be secured.

PATIENT'S/FAMILY'S RIGHTS AND RESPONSIBILITIES

Empowering patients and families to act as their own advocates requires they have a clear understanding of their **rights and responsibilities.** These should be given (in print form) and/or presented (audio/video) to patients and families on admission or as soon as possible:

- **Rights** should include competent, non-discriminatory medical care that respects privacy and allows participation in decisions about care and the right to refuse care. They should have clear understandable explanations of treatments, options, and conditions, including outcomes. They should be apprised of transfers, changes in care plan, and advance directives. They should have access to medical records information about charges.
- **Responsibilities** should include providing honest and thorough information about health issues and medical history. They should ask for clarification if they don't understand information that is provided to them, and they should follow the plan of care that is outlined or explain why that is not possible. They should treat staff and other patients with respect.

ETHICAL ISSUES RELATED TO TREATMENT OF TERMINALLY ILL PATIENTS

There are a number of **ethical concerns** that healthcare providers and families must face when determining the treatments that are necessary and appropriate for a terminally-ill patient. It is the nurse's responsibility to provide support and information to help parents/families make informed decisions. Common treatments (with their advantages and disadvantages) that present dilemmas include:

- **Analgesia:** Provide comfort. Ease the dying process. Increase sedation and decrease cognition and interaction with family. May hasten death.
- **Active treatments (such as antibiotics, chemotherapy):** Prolong life. Relieve symptoms. Reassure family. Prolong the dying process. Side effects may be severe (as with chemotherapy).
- **Supplemental nutrition:** Relieve family's anxiety that patient is hungry. Prolong life. May cause nausea, vomiting. May increase tumor growth with cancer. May increase discomfort.
- **IV fluids for hydration:** Relieve family's anxiety that patient is thirsty. Keep mouth moist. May result in congestive heart failure and pulmonary edema with increased dyspnea. Increased urinary output and incontinence may cause skin breakdown. Prolong dying process.
- **Resuscitation efforts:** Allow family to deny death is imminent. Cause unnecessary suffering and prolong dying process.

Caring Practices

CARING PRACTICES

In the ACCN Synergy model, **caring practices** encompass all nursing activities that respond to the individual patient's and family's needs in a caring, compassionate, and therapeutic environment to promote patient comfort and prevent unnecessary suffering. Caring practices recognize inner strength and its relation to healing and seeks to enhance the dignity of the individual through vigilance, nurturing, and skilled technical and basic nursing practices. Levels of caring practices include:

- **Level 1**: This nurse provides a safe environment and cares for the present basic needs of the patient without focus on future needs and considers death a potential outcome.
- **Level 3**: This nurse provides compassionate care, responding to changes in the patient and acts of kindness while accepting death as a possible outcome and providing measures to ensure good end-of-life care and a peaceful death.
- **Level 5:** This nurse is fully engaged in patient care and understands and interprets patient/family dynamics and needs, ensuring comfort, dignity, and safety while respecting the individual and family.

PROBLEM SOLVING

Problem solving to anticipate or prevent recurrences of patient/family dissatisfaction involves arriving at a hypothesis, testing, and assessing data to determine if the hypothesis holds true. If a problem has arisen, taking steps to resolve the immediate problem is only the first step if recurrence is to be avoided:

- **Define the issue:** Talk with the patient or family and staff to determine if the problem related to a failure of communication or other issues, such as culture or religion.
- **Collect data:** This may mean interviewing additional staff or reviewing documentation, gaining a variety of perspectives.
- **Identify important concepts:** Determine if there are issues related to values or beliefs.
- **Consider reasons for actions:** Distinguish between motivation and intention on the part of all parties to determine the reason for the problem.
- **Make a decision:** A decision on how to prevent a recurrence of a problem should be based on advocacy and moral agency, reaching the best solution possible for the patient and family.

PATIENTS'/FAMILIES' RIGHTS

Patients' (and families') rights in relation to what they should expect from a healthcare organization are outlined in both standards of the Joint Commission and National Committee for Quality Assurance. Rights include:

- Respect for patient, including personal dignity and psychosocial, spiritual, and cultural considerations.
- Response to needs related to access and pain control.
- Ability to make decisions about care, including informed consent, advance directives, and end of life care.
- Procedure for registering complaints or grievances.
- Protection of confidentiality and privacy.
- Freedom from abuse or neglect.
- Protection during research and information related to ethical issues of research.

208

- Appraisal of outcomes, including unexpected outcomes.
- Information about organization, services, and practitioners.
- Appeal procedures for decisions regarding benefits and quality of care.
- Organizational code of ethical behavior.
- Procedures for donating and procuring organs/tissue.

FACILITATING SAFE PASSAGE

Facilitating **safe passage** is part of caring practice that ensures patient safety, in a broad sense, from a variety of perspectives:

- Giving appropriate medications and treatment without errors that endanger the patient's health is essential.
- Providing information to the patient/family about treatments, changes, conditions, and other aspects related to care helps them to cope with the situations as they arise.
- Preventing infection is central to patient safety and includes staff using proper infection control methods, such as handwashing.
- Knowing the person requires the nurse to take the time and effort to understand the needs and wishes of the patient/family.
- Assisting with transitions involves not only helping the patient/family cope with moving from one form of treatment, or one unit to another but also with transitions in health, such as from illness to health or from illness to death.

ADVANCE DIRECTIVES

In accordance to Federal and state laws, individuals have the right to self-determination in health care, including decisions about end of life care through **advance directives** such as living wills and the right to assign a surrogate person to make decisions through a durable power of attorney. Patients should routinely be questioned about an advanced directive as they may present at a healthcare provider without the document. Patients who have indicated they desire a do-not-resuscitate (DNR) order should not receive resuscitative treatments for terminal illness or conditions in which meaningful recovery cannot occur. Patients and families of those with terminal illnesses should be questioned as to whether the patients are Hospice patients. For those with DNR requests or those withdrawing life support, staff should provide the patient palliative rather than curative measures, such as pain control and/or oxygen, and emotional support to the patient and family. Religious traditions and beliefs about death should be treated with respect.

PAIN MANAGEMENT

Promoting a caring and supportive environment means ensuring that the patient is comfortable. According to Joint Commission guidelines and Federal law, all patients have to right to **pain management,** and this applies to all ages. It's not enough to recognize this; procedures must be in place to assure that all staff are committed to reducing pain and that patients/families be apprised of the right and benefits of pain management. There are steps that the institution can take in this process:

- Create an interdisciplinary team to research, provide guidelines, and communicate goals.
- Assess pain management procedures already in place to determine effectiveness or need for change.
- Establish a minimum standard that should be legally followed.
- Clarify responsibility for pain control and imbed this in the standards of practice.
- Provide information about pain control to all levels of care providers.

- Educate patients to understand they are entitled to rapid response.
- Educate staff to institutionalize pain management.

SUPPORTING FAMILIES OF DYING PATIENTS

Families of **dying patients** often do not receive adequate support from nursing staff that feel unprepared for dealing with families' grief and unsure of how to provide comfort, but families may be in desperate need of this support:

- **Before death:**
  - Stay with the family and sit quietly, allowing them to talk, cry, or interact if they desire.
  - Avoid platitudes, "His suffering will be over soon."
  - Avoid judgmental reactions to what family members say or do and realize that anger, fear, guilt, and irrational behavior are normal responses to acute grief and stress.
  - Show caring by touching the patient and encouraging family to do the same.
  - Note: Touching hands, arms, or shoulders of family members can provide comfort, but follow clues of the family.
  - Provide referrals to support groups if available.

- **Time of death:**
  - Reassure family that measures have been taken to ensure the patient's comfort.
  - Express personal feeling of loss, "She was such a sweet woman, and I'll miss her" and allow family to express feelings and memories. Provide information about what is happening during the dying process, explaining death rales, Cheyne-Stokes respirations, etc.
  - Alert family members to imminent death if they are not present. Assist to contact clergy/spiritual advisors.
  - Respect feelings and needs of parents, siblings, and other family.

- **After death:**
  - Encourage parents/family members to stay with the patient as long as they wish to say goodbye.
  - Use the patient's name when talking to the family.
  - Assist family to make arrangements, such as contacting funeral home.
  - If an autopsy is required, discuss with the family and explain timing.
  - If organ donation is to occur, assist the family to make arrangements. Encourage family members to grieve and express emotions.

KÜBLER-ROSS'S FIVE STAGES OF GRIEF

Grief is a normal response to the death or severe illness/abnormality of a patient. How a person deals with grief is very personal, and each will grieve differently. Elisabeth Kübler-Ross identified **five stages of grief** in *On Death and Dying* (1969), which can apply to both patients and family members. A person may not go through each stage but usually goes through two of the five stages:

- **Denial**: Patients/families may be resistive to information and unable to accept that a person is dying/impaired. They may act stunned, immobile, or detached and may be unable to respond appropriately or remember what's said, often repeatedly asking the same questions.
- **Anger**: As reality becomes clear, patient/families may react with pronounced anger, directed inward or outward. Women, especially, may blame themselves and self-anger may lead to severe depression and guilt, assuming they are to blame because of some personal action. Outward anger, more common in men, may be expressed as overt hostility.

- **Bargaining**: This involves if-then thinking (often directed at a deity): "If I go to church every day, then God will prevent this." Patient/family may change doctors, trying to change the outcome.
- **Depression**: As the patient and family begin to accept the loss, they may become depressed, feeling no one understands and overwhelmed with sadness. They may be tearful or crying and may withdraw or ask to be left alone.
- **Acceptance**: This final stage represents a form of resolution and often occurs outside of the medical environment after months. Patients are able to accept death/dying/incapacity. Families are able to resume their normal activities and lose the constant preoccupation with their loved one. They are able to think of the person without severe pain.

MEDICATION ERRORS

There are about 7000 deaths yearly in the United States attributed to **medication errors.** Studies indicate that there are errors in 1 in 5 doses of medication given to patients in hospitals. A caring environment is one in which patient safety is ensured with proper handling and administering of medications:

- Avoid error-prone abbreviations or symbols. The Joint Commission has established a list of abbreviations to avoid, but mistakes are frequent with other abbreviations as well. In many cases, abbreviations and symbols should be avoided altogether or restricted to a limited approved list.
- Prevent errors from illegible handwriting or unclear verbal orders. Handwritten orders should be block printed to reduce chance of error; verbal orders should be repeated back to the physician.
- Institute barcoding and scanners that allow the patient's wristband and medications to be scanned for verification.
- Provide lists of similarly-named medications to educate staff.
- Establish an institutional policy for administering of medications that includes protocols for verification of drug, dosage, and patient as well as educating the patient about the medications.

THERAPEUTIC COMMUNICATION

Therapeutic communication begins with respect for the patient/family and the assumption that all communication, verbal and non-verbal, has meaning. Listening must be done empathetically. Techniques that facilitate communication include:

- **Introduction:** Make a personal introduction and use the patient's name:
  - "Mrs. Brown, I am Susan Williams, your nurse."
- **Encouragement:** Use an open-ended opening statement:
  - "Is there anything you'd like to discuss?"
  - Acknowledge comments: "Yes," and "I understand."
  - Allow silence and observe non-verbal behavior rather than trying to force conversation. Ask for clarification if statements are unclear.
  - Reflect statements back (use sparingly):
    - ❖ Patient: "I hate this hospital."
    - ❖ Nurse: "You hate this hospital?"

- **Empathy:** Make observations: "You are shaking," and "You seem worried."
  - o Recognize feelings:
    - ❖ Patient: "I want to go home."
    - ❖ Nurse: "It must be hard to be away from your home and family."
  - o Provide information as honestly and completely as possible about condition, treatment, and procedures and respond to patient's questions and concerns.

Methods to promote a caring and supportive environment with **therapeutic communication** include:

- **Exploration:** Verbally express implied messages:
  - o Patient: "This treatment is too much trouble."
  - o Nurse: "You think the treatment isn't helping you?"
  - o Explore a topic but allow the patient to terminate the discussion without further probing: "I'd like to hear how you feel about that.
- **Orientation:** Indicate reality:
  - o Patient: "Someone is screaming."
  - o Nurse: "That sound was an ambulance siren."
  - o Comment on distortions without directly agreeing or disagreeing:
    - ❖ Patient: "That nurse promised I didn't have to walk again."
    - ❖ Nurse: "Really? That's surprising because the doctor ordered physical therapy twice a day."
- **Collaboration:** Work together to achieve better results:
  - o "Maybe if we talk about this, we can figure out a way to make the treatment easier for you."
- **Validation:** Seek validation:
  - o "Do you feel better now?" or "Did the medication help you breathe better?"

AVOIDING NON-THERAPEUTIC COMMUNICATION

While using therapeutic communication is important, it is equally important to avoid interjecting **non-therapeutic communication**, which can block effective communication. *Avoid the following:*

- Meaningless clichés: "Don't worry. Everything will be fine." "Isn't it a nice day?"
- Providing advice: "You should…" or "The best thing to do is…." It's better when patients ask for advice to provide facts and encourage the patient to reach a decision.
- Inappropriate approval that prevents the patient from expressing true feeling or concerns:
  - o Patient: "I shouldn't cry about this."
  - o Nurse: "That's right! You're an adult!"
- Asking for explanations of behavior that is not directly related to patient care and requires analysis and explanation of feelings: "Why are you upset?"
- Agreeing with rather than accepting and responding to patient's statements can make it difficult for the patient to change his/her statement or opinion later: "I agree with you," or "You are right."

Methods to promote a caring and supportive environment, avoiding **non-therapeutic communication** include:

- Negative judgments: "You should stop arguing with the nurses."
- Devaluing patient's feelings: "Everyone gets upset at times."
- Disagreeing directly: "That can't be true," or "I think you are wrong."
- Defending against criticism: "The doctor is not being rude; he's just very busy today."
- Subject change to avoid dealing with uncomfortable topics;
  - Patient: "I'm never going to get well."
  - Nurse: "Your family will be here in just a few minutes."
- Inappropriate literal responses, even as a joke, especially if the patient is at all confused or having difficulty expressing ideas:
  - Patient: "There are bugs crawling under my skin."
  - Nurse: "I'll get some buy spray,"
- Challenge to establish reality often just increases confusion and frustration:
  - "If you were dying, you wouldn't be able to yell and kick!"

Response to Diversity

RESPONSE TO DIVERSITY

In the ACCN Synergy model, **response to diversity** is the ability to recognize a wide range of differences (social, cultural, ethnic, racial, economic, language, and religious), to appreciate these differences and incorporate consideration for them into the plan of care. Diverse groups also include the disabled, gay and lesbians, and marginal groups, such as the homeless. Levels of response to diversity include:

- **Level 1:** This nurse can assess diversity with standardized questionnaires and provide care based on personal belief system and past experience, but doesn't seek assistance in dealing adequately with diversity.
- **Level 3:** This nurse takes a much more active role in asking about issues of diversity issues and incorporates needs into the plan of care, teaching the patient about the healthcare system.
- **Level 5:** This nurse considers issues of diversity in all aspects of care and presents patients with alternatives, responding to, anticipating, and integrating consideration of cultural and other differences.

CULTURAL COMPETENCE

Different cultures view health and illness from very different perspectives, and patients often come from a mix of many cultures, so the acute care nurse must be not only accepting of cultural differences but must be sensitive and aware. There are a number of characteristics that are important for a nurse to have **cultural competence:**

- **Appreciating diversity:** This must be grounded in information about other cultures and understanding of their value system.
- **Assessing own cultural perspectives:** Self-awareness is essential to understanding potential biases.
- **Understanding intercultural dynamics:** This must include understanding ways in which cultures cooperate, differ, communicate, and reach understanding.
- **Recognizing institutional culture:** Each institutional unit (hospital, clinic, office) has an inherent set of values that may be unwritten but is accepted by the staff.
- **Adapting patient service to diversity:** This is the culmination of cultural competence as it is the point of contact between cultures.

JEHOVAH'S WITNESSES

Jehovah's Witnesses have traditionally shunned transfusions and blood products as part of their religious belief. In 2004, the *Watchtower,* a Jehovah Witness publication presented a guide for members. When medical care indicates the need for blood transfusion or blood products and the patient and/or family members are practicing Jehovah Witnesses, this may present a conflict. It's important to approach the patient/family with full information and reasons for the transfusion or blood components without being judgmental, allowing them to express their feelings. In fact, studies show that while adults often refuse transfusions for themselves, they frequently allow their children to receive blood products, so one should never assume that an individual would refuse blood products based on the religion alone. Jehovah Witnesses can receive fractionated blood cells, thus allowing hemoglobin-based blood substitutes. The following guidelines are provided to church members:

Basic blood standards for Jehovah Witnesses:

- **Not acceptable:** Whole blood: red cells, white cells, platelets, plasma
- **Acceptable**: Fractions from red cells, white cells, platelets, and plasma

HISPANIC PATIENTS

Many areas of the country have large populations of **Hispanic** and Hispanic-Americans. As always, it's important to recognize that cultural generalizations don't always apply to individuals. Recent immigrants, especially, have cultural needs that the nurse must understand:

- Many Hispanics are Catholic and may like the nurse to make arrangements for a priest to visit.
- Large extended families may come to visit to support the patient and family, so patients should receive clear explanations about how many visitors are allowed, but some flexibility may be required.
- Language barriers may exist as some may have limited or no English skills so translation services should be available around the clock.
- Hispanic culture encourages outward expressions of emotions, so family may react strongly to news about a patient's condition, and people who are ill may expect some degree of pampering, so extra attention to the patient/family members may alleviate some of their anxiety.

Caring for **Hispanic** and Hispanic-American patients requires understanding of cultural differences:

- Some immigrant Hispanics have very little formal education, so medical information may seem very complex and confusing, and they may not understand the implications or need for follow-up care.
- Hispanic culture perceives time with more flexibility than American, so if parents need to be present at a particular time, the nurse should specify the exact time (1:30 PM) and explain the reason rather than saying something more vague, such as "after lunch."
- People may appear to be unassertive or unable to make decisions when they are simply showing respect to the nurse by being deferent.
- In traditional families, the males make decisions, so a woman waits for the father or other males in the family to make decisions about treatment or care.
- Families may choose to use folk medicines instead of Western medical care or may combine the two.
- Children and young women are often sheltered and are taught to be respectful to adults, so they may not express their needs openly.

MIDDLE EASTERN PATIENTS

There are considerable cultural differences among **Middle Easterners,** but religious beliefs about the segregation of males and females are common. It's important to remember that segregating the female is meant to protect her virtue. Female nurses have low status in many countries because they violate this segregation by touching male bodies, so parents may not trust or show respect for the nurse who is caring for their family member. Additionally, male patients may not want to be cared for by female nurses or doctors, and families may be very upset at a female being cared for by a male nurse or physician. When possible, these cultural traditions should be accommodated:

- In Middle Eastern countries, males make decisions, so issues for discussion or decision should be directed to males, such as the father or spouse, and males may be direct in stating what they want, sometimes appearing demanding.
- If a male nurse must care for a female patient, then the family should be advised that *personal care* (such as bathing) will be done by a female while the medical treatments will be done by the male nurse.

Caring for **Middle Eastern** patients requires understanding of cultural differences:

- Families may practice strict dietary restrictions, such as avoiding pork and requiring that animals be killed in a ritual manner, so vegetarian or kosher meals may be required.
- People may have language difficulties requiring a translator, and same-sex translators should be used if at all possible.
- Families may be accompanied by large extended families that want to be kept informed and whom patients consult before decisions are made.
- Most medical care is provided by female relatives, so educating the family about patient care should be directed at females (with female translators if necessary).
- Outward expressions of grief are considered as showing respect for the dead.
- Middle Eastern families often offer gifts to caregivers. Small gifts (candy) that can be shared should be accepted graciously, but for other gifts, the families should be advised graciously that accepting gifts is against hospital policy.
- Middle Easterners often require less personal space and may stand very close.

ASIAN PATIENTS

There are considerable differences among different **Asian** populations, so cultural generalizations may not apply to all, but nurses caring for Asian patients should be aware of common cultural attitudes and behaviors:

- Nurses and doctors are viewed with respect, so traditional Asian families may expect the nurse to remain authoritative and to give directions and may not question, so the nurse should ensure that they understand by having them review material or give demonstrations and should provide explanations clearly, anticipating questions that the family might have but may not articulate.
- Disagreeing is considered impolite. "Yes" may only mean that the person is heard, not that they agree with the person. When asked if they understand, they may indicate that they do even when they clearly do not so as not to offend the nurse.
- Asians may avoid eye contact as an indication of respect. This is especially true of children in relation to adults and younger adults in relation to elders.

Caring for **Asian** patients requires understanding of cultural differences:

- Patients/families may not show outward expressions of feelings/grief, sometimes appearing passive. They also avoid public displays of affection. This does not mean that they don't feel, just that they don't show their feelings.
- Families often hide illness and disabilities from others and may feel ashamed about illness.
- Terminal illness is often hidden from the patient, so families may not want patients to know they are dying or seriously ill.

- Families may use cupping, pinching, or applying pressure to injured areas, and this can leave bruises that may appear as abuse, so when bruises are found, the family should be questioned about alternative therapy before assumptions are made.
- Patients may be treated with traditional herbs.
- Families may need translators because of poor or no English skills.
- In traditional Asian families, males are authoritative and make the decisions.

Facilitation of Learning

FACILITATION OF LEARNING

In the ACCN Synergy model, **facilitation of learning** is the ability to facilitate learning by patient and family/caregivers as well as other health and allied professionals and community members. Facilitation of learning requires needs assessment and preparation of content that is suited for the receiver in terms of delivery and content. Levels of facilitation of learning include:

- **Level 1:** This nurse is able to deliver planned educational content that is disease specific but does not have the ability to assess patient readiness to learn or abilities. The patient/family is considered a passive recipient of knowledge.
- **Level 3:** This nurse is able to individualize treatment according to patient/family needs and has an understanding of different methods of teaching and learning styles. The patient's needs are considered in planning.
- **Level 5:** This nurse has excellent understanding of teaching methods, learning styles, and assessment for learning readiness and develops an educational plan in cooperation and collaboration with others, including patients, families, and other health and allied professionals.

DEVELOPMENT OF GOALS, MEASURABLE OBJECTIVES, AND LESSON PLANS

Once a topic for performance improvement education has been chosen, then **goals, measurable objectives with strategies, and lesson plans** must be developed. A class should stay focused on one area rather than trying to cover many things. For example:

- **Goal:** Increase compliance with hand hygiene standards in ICU.
- **Objectives:** Develop series of posters and fliers by June 1.
  - Observe 100% compliance with hand hygiene standards at 2 weeks, 1-month, and 2-month intervals after training is completed.
- **Strategies:** Conduct 4 classes at different times over a one-week period, May 25-31.
  - Place posters in all nursing units, staff rooms, and utility rooms by January 3.
  - Develop PowerPoint presentation for class and Intranet/Internet for access by all staff by May 25.
  - Utilize handwashing kits.
- **Lesson plans:**
  - Discussion period: Why do we need 100% compliance?
  - PowerPoint: The case for hand hygiene.
  - Discussion: What did you learn?
  - Demonstration and activities to show effectiveness
  - Handwashing technique.

APPROACHES TO TEACHING

There are many **approaches to teaching**, and the nurse educator must prepare, present, and coordinate a wide range of educational workshops, lectures, discussions, and one-on-one instructions on any chosen topic. All types of classes will be needed, depending upon the purpose and material:

- **Educational workshops** are usually conducted with small groups, allowing for maximal participation and are especially good for demonstrations and practice sessions.
- **Lectures** are often used for more academic or detailed information that may include questions and answers but limits discussion. An effective lecture should include some audiovisual support.
- **Discussions** are best with small groups so that people can actively participate. This is a good method for problem solving.
- **One-on-one instruction** is especially helpful for targeted instruction in procedures for individuals.
- **Computer/Internet modules** are good for independent learners.

Participants should be asked to evaluate the presentations in the forms of surveys or suggestions, but ultimately the program is evaluated in terms of patient outcomes.

USE OF VIDEOS

Videos are a useful adjunct to teaching as they reduce the time needed for one-on-one instruction (increasing cost-effectiveness). Passive presentation of videos, such as in the waiting area, has little value, but focused viewing in which the nurse discusses the purpose of the video presentation prior to viewing and then is available for discussion after viewing can be very effective. Patients and/or families are often nervous about learning patient care and are unsure of their abilities, so they may not focus completely when the nurse is presenting information. Allowing the patients/families to watch a video demonstration or explanation first and allowing them to stop or review the video presentation can help them to grasp the fundamentals before they have to apply them, relieving some of the anxiety they may be experiencing. Videos are much more effective than written materials for those with low literacy or poor English skills. The nurse should always be available to answer questions and discuss the material after the patients and their families finish viewing.

READABILITY

Studies have indicated that learning is more effective if oral presentations and/or demonstrations are supplemented with reading materials, such as handouts. **Readability** (the grade level of material) is a concern because many patients and families may have limited English skills or low literacy, and it can be difficult for the nurse to assess people's reading level. The average American reads effectively at the 6th to 8th grade level (regardless of education achieved), but many health education materials have a much higher readability level. Additionally, research indicates that even people with much higher reading skills learn medical and health information most effectively when the material is presented at the 6th to 8th grade readability level. Therefore, patient education materials (and consent forms) should not be written at higher than 6th to 8th grade level. Readability index calculators are available on the Internet to give an approximation of grade level and difficulty for those preparing materials without expertise in teaching reading.

INSTRUCTING AND ADVISING STAFF ON CHANGES IN POLICIES, PROCEDURES, OR WORKING STANDARDS

Changes in policies, procedures, or working standards are common and, the quality professional is responsible for educating the staff about changes related to processes, which should be communicated to staff in an effective and timely manner:

- **Policies** are usually changed after a period of discussion and review by administration and staff, so all staff should be made aware of policies under discussion. Preliminary information should be disseminated to staff regarding the issue during meetings or through printed notices.
- **Procedures** may be changed to increase efficiency or improve patient safety often as the result of surveillance and data about outcomes. Procedural changes are best communicated in workshops with demonstrations. Posters and handouts should be available as well.
- **Working standards** are often changed because of regulatory or accrediting requirements and this information should be covered extensively in a variety of different ways: discussions, workshops, handouts so that the implications are clearly understood.

LEARNING STYLES

Not all people are aware of their preferred **learning style.** A range of teaching materials/methods that relate to all 3 learning preferences (visual, auditory, kinesthetic) and are appropriate for different ages should be available. Part of assessment for teaching involves choosing the right approach based on observation and feedback. Often presenting learners with different options gives a clue to their preferred learning style. Some people have a combined learning style:

Visual learners: Learn best by seeing and reading:

- Provide written directions, picture guides, or demonstrate procedures. Use charts and diagrams.
- Provide photos, videos.

Auditory learners: Learn best by listening and talking:

- Explain procedures while demonstrating and have learner repeat.
- Plan extra time to discuss and answer questions.
- Provide audiotapes.

Kinesthetic learners: Learn best by handling, doing, and practicing:

- Provide hands-on experience throughout teaching.
- Encourage handling of supplies/equipment.
- Allow learner to demonstrate.
- Minimize instructions and allow person to explore equipment and procedures.

PRINCIPLES OF ADULT LEARNING

Adults have a wealth of life and/or employment experiences. Their attitudes toward education may vary considerably. There are, however, some **principles of adult learning** and typical characteristics of adult learners that an instructor should consider when planning strategies for teaching parents, families, or staff:

- **Practical and goal-oriented:**
  - o Provide overviews or summaries and examples.
  - o Use collaborative discussions with problem-solving exercises.
  - o Remain organized with the goal in mind.
- **Self-directed:**
  - o Provide active involvement, asking for input.
  - o Allow different options toward achieving the goal.
  - o Give them responsibilities.
- **Knowledgeable:**
  - o Show respect for their life experiences/ education.
  - o Validate their knowledge and ask for feedback.
  - o Relate new material to information with which they are familiar.
- **Relevancy-oriented:**
  - o Explain how information will be applied.
  - o Clearly identify objectives.
- **Motivated:** Provide certificates of professional advancement and/or continuing education credit for staff when possible.

BLOOM'S TAXONOMY AND 3 TYPES OF LEARNING

Bloom's taxonomy outlines behaviors that are necessary for learning, and this can apply to healthcare. The theory describes 3 types of learning.

Cognitive: Learning and gaining intellectual skills to master 6 categories of effective learning: Knowledge, Comprehension, Application, Analysis, Synthesis, Evaluation

Affective: Recognizing 5 categories of feelings and values from simple to complex. This is slower to achieve than cognitive learning:

- Receiving phenomena: Accepting need to learn
- Responding to phenomena: Taking active part in care
- Valuing: Understanding value of becoming independent in care
- Organizing values: Understanding how surgery/treatment has improved life
- Internalizing values: Accepting condition as part of life, being consistent and self-reliant

Psychomotor: Mastering 7 categories of motor skills necessary for independence. This follows a progression from simple to complex:

- Perception: Uses sensory information to learn tasks
- Set: Shows willingness to perform tasks
- Guided response: Follows directions
- Mechanism: Does specific tasks
- Complex overt response: Displays competence in self-care
- Adaptation: Modifies procedures as needed
- Origination: Creatively deals with problems

BEHAVIOR MODIFICATION AND COMPLIANCE RATE

Education, like all interventions, must be evaluated for **effectiveness**. Two determinants of effectiveness include:

- **Behavior modification** involves thorough observation and measurement, identifying behavior that needs to be changed and then planning and instituting interventions to modify that behavior. The nurse can use a variety of techniques, including demonstrations of appropriate behavior, reinforcement, and monitoring until new behavior is adopted consistently. This is especially important when longstanding procedures and habits of behavior are changed.
- **Compliance rates** are often determined by observation, which should be done at intervals and on multiple occasions, but with patients, this may depend on self-reports. Outcomes is another measure of compliance; that is, if education is intended to improve patient health and reduce risk factors and that occurs, it is a good indication that there is compliance. Compliance rates are calculated by determining the number of events/procedures and degree of compliance.

LEARNER OUTCOMES

When the quality professional plans an educational offering, whether it be a class, an online module, a workshop, or educational materials, the professional should identify **learner outcomes,** which should be conveyed to the learners from the very beginning so that they are aware of the expectations. The subject matter of the educational material and the learner outcomes should be directly related. For example, if the quality professional is giving a class on decontamination of the environment, then a learner outcome might be: "Identify the difference between disinfectants and antiseptics." There may be one or multiple learner outcomes, but part of the assessment at the end of the learning experience should be to determine if, in fact, the learner outcomes have been achieved. A survey of whether or not the learners felt that they had achieved the learner outcomes can give valuable feedback and guidance to the quality professional.

ONE-ON-ONE INSTRUCTION AND GROUP INSTRUCTION FOR PATIENT/FAMILY EDUCATION

Both one-on-one instruction and group **instruction** have a place in patient/family education.

- **One-on-one instruction** is the most costly for an institution because it is time intensive. However, it allows the patient and family more interaction with the nurse instructor and allows them to have more control over the process by asking questions or having the instructor repeat explanations or demonstrations. One-on-one instruction is especially valuable when patients and families must learn particular skills, such as managing dialysis, or if confidentiality is important.
- **Group instruction** is the less costly because the needs of a number of people can be met at one time. Group presentations are more planned and usually scheduled for a particular time period (an hour, for example), so patients and families have less control. Questioning is usually more limited and may be done only at the end. Group instruction allows patients/families with similar health problems to interact. Group instruction is especially useful for general types of instruction, such as managing diet or other lifestyle issues.

Mometrix

READINESS TO LEARN

The patient/family's **readiness to learn** should be assessed because if they are not ready, instruction is of little value. Often readiness is indicated when the patient/family asks questions or shows and interest in procedures. There are a number of factors related to readiness to learn:

- **Physical factors:** There are a number of physical factors than can affect ability. Manual dexterity may be required to complete a task, and this varies by age and condition. Hearing or vision deficits may impact ability. Complex tasks may be too difficult for some because of weakness or cognitive impairment, and modifications of the environment may be needed. Health status, age, and gender may all impact the ability to learn.
- **Experience:** People's experience with learning can vary widely and is affected by their ability to cope with changes, their personal goals, motivation to learn, and cultural background. People may have widely divergent ideas about what constitutes illness and/or treatment. Lack of English skills may make learning difficult and prevent people from asking questions.
- **Mental/emotional status:** The support system and motivation may impact readiness. Anxiety, fear, or depression about condition can make learning very difficult because the patient/family cannot focus on learning, so the nurse must spend time to reassure the patient/family and wait until they are emotionally more receptive.
- **Knowledge/education:** The knowledge base of the patient/family, their cognitive ability, and their learning styles all affect their readiness to learn. The nurse should always begin by assessing what knowledge the patient/family already has about their disease, condition, or treatment and then build form that base. People with little medical experience may lack knowledge of basic medical terminology, interfering with their ability and readiness to learn.

Collaboration

COLLABORATION

In the ACCN Synergy model, **collaboration** is a team approach of working with a variety of others (physicians, nurses, dietitians, therapist, families, social workers, community leaders and members, clergy, intra- and inter-disciplinary teams) in a cooperative manner, using good therapeutic communication skills, to ensure that each person is contributing optimally toward reaching patient goals and positive outcomes. Collaboration requires mutual respect, professional maturity, common purpose, and a positive sense of self. Levels of collaboration include:

- **Level 1:** This nurse participates in collaborative activities, learns from others, including mentors, and respects the input of others.
- **Level 3:** This nurse not only participates in collaborative activities but also initiates them and actively seeks learning opportunities.
- **Level 5:** This nurse takes a leadership role in collaborative activities by mentoring and teaching others while still seeking learning opportunities and actively seeks additional resources as needed.

NECESSARY COMMUNICATION SKILLS

Collaboration requires a number of **communication skills** that differ from those involved in communication between nurse and patient. These skills include:

- **Using an assertive approach:** It's important for the nurse to honestly express opinions and to state them clearly and with confidence, but the nurse must do so in a calm non-threatening manner.
- **Making casual conversation:** It's easier to communicate with people with whom one has a personal connection. Asking open-ended questions, asking about other's work, or commenting on someone's contributions helps to establish a relationship. The time before meetings, during breaks, and after meetings presents an opportunity for this type of conversation.
- **Being competent in public speaking:** Collaboration requires that a nurse be comfortable speaking and presenting ideas to groups of people, and doing so helps the person to gain credibility. This is a skill that must be practiced.
- **Communicating in writing:** The written word remains a critical component of communication, and the nurse should be able to communicate clearly and grammatically.

SKILLS NEEDED FOR COLLABORATION

Nurses must learn the set of **skills needed for collaboration** in order to move nursing forward. Nurses must take an active role in gathering data for evidence-based practice to support nursing's role in health care and must share this information with other nurses and health professionals in order to plan staffing levels and to provide optimal care to patients. Increased and adequate staffing has consistently been shown to reduce adverse outcomes, but there is a well-documented shortage of nurses in the United States, and more than half of current RNs work outside the hospital. Increased patient loads not only increase adverse outcomes but also increase job dissatisfaction and burnout. In order to manage the challenges facing nursing, nurses must develop skills needed for collaboration:

- Be willing to compromise.
- Communicate clearly.
- Identify specific challenges and problems.
- Focus on the task.
- Work with teams.

DELEGATION OF TASKS TO UNLICENSED ASSISTIVE PERSONNEL

The scope of nursing practice includes **delegation of tasks** to unlicensed assistive personnel, providing those personnel have adequate training and knowledge to carry out the tasks. Delegation should be used to manage the workload and to provide adequate and safe care. The nurse who delegates remains accountable for patient outcomes and for supervision of the person to whom the task was delegated, so the nurse must consider the following:

- Whether knowledge, skills, and training of the unlicensed assistive personnel provides the ability to perform the delegated task.
- Whether the patient's condition and needs have been properly evaluated and assessed.
- Whether the nurse is able to provide ongoing supervision.

Delegation should be done in a manner that reduces liability by providing adequate communication. This includes specific directions about the task, including what needs to be done, when, and for how long. Expectations related to consultation, reporting, and completion of tasks should be clearly defined. The nurse should be available to assist if necessary.

FIVE RIGHTS OF DELEGATION

Prior to delegating tasks, the nurse should assess the needs of the patients and determine the task that needs to be completed, assure that he/she can remain accountable and can supervise the task appropriately and evaluate effective completion. The **5 rights of delegation** include:

- **Right task:** The nurse should determine an appropriate task to delegate for a specific patient. This would not include tasks that require assessment or planning.
- **Right circumstance:** The nurse has considered the setting, resources, time factors, safety factors, and all other relevant information to determine the appropriateness of delegation. A task that is usually in one's scope (such as feeding a patient) may require assessment that makes it inappropriate to delegate (feeding a new stroke patient).
- **Right person:** The nurse is in the right position to choose the right person (by virtue of education/skills) to perform a task for the right patient.
- **Right direction:** The nurse provides a clear description of the task, the purpose, any limits, and expected outcomes.
- **Right supervision:** The nurse is able to supervise, intervene as needed, and evaluate performance of the task.

DELEGATION OF TASKS IN TEAMS

On major responsibility of leadership and management in performance improvement teams is using **delegation** effectively. The purpose of having a team is so that the work is shared, and leaders can cripple themselves by taking on too much of the workload. Additionally, failure to delegate shows an inherent distrust in team members. Delegation includes:

- Assessing the skills and available time of the team members, determining if a task is suitable for an individual.
- Assigning tasks, with clear instructions that include explanation of objectives and expectations, including a timeline.
- Ensuring that the tasks are completed properly and on time by monitoring progress but not micromanaging.
- Reviewing the final results and recording outcomes.

Because the leader is ultimately responsible for the delegated work, mentoring, monitoring, and providing feedback and intervention as necessary during this process is a necessary component of leadership. While delegated tasks may not always be completed successfully, they represent an opportunity for learning.

CREATING A COMMON VISION OF CARE

Facilitating the creation of a **common vision** for care within the healthcare system begins with the organization/facility, working collaboratively to create teams and an organization focused on serving the patient/family. A common vision should be the ideal in any organization, but achieving such a goal requires a true collaborative effort:

- Inclusion of all levels of staff across the organization/facility, both those in nursing and non-nursing positions.
- Consensus building through discussions, inservice, and team meetings to bring about convergence of diverse viewpoints.
- Facilitation that values creativity and provides encouragement during the process.
- Vision statement incorporating the common vision that accessible to all staff.
- Recognition that a common vision is an organic concept that may evolve over time and should be reevaluated regularly and changed as needed to reflect the needs of the organization, patients, families, and staff.

TEAMBUILDING

Leading, facilitating, and participating in performance improvement teams requires a thorough understanding of the dynamics of **team building:**

- **Initial interactions:** This is the time when members begin to define their roles and develop relationships, determining if they are comfortable in the group.
- **Power issues:** The members observe the leader and determine who controls the meeting and how control is exercised, beginning to form alliances.
- **Organizing:** Methods to achieve work are clarified and team members begin to work together, gaining respect for each other's contributions and working toward a common goal.
- **Team identification:** Interactions often become less formal as members develop rapport, and members are more willing to help and support each other to achieve goals.
- **Excellence:** This develops through a combination of good leadership, committed team members, clear goals, high standards, external recognition, spirit of collaboration, and a shared commitment to the process.

EFFECTIVE TEAM MEETINGS

Leading and facilitating improvement teams requires utilizing good **techniques for meetings**. Considerations include:

- **Scheduling**: Both the time and the place must be convenient and conducive to working together, so the leader must review the work schedules of those involved, finding the most convenient time. Venues or meeting rooms should allow for sitting in a circle or around a table to facilitate equal exchange of ideas. Any necessary technology, such as computers or overhead projectors, or other equipment, such as whiteboards, should be available.
- **Preparation**: The leader should prepare a detailed agenda that includes a list of items for discussion.
- **Conduction**: Each item of the agenda should be discussed, soliciting input from all group members. Tasks should be assigned to individual members based on their interest and part in the process in preparation for the next meeting. The leader should summarize input and begin a tentative future agenda.
- **Observation**: The leader should observe the interactions, including verbal and non-verbal communication, and respond to these.

LEADING AND FACILITATING COORDINATION OF INTRA-AND INTER-DISCIPLINARY TEAMS

There are a number of skills that are needed to lead and facilitate coordination of **intra- and inter-disciplinary teams:**

- Communicating openly is essential with all members being encouraged to participate as valued members of a cooperative team.
- Avoiding interrupting or interpreting the point another is trying to make allows free flow of ideas.
- Avoiding jumping to conclusions, which can effectively shut off communication.
- Active listening requires paying attention and asking questions for clarification rather than to challenge other's ideas.
- Respecting others opinions and ideas, even when opposed to one's own, is absolutely essential.
- Reacting and responding to facts rather than feelings allows one to avoid angry confrontations and diffuse anger.
- Clarifying information or opinions stated can help avoid misunderstandings.
- Keeping unsolicited advice out of the conversation shows respect for others and allows them to solicit advice without feeling pressured.

LEADERSHIP STYLES

Leadership styles often influence the perception of leadership values and commitment to collaboration. There are a number of different leadership styles:

- **Charismatic:** Depends upon personal charisma to influence people, and may be very persuasive, but this type leader may engage "followers" and relate to one group rather than the organization at large, limiting effectiveness.
- **Bureaucratic:** Follows organization rules exactly and expects everyone else to do so. This is most effective in handling cash flow or managing work in dangerous work environments. This type of leadership may engender respect but may not be conducive to change.

- **Autocratic:** Makes decisions independently and strictly enforces rules, but team members often feel left out of process and may not be supportive. This type of leadership is most effective in crisis situations, but may have difficulty gaining commitment of staff
- **Consultative:** Presents a decision and welcomes input and questions although decisions rarely change. This type of leadership is most effective when gaining the support of staff is critical to the success of proposed changes.
- **Participatory:** Presents a potential decision and then makes final decision based on input from staff or teams. This type of leadership is time-consuming and may result in compromises that are not entirely satisfactory to management or staff, but this process is motivating to staff who feel their expertise is valued.
- **Democratic:** Presents a problem and asks staff or teams to arrive at a solution although the leader usually makes the final decision. This type of leadership may delay decision-making, but staff and teams are often more committed to the solutions because of their input.
- **Laissez-faire ("Free Reign"):** Exerts little direct control but allows employees/ teams to make decisions with little interference. This may be effective leadership if teams are highly skilled and motivated, but in many cases, this type of leadership is the product of poor management skills and little is accomplished because of this lack of leadership.

RESISTANCE TO ORGANIZATIONAL CHANGE

Performance improvement processes cannot occur without organizational change, and **resistance to change** is common for many people, so coordinating collaborative processes requires anticipating resistance and taking steps to achieve cooperation. Resistance often relates to concerns about job loss, increased responsibilities, and general denial or lack of understanding and frustration. Leaders can prepare others involved in the process of change by taking these steps:

- Be honest, informative, and tactful, giving people thorough information about anticipated changes and how the changes will affect them, including positives.
- Be patient in allowing people the time they need to contemplate changes and express anger or disagreement.
- Be empathetic in listening carefully to the concerns of others.
- Encourage participation, allowing staff to propose methods of implementing change, so they feel some sense of ownership.
- Establish a climate in which all staff members are encouraged to identify the need for change on an ongoing basis.
- Present further ideas for change to management.

CONFLICT RESOLUTION

Conflict is an almost inevitable product of teamwork, and the leader must assume responsibility for **conflict resolution.** While conflicts can be disruptive, they can produce positive outcomes by forcing team members to listen to different perspectives and opening dialogue. The team should make a plan for dealing with conflict resolution. The best time for conflict resolution is when differences emerge but before open conflict and hardening of positions occur. The leader must pay close attention to the people and problems involved, listen carefully, and reassure those involved that their points of view are understood. Steps to conflict resolution include:

- Allow both sides to present their side of conflict without bias, maintaining a focus on opinions rather than individuals.
- Encourage cooperation through negotiation and compromise.
- Maintain the focus, providing guidance to keep the discussions on track and avoid arguments.
- Evaluate the need for re-negotiation, formal resolution process, or third party.
- Utilize humor and empathy to diffuse escalating tensions.
- Summarize the issues, outlining key arguments.
- Avoid forcing resolution if possible.

NURSE AND PATIENT/FAMILY COLLABORATION

One of the most important forms of **collaboration** is that between the nurse and the patient/family, but this type of collaboration is often overlooked. Nurses and others in the healthcare team must always remember that the point of collaborating is to improve patient care, and this means that the patient and patient's family must remain central to all planning. For example, including family in planning for a patient takes time initially, but sitting down and asking the patient and family, "What do you want?" and using the Synergy model to evaluate patient's (and family's) characteristics can provide valuable information that saves time in the long run and facilitates planning and expenditure of resources. Families, and even young children, often want to participate in care and planning and feel validated and more positive toward the medical system when they are included.

COLLABORATION WITH EXTERNAL AGENCIES

The critical care nurse must initiate and facilitate collaboration with **external agencies** because many have direct impacts on patient care and needs:

- Industry can include other facilities sharing interests in patient care or pharmaceutical companies. It's important for nursing to have a dialog with drug companies about their products and how they are used in specific populations because many medications are prescribed to women, children, or the aged without validating studies for dose or efficacy.
- Payers have a vested interest in containing health care costs, so providing information and representing the interests of the patient is important.
- Community groups may provide resources for patients and families, both in terms of information and financial or other assistance.
- Political agencies are increasingly important as new laws are considered about nurse-patient ratios and infection control in many states.
- Public health agencies are partners in health care with other facilities and must be included, especially in issues related to communicable disease.

Systems Thinking

SYSTEMS THINKING

In the ACCN Synergy model, **systems thinking** is having the background knowledge and practical tools to manage both environmental and system resources, within and outside of the healthcare system, in order to solve problems for the patient/family and meet their needs. Solving problems requires a holistic view of the interrelationships and understanding of how structures, patterns, and events affect outcomes. Levels of systems thinking include:

- **Level 1:** This nurse views himself/herself as the primary resource to meet the needs of the patient within the confines of the unit and doesn't recognize the need to negotiate.
- **Level 3:** This nurse looks beyond the unit and personal contributions to care to view the patient's progress through the entire system and sees the need to negotiate with others to provide the best resources available although may lack the skills needed to do so.
- **Level 5:** This nurse is expert at understanding the organization holistically and uses a number of different strategies to negotiate with others and assist the patient with progress through the system.

PATIENT CHARACTERISTICS

The Synergy method for patient care recognizes that there are a number of **patient characteristics** that must be considered if a nurse's competencies are to match those of the patient/family:

- **Resiliency** is the ability to recover from a devastating illness and regain a sense of stability, both physically and emotionally. Things that often support resiliency are faith, a positive sense of hope, and a supportive network of friends and family.
- **Vulnerability** are those factors putting a person at increased risk and interfering with recovery and/or compliance, such as anxiety, fear, lack of support, chronic illness, prejudice, and lack of information.
- **Stability** allows a patient/family to maintain a state of equilibrium (physically and/or emotionally) despite illness and challenges. Important factors include relief from stress, conflicts, or emotional burdens, motivation, and values.
- **Complexity** occurs when more than one system is involved, and these can be internal (cardiac and renal systems) or external (addicted and homeless) or some combination (ill with poor family dynamics).

BARRIERS TO SYSTEM THINKING

Barriers to system thinking can arise with the individual, the department, or the administrative level:

- **Identification with role rather than purpose:** People see themselves from the perspective of their role in the system, as nurse or physician, and are not able to step outside their preconceived ideas to view situations holistically or to accept the roles of others. They may lack the ability to look at situations as human beings first, and professionals second.
- **Feelings of victimization:** People may blame the organization or the leadership for personal shortcomings or feel that there is nothing that they can do to improve or change situations. A feeling of victimization may permeate an institution to the point that meaningful communication cannot take place, and people are not open to change.
- **Relying on past experience:** New directions require new solutions, so being mired in the past or relying solely on past experience can prevent progress.

- **Autocratic views:** Some feel that their perceptions and practices are the only ones that are acceptable and often have a narrow focus so that they cannot view the system as a whole but focus on short-term outcomes. They fail to see that there are many aspects to a problem, affecting many parts of the system.
- **Failure to adapt:** Change is difficult for many individuals and institutions, but the medical world is changing rapidly, and this requires adaptability. Those who fail to adapt may feel threatened by changes and unsure of their ability to relearn new concepts, principles, and procedures.
- **Weak consensus**: Groups that arrive at easy or weak consensus without delving into important issues may delude themselves into believing that they have solved problems and remain fixed and often ignored rather than moving forward.

IMPACT OF SOCIAL, POLITICAL, REGULATORY, AND ECONOMIC FORCES ON DELIVERY OF CARE

The **delivery of care** is impacted by numerous forces:

- **Social forces** are increasing demand for access to treatment and medical services, both traditional and complementary. As society views equitable medical care as a right, then delivery of care must be available to all.
- **Political forces** affect medical care as the Federal and state governments increasingly become purchasers of medical care, imposing their guidelines and limitations on the medical system.
- **Regulatory forces** may be local, state, or Federal and can have a profound effect of delivery of care and services, differing from one state or region to another.
- **Economic forces**, such as managed care or cost-containment committees, try to contain costs to insurers and facilities by controlling access to and duration of treatment, and limiting products. Economic pressure is working to prevent duplication of services in a geographical area, and providers are creating networks to purchase supplies and equipment directly.

CONCEPTS OF SYSTEMS THINKING

The promotion of organizational values and commitment requires that the organization embody systems thinking and the associated concepts. **Systems thinking** focuses on how systems interrelate, with each part affecting the entire system: Concepts include:

- **Individual responsibility**: Individuals are encouraged to establish their own goals within the organization and to work toward a purpose.
- **Learning process:** The internalized beliefs of the staff are respected while building upon these beliefs to establish a mindset based on continuous learning and improvement.
- **Vision**: A sharing of organizational vision helps staff to understand the purpose of change and builds commitment.
- **Team process:** Teams are assisted to develop good listening and collaborative skills so that there is an increase in dialogue and an ability to reach consensus.
- **Systems thinking:** Staff members are encouraged to understand the interrelationship of all members of the organization and to appreciate how any change affects the whole.

STEPS TO SYSTEMS THINKING

An approach to systems thinking is especially valuable in organizations in which there is lack of consensus, effective change is stalemated, and standards are inconsistent. Systems thinking is a critical thinking approach to problem solving that takes an organization-wide perspective. Steps include:

1. **Define the issue:** Describe the problem in detail without judgment or solutions.
2. **Describe behavior patterns:** This includes listing factors related to the problem, using graphs to outline possible trends.
3. **Establish cause-effect relationships:** This may include using the Five Whys or other root cause analysis or feedback loops.
4. **Define patterns of performance/behavior:** Determine how variables affect outcomes and the types of patterns of behavior currently taking place.
5. **Find solutions:** Discuss possible solutions and outcomes.
6. **Institute performance improvement activities:** Make changes and then monitor for changes in behavior.

INTEGRATION OF KEY QUALITY CONCEPTS WITHIN THE ORGANIZATION

There are a number of **key concepts** related to quality that must be communicated to all members of an organization through inservice, workshops, newsletters, fact sheets, and team meetings. Quality care/performance should be:

- **Appropriate** to needs and in keeping with best practices.
- **Accessible** to the individual despite financial, cultural, or other barriers.
- **Competent**, with practitioners being well-trained and adhering to standards.
- **Coordinated** among all healthcare providers.
- **Effective** in achieving outcomes based on the current state of knowledge.
- **Efficient** in methods of achieving the desired outcomes.
- **Preventive**, allowing for early detection and prevention of problems.
- **Respectful** and caring with consideration of the individual needs given primary importance.
- **Safe** so that the organization is free of hazards or dangers that may put patients or others at risk.

Clinical Inquiry

CLINICAL INQUIRY

In the ACCN Synergy model, **clinical inquiry** is a continual process of questioning and evaluating practice in order to provide innovative and outstanding care through application of the results of research and experience. Clinical inquiry requires a desire to acquire new knowledge, openness to accepting advice from mentors and other health and allied professionals, competency in identifying clinical problems, and the ability search the literature for research, critical skills to interpret research findings, and to willingness and ability to design and participate in research. Levels of clinical inquiry include:

- **Level 1:** This nurse recognizes problems and seeks advice, follows industry standards and guidelines, and seeks further knowledge.
- **Level 3:** This nurse questions industry standards and guidelines as well as current practice and utilizes research and education to improve patient care.
- **Level 5:** This nurse is able to deviate from industry standards and guidelines when necessary for the individual patients and utilizes literature review and clinical research to gain knowledge, establish new practices, and improve patient care.

STEPS TO EVIDENCE-BASED GUIDELINES

Steps to **evidence-based practice guidelines** include:

- **Focus on the topic/methodology:** This includes outlining possible interventions/treatments for review, choosing patient populations and settings and determining significant outcomes. Search boundaries (such as types of journals, types of studies, dates of studies) should be determined.
- **Evidence review:** This includes review of literature, critical analysis of studies, and summarizing of results, including pooled meta-analysis.
- **Expert judgment:** Recommendations based on personal experience from a number of experts may be utilized, especially if there is inadequate evidence based on review, but this subjective evidence should be explicated acknowledged.
- **Policy considerations:** This includes cost-effectiveness, access to care, insurance coverage, availability of qualified staff, and legal implications.
- **Policy:** A written policy must be completed with recommendations. Common practice is to utilize letter guidelines, with "A" the most highly recommended, usually based the quality of supporting evidence.
- **Review:** The completed policy should be submitted to peers for review and comments before instituting the policy.

STEPS TO DEVELOPMENT OF CLINICAL/CRITICAL PATHWAYS

Clinical/critical pathway development is done by those involved in direct patient care. The pathway should require no additional staffing and cover the entire scope of an illness. Steps include:

1. Selection of patient group and diagnosis, procedures, or conditions, based on analysis of data and observations of wide variance in approach to treatment and prioritizing organization and patient needs.
2. Creation of interdisciplinary team of those involved in the process of care, including physicians to develop pathway.
3. Analysis of data includes literature review and study of best practices to identify opportunities for quality improvement.
4. Identification of all categories of care, such as nutrition, medications, nursing.
5. Discussion, reaching consensus.
6. Identifying the levels of care and number of days to be covered by the pathway.
7. Pilot testing and redesigning steps as indicated.
8. Educating staff about standards.
9. Monitoring and tracking variances in order to improve pathways.

BASIC RESEARCH CONCEPTS

The nurse must be taught and understand the process of critical analysis and know how to conduct a survey of the literature. **Basic research concepts** include:

- **Survey of valid sources:** Information from a juried journal and an anonymous website or personal website are very different sources, and evaluating what constitutes a valid source of data is critical.
- **Evaluation of internal and external validity:** Internal validity shows a cause and effect relationship between two variables, with the cause occurring before the effect and no intervening variable. External validity occurs when results hold true in different environments and circumstances with different populations.
- **Sample selection and sample size:** Selection and size can have a huge impact on the results, but a sample that is too small may lack both internal and external validity. Selection may be so narrowly focused that the results can't be generalized to others groups.

CRITICAL READING OF RESEARCH ARTICLES

There are a number of steps to **critical reading** to evaluate research:

- **Consider the source** of the material. If it is in the popular press, it may have little validity compared to something published in a peer-reviewed journal.
- **Review the author's credentials** to determine if a person is an expert in the field of study.
- **Determine thesis**, or the central claim of the research. It should be clearly stated.
- **Examine the organization** of the article, whether it is based on a particular theory, and the type of methodology used.
- **Review the evidence** to determine how it is used to support the main points. Look for statistical evidence and sample size to determine if the findings have wide applicability.
- **Evaluate** the overall article to determine if the information seems credible and useful and should be communicated to administration and/or staff.

INTERNAL AND EXTERNAL VALIDITY, GENERALIZABILITY, AND REPLICATION

Many research studies are most concerned with **internal validity** (adequate unbiased data properly collected and analyzed within the population studied), but studies that determine the efficacy of procedures or treatments, for example, should have **external validity** as well; that is, the results should be **generalizable** (true) for similar populations. **Replication** of the study with different subjects, researchers, and under different circumstances should produce similar results. For various reasons, some people may be excluded from a study so that instead of randomized subjects, the subjects may be highly selected so when data is compared with another population in which there is less or more selection, results may be different. The selection of subjects, in this case, would interfere with external validity. Part of the design of a study should include considerations of whether or not it should have external validity or whether there is value for the institution based solely on internal validation.

SELECTION AND INFORMATION BIAS

Selection bias occurs when the method of selecting subjects results in a cohort that is not representative of the target population because of inherent error in design. For example, if all patients who develop urinary infections are evaluated per urine culture and sensitivities for microbial resistance, but only those patients with clinically-evident infections are included, a number of patients with sub-clinical infections may be missed, skewing the results. Selection bias is only a concern when participants in studies are specifically chosen. Many surveillance studies do not involve selection of subjects.

Information bias occurs when there are errors in classification, so an estimate of association is incorrect. Non-differential misclassification occurs when there is similar misclassification of disease or exposure among both those who are diseased/exposed and those who are not. Differential misclassification occurs when there is a differing misclassification of disease or exposure among both those who are diseased/exposed and those who are not.

QUALITATIVE AND QUANTITATIVE DATA

Both **qualitative and quantitative data** are used for analysis, but the focus is quite different:

- **Qualitative data**: Data are described verbally or graphically, and the results are subjective, depending upon observers to provide information. Interviews may be used as a tool to gather information, and the researcher's interpretation of data is important. Gathering this type of data can be time-intensive, and it can usually not be generalized to a larger population. This type of information gathering is often useful at the beginning of the design process for data collection.
- **Quantitative data**: Data are described in terms of numbers within a statistical format. This type of information gathering is done after the design of data collection is outlined, usually in later stages. Tools may include surveys, questionnaires, or other methods of obtaining numerical data. The researcher's role is objective.

HYPOTHESIS AND HYPOTHESIS TESTING

A **hypothesis** should be generated about the probable cause of the disease/infection based on the information available in laboratory and medical records, epidemiologic study, literature review, and expert opinion. A hypothesis, for example, should include the infective agent, the likely source, and the mode of transmission: "Wound infections with *Staphylococcus aureus* were caused by reuse and inadequate sterilization of single-use irrigation syringes used during wound care in the ICU."

Hypothesis testing includes data analysis, laboratory findings, and outcomes of environmental testing. It usually includes case control studies, with 2-4 controls picked for each case of infection. They may be matched according to age, sex, or other characteristics, but they are not infected at the time they are picked for the study. Cohort studies, whose controls are picked based on having or lacking exposure, may also be instituted. If the hypothesis cannot be supported, then a new hypothesis or different testing methods may be necessary.

OUTCOMES EVALUATION AND EVIDENCE-BASED PRACTICE

Outcomes evaluation is an important component of evidence-based practice, which involves both internal and external research. All treatments are subjected to review to determine if they produce positive outcomes, and policies and protocols for outcomes evaluation should be in place. Outcomes evaluation includes the following:

- **Monitoring** over the course of treatment involves careful observation and record keeping that notes progress, with supporting laboratory and radiographic evidence as indicated by condition and treatment.
- **Evaluating** results includes reviewing records as well as current research to determine if outcomes are within acceptable parameters.
- **Sustaining** involves discontinuing treatment, but continuing to monitor and evaluate.
- **Improving** means to continue the treatment but with additions or modifications in order to improve outcomes.
- **Replacing** the treatment with a different treatment must be done if outcomes evaluation indicates that current treatment is ineffective.

CCRN Practice Test

1. Therapeutic hypothermia is ordered for a patient who was resuscitated from a cardiac arrest associated with ventricular tachycardia. What is the optimal temperature range that should be maintained for therapeutic hypothermia?

  a. 26 -30 °C (78.8-86 °F)
  b. 30-34 °C (86-93.2 °F)
  c. 32-36 °C (89.6-96.8 °F)
  d. 34-37 °C (93.2-98.6 °F)

2. Which electrolyte imbalance is the most life threatening for patients with renal failure?

  a. hypernatremia
  b. hyponatremia
  c. hypokalemia
  d. hyperkalemia

3. A patient who is undergoing rehabilitation after severe traumatic injuries is depressed about his condition and concerned about his ability to live independently. What is the most effective strategy for the nurse to help improve the patient's motivation?

  a. provide positive feedback about tasks he is able to complete
  b. assist him in developing a list of long-term goals
  c. compare his present abilities to his abilities immediately after the injury
  d. tell him that everyone feels the same way during therapy

4. A non-diabetic patient with a Foley catheter develops sudden onset of increased temperature (39 °C); a heart rate of 108/min; a respiratory rate of 32/min; peripheral edema with decreased capillary refill; serum glucose of 160 mg/dL; WBC of 16,000; platelet count of 95,000; blood pressure of 86/52 mmHg; urinary output of 0.2 mL/kg/hr; and flushed skin. The most likely diagnosis is

  a. bacteremia.
  b. pyelonephritis.
  c. sepsis.
  d. kidney failure.

5. A nurse believes that a clinical pathway for treatment of hospitalized asthma patients would help to standardize care and improve patient outcomes. What type of team should be involved in development of the clinical pathway?

  a. nurses and physicians
  b. respiratory therapists and physicians
  c. interdisciplinary team
  d. physicians only

6. Which of the following is an example of a well-written learning objective?

a. "After attending a workshop about hypertension, the patient will be able to state 4 causes for high blood pressure."

b. "The patient will understand how to monitor blood sugar."

c. "The nurse will provide a demonstration on use of the BiPAP machine."

d. "After instruction about infection prevention, the patient will understand infection control procedures."

7. Following brain surgery, a patient's intracranial pressure has increased. What $PaCO_2$ level is optimal to control increased ICP?

a. 35-38 mmHg

b. 38-45 mmHg

c. 24-27 mmHg

d. 27-32 mmHg

8. An alert elderly patient has multiple bruises on the chest, back, abdomen, and both arms in various stages of healing and seems fearful and withdrawn when her daughter, who is her caregiver, is present. When questioned about the bruising, the patient states she "fell." The nurse should

a. question the daughter about the bruising.

b. report the observations to adult protective services.

c. ask the hospital social worker to speak with the patient.

d. report observations to administration.

9. A 38-year-old patient with acute respiratory distress syndrome (ARDS) is placed on mechanical ventilation. The optimal setting for tidal volume for ARDS is usually

a. 12 mL/kg predicted body weight.

b. 10 mL/kg predicted body weight.

c. 6-8 mL/kg predicted body weight.

d. 4-5 mL/kg predicted body weight.

10. A 36-year-old patient with Guillain-Barré syndrome is hospitalized with ascending paralysis and acute respiratory distress. The patient is stabilized and placed on mechanical ventilation. Which treatment is most indicated to reduce symptoms?

a. IV Ig or plasmapheresis

b. corticosteroids

c. antiviral medications

d. immunoadsorption

11. A patient with a history of previous myocardial infarction presents with dyspnea and audible basilar rales as well as 2+ peripheral edema. The patient's respiratory rate is 34/min and heart rate is 104/min with lateral displacement of the apical beat. Blood pressure is 162/94 mmHg. Despite administration of 100% oxygen, the patient's oxygen saturation level is 92% and the patient reports that he feels very short of breath and insists on sitting in tripod position. Which intervention is most indicated to relieve the patient's dyspnea?

    a. morphine sulfate
    b. furosemide IV
    c. CPAP or BiPAP
    d. endotracheal intubation with mechanical ventilation

12. A patient who suffered penetrating chest trauma is recovering from surgical repair but complains of increasing chest pain and dyspnea and appears cyanotic. Pulse is 110 bpm, BP is 80/48 mmHg, and pulsus paradoxus is evident. When auscultating the heart, the nurse notes a mill wheel murmur and shifting tympany when percussing the heart with the patient supine and then sitting upright. Hamman's sign is negative. The most likely cause is

    a. pneumomediastinum.
    b. pneumopericardium.
    c. cardiac tamponade.
    d. pneumothorax.

13. A 68-year-old man with a history of alcoholism has developed sudden onset of severe epigastric pain radiating to the back after eating. The pain is exacerbated when the patient lies flat or walks. He is pale and tachycardic and has nausea and vomiting and a temperature of 39 °C. Physical examination shows the upper abdomen is tender but not rigid and without guarding. The most likely cause of these symptoms is

    a. hepatitis.
    b. acute cholecystitis.
    c. small bowel obstruction.
    d. pancreatitis.

14. A patient who is 24 hours postoperative after a pulmonary lobectomy requests pain medication for severe pain, but when the nurse brings the opioid medication a few minutes later, the nurse finds the patient laughing and talking with family. The nurse should

    a. give the patient the opioid medication.
    b. ask the patient if she still needs the pain medication.
    c. withhold the pain medication altogether.
    d. exchange the opioid for acetaminophen.

15. A patient who is restless pulls out his chest tube when trying to get out of bed independently, and no dressing supplies are available at bedside. What immediate action is indicated?

    a. call for assistance and dressing supplies
    b. hold a folded washcloth against the insertion site
    c. cover the insertion site with Vaseline gauze
    d. ask the patient to place his hand over insertion site and go for dressings

16. During the post-surgical period following a bowel resection, a patient develops sudden dyspnea with tachypnea, chest pain, anxiety, fever, and cough. Which of the following tests is most indicated to diagnose pulmonary embolus?

    a. arterial blood gas
    b. D-dimer
    c. CT-PA
    d. chest radiograph

17. A patient with a history of heart failure and supraventricular dysrhythmias has been maintained on digoxin but has developed bradycardia (48 bpm), headache, fatigue, nausea, diarrhea, and green halo vision. The physician has ordered serum digoxin, electrolyte levels, and continuous ECG monitoring. Which of the following electrolyte values would be most concerning?

    a. potassium of 3.2 mEq/L
    b. potassium of 5 mEq/L
    c. sodium 140 mEq/L
    d. magnesium 2 mEq/L

18. Which of the following reactions after a bee sting indicates the patient is at high risk for anaphylaxis?

    a. severe pain at site of sting
    b. itching localized hives about sting site.
    c. swelling extends beyond sting site, involving an entire limb
    d. urticaria, edema, and itching in areas distant from sting

19. A patient is brought to the emergency department with suspected substance abuse. The patient exhibits euphoria, restlessness, hyperactivity, tachycardia, hypertension, dilated pupils, and rhinitis. Which of the following substances did the patient most likely use?

    a. barbiturate (Valium)
    b. heroin
    c. cocaine
    d. amphetamines

20. A patient with paroxysmal supraventricular tachycardia has received IV adenosine in order to slow the heart rate and convert to a sinus rhythm. Following administration of the drug, the nurse should carefully monitor the patient for

    a. ventricular fibrillation.
    b. transient asystole.
    c. premature ventricular contractions.
    d. facial flushing.

21. With chronic kidney disease, potassium-sparing diuretics are recommended for

    a. patients with persistent hypokalemia.
    b. all patients with chronic kidney disease.
    c. patients with hyporeninemic hypoaldosteronism.
    d. patients who cannot tolerate hydrochlorothiazide.

22. A patient has been admitted with unstable angina but without cardiac enzyme elevation. During periods when the patient is pain-free, the nurse notes the following 12-lead ECG changes (Wellens syndrome): Slight elevation of ST segments in leads V1 and V3; terminal T-wave inversion in V2 to V3; and intact R waves. This patient is at risk for

    a. ventricular arrhythmias.
    b. acute posterior wall myocardial infarction.
    c. atrial fibrillation.
    d. acute anterior wall myocardial infarction.

23. A patient with valvular diseases has continuous ECG monitoring and shows the following ECG tracing:

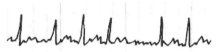

Which of the following best describes this pattern?

    a. atrial flutter
    b. atrial fibrillation
    c. premature ventricular contractions
    d. premature atrial contractions

24. A patient has a chest tube in place and all connections are tight, but bubbling is occurring in the water seal container. What initial action is indicated?

    a. no initial action is indicated because this is a normal finding
    b. immediately change the drainage system
    c. clamp the drainage tube close to chest tube and observe water seal
    d. listen for the sound of hissing

25. A patient with myasthenia gravis develops sudden exacerbation of these symptoms: extreme weakness, inability to hold up their head, missing gag reflex. The patient is anxious, dyspneic, and tachypneic. Which of the following diagnostic tests is best to differentiate between myasthenic and cholinergic crises?

    a. Tensilon test
    b. MRI
    c. ice pack test
    d. electromyography

26. A patient with bradyarrhythmia has not responded to pharmaceutical intervention (atropine) and is experiencing hemodynamic instability, so transcutaneous pacing has been initiated. The rate of pacing is usually set at

    a. 80 to 90 bpm
    b. 70 to 80 bpm
    c. 60 to 70 bpm
    d. 50 to 60 bpm

27. The most common cause of hospital-associated pneumonia (HAP) is

    a. mechanical ventilation.

    b. bed rest in a supine position.

    c. previous antibiotic therapy.

    d. poor hand-washing practices.

28. What precaution should be used when administering IV mannitol solution to patients in order to control increased intracranial pressure?

    a. chill solution prior to administration.

    b. administer solution through a filter.

    c. heat solution prior to administration.

    d. administer a test dose to determine response.

29. Which of the following is an indication for intubation and mechanical ventilation for a patient presenting with possible status asthmaticus?

    a. ABGs showing hypocapnia and respiratory alkalosis

    b. pulsus paradoxus of 20 mmHg

    c. peak expiratory flow rate 38% of predicted

    d. FEV1 25% of predicted

30. The pacing mode that is most commonly used with temporary transvenous pacing is

    a. DDD.

    b. AOO.

    c. VDD.

    d. VVI.

31. A patient with severe urinary tract infection and bacteremia begins to develop petechiae and purpura and is bleeding at the IV site. The patient passes bloody diarrhea. BP is 64/48 mmHg and pulse is 122/min. Recent laboratory findings include increased WBC count, decreased platelet count, and fragmented RBCs. Which further laboratory testing should the nurse anticipate?

    a. liver function tests

    b. kidney function tests

    c. DIC panel

    d. arterial blood gases

32. A 72-year-old man underwent a total knee replacement. Prior to surgery he was alert, responsive, and oriented, but 24 hours after surgery he is having fluctuating periods of confusion with sudden changes in consciousness, inability to sustain attention, disorientation, and visual hallucinations. The most effective pharmaceutical intervention is

    a. lorazepam (Ativan).

    b. benztropine (Cogentin).

    c. chlordiazepoxide (Librium).

    d. paroxetine (Paxil).

33. An older adult who recently traveled in an area endemic to West Nile virus presents with poliomyelitis-like symptoms, including fever, headache, flaccid quadriplegic paralysis, bladder dysfunction, and cranial nerve involvement. What complication should the nurse anticipate most?

a. heart failure
b. respiratory failure
c. disseminated intravascular coagulation
d. deep vein thrombosis/pulmonary embolism

34. A patient with post-surgical left ventricular failure and low cardiac output has an intra-aortic balloon pump (IABP) inserted. At which point in the cardiac cycle should inflation occur?

a. end of diastole
b. beginning of systole
c. end of systole
d. beginning of diastole

35. When preparing written materials for patient education, the maximum word length for a sentence should be

a. 30.
b. 25.
c. 20.
d. 15.

36. A patient with cardiac ischemia develops a hypertensive crisis with blood pressure of 240/130 mmHg. Which initial pharmaceutical treatment is usually indicated?

a. sodium nitroprusside
b. short-acting beta-blockers (labetalol or esmolol)
c. furosemide
d. alpha blocker

37. The nurse is reviewing the medication list with a 76-year-old patient who takes multiple drugs for heart disease and COPD, including warfarin and theophylline. Which of the following OTC drugs that the patient reports using regularly is likely to be the most problematic?

a. acetaminophen
b. cimetidine
c. docusate sodium stool softener
d. topical cortisone cream

38. A patient with a tracheostomy is to receive the Passy-Muir valve to facilitate communication and improve swallowing. What change must be made when placing the valve on the tracheostomy tube?

a. cuff deflated
b. cuff inflation increased
c. no changes necessary
d. cuff inflation decreased by approximately 50%

39. A patient who is taking metformin for diabetes mellitus, type 2, is also taking metoprolol for junctional tachycardia and has been prescribed hydrochlorothiazide for persistent elevated blood pressure. What is the primary concern with this drug combination?

    a. increased tachycardia
    b. hyperglycemia
    c. renal failure
    d. muscle cramps

40. A patient with SIRS is at risk for developing MODS. Which organ system is usually the first to fail?

    a. cardiac
    b. renal
    c. hepatic
    d. pulmonary

41. The physician has ordered position therapy for a patient with acute lung injury (ALI) in order to improve oxygenation. Which position is most likely to improve oxygenation and ventilation/perfusion matching and decrease shunting?

    a. supine, flat
    b. supine with head of bed elevated
    c. right or left side lying (most damaged lung in dependent position)
    d. prone

42. If a patient is receiving oxygen therapy with a mask with a reservoir bag and the flow rate is set at 6, what is the estimated FiO_2?

    a. 40%
    b. 50%
    c. 60%
    d. 100%

43. A patient with bronchogenic small (oat) cell carcinoma exhibits lethargy, anorexia, nausea, and vomiting. Urinary output is diminished, and urine specific gravity is increased. Serum sodium is 122 mEq/L, and the patient is beginning to have difficulty concentrating and exhibiting confusion. Based on these observations, the most likely cause is

    a. diabetes insipidus.
    b. hypothyroidism.
    c. renal metastasis.
    d. syndrome of inappropriate secretion of antidiuretic hormone.

44. A patient with a history of COPD and heavy smoking is admitted with respiratory distress, using accessory muscles for breathing. The assessment findings include a heart rate of 122/min; a blood pressure of 86/42 mmHg; SpO_2 of 80%; diminished lung sounds, especial on the left; tracheal deviation on the right; and increased venous distention. Based on these findings, the most likely cause is

    a. viral pneumonia.
    b. pleural effusion.
    c. aspiration pneumonia.
    d. tension pneumothorax.

45. The three characteristics most often associated with cardiogenic shock include

a. increased preload, increased afterload, and decreased contractility.
b. decreased preload, decreased afterload, and decreased contractility.
c. increased preload, increased afterload, and increased contractility.
d. increased preload, decreased afterload, and decreased contractility.

46. When auscultating heart sounds, the nurse notes an ejection click, a brief high-pitched sound that occurs immediately after S1. This heart sound is associated with

a. left ventricular failure.
b. aortic valve stenosis.
c. pericarditis.
d. mitral valve stenosis.

47. An elderly Chinese woman with inoperative metastatic liver cancer believes she has a "liver infection" that will improve with time. Her family members have asked that the patient be shielded from the truth because of her fear of cancer, and the physician has agreed. The best action for the nurse is to

a. take the issue to the ethics committee.
b. tell the patient the truth.
c. respect the family's wishes.
d. report the physician to administration.

48. A patient with bleeding esophageal varices has undergone balloon tamponade to control sudden onset of bleeding before more definitive therapy can be carried out. What is the maximum period of time that balloon tamponade can be maintained?

a. 4 hours
b. 8 hours
c. 12 hours
d. 24 hours

49. A patient with atrial fibrillation is to undergo cardioversion. What pharmaceutical intervention is usually prescribed three weeks prior to cardioversion?

a. digoxin
b. loop diuretic
c. anticoagulant
d. beta blocker

50. A patient receiving total parental nutrition (TPN) exhibits signs of dehydration (dry mucous membranes, decreased ski turgor), increased BUN, and increased urinary specific gravity. The most likely complication resulting in these findings is

a. hypoglycemia.
b. hyperammonemia.
c. azotemia.
d. deficiency of essential fatty acids.

51. A patient who has undergone open-heart surgery and cardiopulmonary bypass (CPB) has an amylase level of 1100 in the early post-surgical period. This indicates

    a. increased risk of myocardial infarction.
    b. increased risk of hypertensive crisis.
    c. a normal value after CPB.
    d. increased risk of pancreatitis.

52. An 80-year-old patient who lives alone is generally in good health but has shown a steady decline with evidence of malaise, lack of appetite, and weight loss. Laboratory tests and physical examination show no abnormalities other than slight anemia and mild hypertension. The patient is able to carry out ADLs but shows little interest in other activities and has withdrawn from social interactions. Which of the following assessments is most indicated?

    a. Index of Independence of Activities of Daily Living (Katz Index)
    b. Confusion Assessment Method
    c. Palliative Performance Scale
    d. Geriatric Depression Scale

53. When assessing jugular venous pressure, the normal height of the jugular vein pulsation above the sternal angle is less than or equal to

    a. 2 cm.
    b. 4 cm.
    c. 5 cm.
    d. 6 cm.

54. A 50-year-old female patient who has recovered from a recent myocardial infarction is prescribed clopidogrel bisulfate to reduce the risk of thrombus formation. Which statement by the patient indicates the need for further education about the drug?

    a. "I check my skin for signs of bruising when I shower."
    b. "I take acetaminophen for my arthritis pain."
    c. "I take red clover supplement to help reduce hot flashes."
    d. "I can take the pill before or after breakfast."

55. When assisting with insertion of a pulmonary artery catheter, the nurse should inflate the balloon when the catheter

    a. reaches the right atrium.
    b. enters the right ventricle.
    c. enters the pulmonary artery.
    d. reaches the superior vena cava.

56. A patient with alcoholism is admitted after an episode of prolonged binge drinking. He has been a heavy drinker, drinking over a pint of distilled alcoholic beverage daily for over 20 years. His blood alcohol level on admission is 0.3. Which of the following symptoms indicates onset of delirium tremens?

    a. impaired judgment, slurred speech, and unsteady gait
    b. nausea, vomiting, and anxiety
    c. audio and visual hallucinations, agitation, and tremor
    d. global confusion, fever, tachycardia, and, hallucinations

57. A patient with a pulmonary artery catheter in place is restless and moving about. The waveform indicates spontaneous wedging, suggesting that the catheter may have migrated and may result in pulmonary artery infarction. What is the initial intervention?

    a. turn the patient onto the opposite side of the catheter placement
    b. flush all air from the system
    c. inflate and deflate the balloon
    d. withdraw catheter into right atrium

58. A patient has recently been diagnosed with celiac disease after tests to determine the cause of chronic weight loss, anemia, diarrhea, rash, bone pain, and irregular menses. When discussing dietary interventions, the nurse tells the patient that celiac disease may result in malabsorption of

    a. vitamin B_{12}.
    b. folate and iron.
    c. vitamin C.
    d. vitamin D.

59. Following an automobile accident with abdominal trauma, intra-abdominal pressure is monitored for compartment syndrome. Which of the following intra-abdominal pressures is the minimum pressure that generally indicates the need for surgical decompression?

    a. 5 mmHg
    b. 13 mmHg
    c. 20 mmHg
    d. 26 mmHg

60. What pressure setting is usually used initially when titrating CPAP?

    a. 1 cmH$_2$O
    b. 5 cmH$_2$O
    c. 10 cmH$_2$O
    d. 20 cmH$_2$O

61. If a patient's cardiac output is 5.6 L/min and the heart rate is 80/min, the stroke volume is

    a. 0.7 mL
    b. 7 mL
    c. 70 mL
    d. 700 mL

62. A 72-year-old male patient with an acute MI and left ventricular failure has a pulmonary artery catheter in place for hemodynamic monitoring and is developing cardiogenic shock. Hemodynamics include a blood pressure (BP) of 90/60 mmHg, a heart rate (HR) of 120/min, MAP of 70, SV of 25 mL/min, RAP of 8 mmHg, PAP of 36/24 mmHg, PAWP of 20 mmHg, CO of 3 L/min, CI of 1.5 L/min/m^2, and SVR of 1626 dynes/sec cm^{-5}. The patient receives oxygen, dobutamine, and nitroprusside. What hemodynamic changes should the nurse expect as a positive response?

    a. increased CO and SV and decreased HR, SVR, and PAWP
    b. decreased HR and increased CO and PAWP
    c. increased CO, SV, SVR, and PAWP and decrease HR
    d. increased HR, CO, SV, and decrease PAWP and SVR

63. A patient is hospitalized with a transmural Q-wave myocardial infarction. In how many hours will the CK level peak?

    a. 3
    b. 14
    c. 27
    d. 45

64. Which of the following changes in fluid intelligence are associated with age?

    a. decreased test anxiety
    b. altered time perception
    c. decreased long-term memory
    d. decreased reaction time

65. A patient whose intermittent claudication had progressed to rest pain and had not responded to conservative treatment has undergone a fem-pop bypass. The patient complains of numbness and tingling on the anterior and medial aspect of the leg. This suggests

    a. damage to the femoral nerve.
    b. occlusion of the femoral artery.
    c. normal postoperative sensation.
    d. bypass occlusion.

66. Which of the following drugs puts the patient with diabetes mellitus, type 2, most at risk for episodes of acute hypoglycemia?

    a. metformin (Glucophage)
    b. rosiglitazone (Avandia)
    c. exenatide (Byetta)
    d. glipizide (Glucotrol)

67. A patient with bilateral lung transplants has developed recurrent respiratory infections and increased exercise intolerance with a decline in FEV1. The patient is diagnosed with bronchiolitis obliterans. Which of the follow treatment options is most likely to be taken?

    a. no treatment
    b. increased immunosuppression
    c. decreased immunosuppression
    d. antibiotics

68. A patient who is taking warfarin is scheduled for cardiac catheterization. How long prior to the catheterization should the patient discontinue the warfarin?

    a. 24 hours
    b. two to three days
    c. one week
    d. two weeks

69. A patient has been hospitalized with nausea and vomiting but minimal abdominal distention. The patient has not passed flatus in 14 hours, and abdominal x-ray shows dilated small bowel loops and no colonic or rectal gas. The patient's CBC and electrolytes are within normal limits. Based on these findings, the nurse should suspect that the primary initial intervention will be

    a. contrast studies.
    b. NG suction.
    c. exploratory surgery.
    d. observation.

70. A patient with chronic heart failure develops severe dyspnea, cough with frothy slightly blood-tinged sputum, cyanosis, and diaphoresis. The nurse notes wheezing, rales, and rhonchi throughout the lung fields. Which initial intervention is indicated?

    a. administer morphine sulfate subcutaneously or IV
    b. sit patient upright and administer 100% oxygen with mask
    c. provide antibiotic therapy
    d. administer furosemide IV

71. Following percutaneous transluminal coronary angioplasty with right femoral access, the patient complains of right back and flank pain and non-specific complaints of feeling weak and dizzy. Her heart rate increases to 112/min and blood pressure is 78/52 mmHg. Based on these findings, the nurse should suspect

    a. cardiac tamponade.
    b. allergic reaction.
    c. myocardial infarction.
    d. retroperitoneal hemorrhage.

72. A patient who experienced chest trauma during an automobile accident shows signs of non-hemorrhagic cardiac tamponade and is to undergo pericardiocentesis. What position should the nurse place the patient in for the procedure?

    a. supine, flat
    b. right lateral side lying
    c. upright at 45 degrees
    d. upright at 90 degrees

73. The nurse is conducting stimulation threshold testing for a patient with a temporary pacemaker. Consistent capture is regained at 2 mA. Based on this finding, the output should be set at

    a. 1-2 mA.
    b. 2-3 mA.
    c. 3-4 mA.
    d. 4-6 mA.

74. A patient with Marfan syndrome is admitted with substernal pain, cough, strider, distention of neck veins, and edema of the upper extremities. The most likely cause is

    a. tricuspid regurgitation.
    b. thoracic aortic aneurysm.
    c. pulmonic regurgitation.
    d. aortic stenosis.

75. A patient suffered smoke inhalation when a fire occurred while he was sleeping. Burned materials included wool carpets, furniture with polyurethane foam, and household plastics. The patient is hypotensive and has altered mental status. Physical examination shows evidence of soot in the nares and mouth. Which of the following antidotes is most indicated?

   a. hydroxocobalamin
   b. sodium nitrite
   c. atropine
   d. oxygen therapy

76. A patient with anoxic encephalopathy resulting from fat embolism exhibits flexor (decorticate) posturing. This indicates damage to which part of the brain?

   a. upper pons
   b. brainstem
   c. midbrain
   d. hemispheres

77. A patient with unstable angina has continuous cardiac monitoring. Which of the following findings places the patient at highest risk for fatal or non-fatal myocardial infarction?

   a. appearance of pathologic Q waves
   b. T-wave inversion greater than 0.2 mV
   c. transient ST-segment changes greater than 0.05 mV
   d. slight elevation of Troponin T, between 0.01 and 0.1 ng/mL

78. A patient with valvular disease has right ventricular hypertrophy and exhibits mild cyanosis, angina, dyspnea, heart murmur, and episodes of fainting. These signs and symptoms are characteristic of

   a. pulmonic stenosis.
   b. aortic stenosis.
   c. mitral valve regurgitation.
   d. mitral stenosis.

79. Indications of primary graft dysfunction in lung transplant recipients include

   a. frequent oxygen desaturation.
   b. chest pressure.
   c. fever.
   d. cough.

80. A patient becomes very resistant and uncooperative during dressing changes, often yelling at the nurse, "You're hurting me!" even though the wound care is minimal. What is the best response to the patient?

   a. "I'm being as gentle as I can."
   b. "You had pain medication an hour ago, so you should not be having pain."
   c. "What would you like for me to do differently?"
   d. "Let's talk about how we can work together to make this easier for you."

81. Normal value for mixed venous oxygen saturation (SvO$_2$) is

    a. 96 to 100%.
    b. 60 to 80%.
    c. 45 to 65%.
    d. 75 to 95%.

82. Forty-eight hours after a subtotal gastrectomy, the patient's pulse has increased from a baseline of 72 to 118/min and blood pressure has fallen from 138/88 to 72/48 mmHg. Urinary output has diminished, and the patient's skin is cold and clammy. The nurse suspects hemorrhage. Which of the following findings is most indicative of extragastric hemorrhage?

    a. abdominal pain
    b. increased bilirubin
    c. melena
    d. clear NG aspirant

83. A patient has undergone a subtotal gastrectomy for gastric cancer and is recovering well and progressing from clear liquids to full liquids and soft foods. What nutritional strategy is most likely to prevent or minimize dumping syndrome?

    a. low fat, high protein, high carbohydrate
    b. high fat, high protein, low carbohydrate
    c. low fat, high protein, low carbohydrate
    d. low fat, low protein, high carbohydrate

84. A patient receiving maintenance lithium at 300 mg three times daily for bipolar disorder has developed vomiting, diarrhea, tinnitus, and tremors. The patient's blood level is 1.8 mEq/L. The initial response should be to

    a. withhold lithium.
    b. increase lithium dosage.
    c. decrease lithium dosage.
    d. maintain lithium dosage and provide an antipsychotic medication.

85. A patient has been receiving unfractionated heparin for five days and has onset of pain in left leg with unilateral edema, erythema, and pain on passive dorsiflexion. Prior to administration of heparin, the patient's platelet count was 160,000 but it is now 104,000 (a 35% reduction). The nurse should expect to

    a. continue unfractionated heparin at same dose.
    b. continue unfractionated heparin at higher dose.
    c. discontinue unfractionated heparin and administer lepirudin or argatroban.
    d. discontinue unfractionated heparin and replace with low-molecular weight heparin.

86. The primary problem with basing research on qualitative data is that qualitative data are

    a. difficult to interpret.
    b. subjective.
    c. uninteresting.
    d. difficult to describe graphically.

87. A patient with an AVM had evidence of reperfusion bleeding during partial embolization, but the patient stabilized. During the postoperative period, the most critical concern is

    a. maintaining blood pressure within established parameters.
    b. monitoring arterial blood gases (ABGs).
    c. monitoring electrolytes.
    d. maintaining fluid balance.

88. A 30-year-old patient is admitted to critical care with second and third degree burns to the right arm (posterior and anterior surfaces), left anterior arm, anterior face, and anterior chest. Utilizing the Rule of 9s, what percentage of total body surface area is injured?

    a. 40.5%.
    b. 22.5%
    c. 36%
    d. 27%.

89. A 40-year-old female patient complains of frequent epistaxis and blood in her urine. Petechial hemorrhages are noted on the lower legs and oral mucosa. A CBC shows that RBCs and WBCs are normal, but the platelet count is 40,000. The patient is diagnosed with idiopathic thrombocytopenia purpura. Based on the patient's symptoms, which of the following treatments is the patient most likely to receive?

    a. observation only
    b. IV Ig immunoglobulin
    c. corticosteroids (oral)
    d. splenectomy

90. A 56-year-old patient with COPD has arterial blood gases done on admission. ABGs are as follows: PaO_2 of 88 mmHg, pH of 7.28, $PaCO_2$ of 48 mmHg, and HCO_3^- of 23 mEq/L. Based on this profile, the patient is in

    a. compensated respiratory acidosis.
    b. uncompensated respiratory acidosis.
    c. compensated metabolic acidosis.
    d. uncompensated metabolic acidosis.

91. A patient with diabetic ketoacidosis shows evidence of hypovolemic shock. What IV fluid is utilized initially to reverse dehydration?

    a. 1-1.5 L of 0.9% normal saline
    b. 3-4 L of 0.9% normal saline
    c. 1-2 L of 0.45% sodium chloride
    d. 1-2 L of 5% dextrose with 45% sodium chloride

92. Following a craniotomy for removal of a meningioma anterior to the pituitary gland and optic chiasm, the patient develops pronounced diuresis and thirst. Laboratory findings include: serum sodium level of 150, serum osmolality of 304, urine osmolality of 290, and urine specific gravity of 1.004. Based on the patient's condition and laboratory findings, which pharmaceutical intervention is most indicated?

    a. hypertonic saline solution
    b. thiazide diuretics
    c. desmopressin acetate
    d. demeclocycline

93. The primary difference between hyperglycemic hyperosmolar nonketotic syndrome (HHNK) and diabetes ketoacidosis (DKA) is that

    a. treatment options for HHNK and DKA are different.
    b. HHNK does not involve breakdown of fat and DKA does.
    c. HHNK involves overhydration and DKA dehydration.
    d. insulin level is lower in HHNK than in DKA.

94. Which of the following is an example of informal collaboration?

    a. team members discussing the best method of meeting a patient's needs
    b. a nurse reporting a patient's concerns about upcoming surgery to the physician
    c. a nurse asking a nurse on another unit about his experience with a procedure
    d. a nurse asking another team member to assist with moving a patient

95. The nurse is reviewing preoperative laboratory values. The nurse should alert the physician to which of the following values?

    a. glucose level of 98 mg/dL
    b. blood, urea, nitrogen (BUN) level of 26 mg/dL
    c. creatinine level of 0.79 mg/dL
    d. calcium level of 9.2 mg/dL

96. A patient has been stabilized after rupture of a cerebral aneurysm with a grade II subarachnoid hemorrhage and is scheduled for surgical repair within 24 hours of the rupture. However, the patient tells the nurse that he wants to wait until his family arrives from overseas in four days. Which of the following is the best response?

    a. "You should discuss that with your surgeon."
    b. "Delaying surgery could be very dangerous."
    c. "I'm sure your family will understand that you needed to have the surgery."
    d. "The risk of re-bleeding increases every day, putting you at grave risk if you delay."

97. While hospitalized for a stroke, a patient vomited and aspirated some of the gastric contents before the nurse could change the patient's position to prevent aspiration. The initial intervention should be to

    a. administer oxygen.
    b. conduct a bronchoalveolar lavage.
    c. suction the upper airway.
    d. provide prophylactic antibiotics.

98. The first-line treatment for obstructive sleep apnea is

    a. BiPAP.
    b. CPAP.
    c. APAP.
    d. BiPAP ST.

99. Following a traumatic brain injury, a patient is to have eight-minute apnea testing to aid in the determination of brain death. Four minutes after the ventilator is disconnected, the patient develops cardiac dysrhythmias. What nursing action is indicated?

    a. obtain a blood sample for ABGs and reconnect the ventilator
    b. obtain ECG tracing and continue monitoring for four more minutes
    c. obtain a blood sample for ABGs and an ECG tracing and continuing monitoring for four more minutes
    d. continue monitoring for four more minutes and then obtain blood sample for ABGs

100. When asking a patient to sign a consent form for a procedure, the most important factor is the

    a. explanation of the procedure.
    b. patient's ability to give informed consent.
    c. reasons for the procedure.
    d. explanation of possible complications.

101. Which of the following modes of ventilation provides a specified volume of air and rate with no triggering required of the patient and respiratory response decreased through medication (such as pancuronium bromide or morphine)?

    a. synchronized intermittent mandatory ventilation (SIMV)
    b. assist control ventilation (ACV)
    c. pressure support ventilation (PSV)
    d. controlled mandatory ventilation (CMV)

102. A patient who was in a car accident 48 hours ago presents with bilateral periorbital ecchymosis. The patient complains of a salty taste in their mouth. The most likely cause of these symptoms is

    a. eye trauma.
    b. diastatic skull fracture.
    c. Le Fort skull fracture.
    d. basal skull fracture.

103. A patient has been diagnosed with metastatic ovarian cancer with a short life expectancy, but she tells the nurse that she believes that she can cure herself with positive thinking. Which of the following is the best response?

    a. "I've heard that positive thinking has cured some people of cancer."
    b. "The mind can be powerful."
    c. "There's no evidence to support positive thinking as a cure."
    d. "Whatever makes you feel better is ok."

104. Considering ventilator management, in order to avoid toxicity, the fraction of inspired oxygen (FiO$_2$) should usually be maintained at less than

    a. 21%.
    b. 40%.
    c. 60%.
    d. 80%.

105. An 18-year-old man who identifies as gay is hospitalized under his parents' insurance. The patient insists that his male partner visit him, but his parents have left a note at the nursing desk advising the staff that the partner is not allowed to visit. What is the best action for the nurse?

    a. advise the partner that he cannot visit the patient
    b. advise the patient that his partner is not allowed to visit
    c. call the parents and advise them that they cannot prevent visits
    d. ignore the parents because they have no standing

106. A patient who sustained a head injury is to have a lumbar puncture to determine if there is CNS bleeding. Which of the following is the most important prior to the lumbar puncture?

    a. CT of the brain
    b. EEG
    c. hemoglobin and hematocrit
    d. coagulation studies

107. In order to avoid protein depletion in trauma patients, how much protein should be provided to the patient each day?

    a. 1.0 to 1.5 g/kg
    b. 1.5 to 2.0 g/kg
    c. 2.0 to 2.5 g/kg
    d. 2.5 to 3.0 g/kg

108. Following a subarachnoid hemorrhage, a patient complains of increasing headache and slight nausea and a CTA shows hydrocephalus. The patient remains awake and responsive. The most likely initial treatment is

    a. lumbar puncture for drainage.
    b. serial lumbar punctures for drainage.
    c. observation.
    d. ventriculostomy or ventriculoperitoneal shunt.

109. After an extended stay in the critical care unit, a patient is to be transferred to a general medical-surgical unit. The patient has developed a trusting relationship with her nurse and is upset about the transfer. The patient begs the nurse to intervene so she can stay in the critical care unit. The best solution for the nurse is to

    a. tell the patient that the nurses on the other unit will take good care of her.
    b. tell the patient the nurse will accompany her to the other unit and introduce her.
    c. ask the physician if the patient can stay longer in the critical care unit.
    d. tell the patient that the nurse will stop by every day to visit her.

110. A patient who has been prescribed oral phenytoin (Dilantin) for seizure control should be advised to

    a. limit alcohol intake to two to three drinks daily.
    b. have weekly blood tests.
    c. maintain superior dental care.
    d. stop the drug immediately if adverse effects occur.

111. Following a craniotomy, the patient is carefully monitored for increasing intracranial pressure. Intracranial hypertension occurs when intracranial pressure (ICP) is greater than

 a. 12 mmHg.
 b. 15 mmHg.
 c. 20 mmHg.
 d. 25 mmHg.

112. A patient receiving continuous renal replacement therapy (CCRT) exhibits increased heart rate, decreased blood pressure, and ECG abnormalities. The nurse should suspect

 a. electrolyte imbalance.
 b. bleeding.
 c. too much or too little dialysate.
 d. problem unrelated to CCRT.

113. The nurse is assessing a patient with suspected ischemic stroke using the NIH stroke scale. The patient speaks only Spanish but no interpreter is available. Only the word list and reading for the assessment are available in Spanish. However, the patient's 13-year-old granddaughter is present and is bilingual. The nurse should

 a. delay the assessment until an interpreter is available.
 b. ask the granddaughter to translate.
 c. omit the sections of the assessment that require verbal directions or responses.
 d. complete the assessment in English using pictures, motions, and pantomime to aid in the patient's comprehension.

114. A patient who has experienced an ischemic stroke arrives at the emergency department in the 3 to 4.5-hour window of time after the stroke. Which of the following would exclude the patient from treatment with recombinant tPA?

 a. age of 81 years
 b. score of 24 on the NIH stroke scale
 c. history of diabetes
 d. history of major surgery 3 months previously

115. Which of the following conditions is most commonly associated with acute renal failure?

 a. respiratory acidosis
 b. respiratory alkalosis
 c. metabolic alkalosis
 d. metabolic acidosis

116. A patient involved in a traumatic motorcycle accident has fractured ribs 9 and 10 on the left side. Injury to which of the following underlying structures is of most concern?

 a. pancreas
 b. spleen
 c. diaphragm
 d. intestines

117. When planning patient education, the nurse realizes that most adults experience low energy in the

    a. early morning.

    b. late morning.

    c. afternoon.

    d. evening.

118. Which of the following defense mechanisms is a patient utilizing if the patient yells at his spouse after receiving bad news from the physician about his condition?

    a. projection

    b. reaction formation

    c. sublimation

    d. displacement

119. A patient who is legally blind is to use a BiPAP machine when he is discharged. The best method to ensure the patient uses the equipment properly is to

    a. provide instructions in brail or audiotapes.

    b. allow the patient to handle and manipulate the equipment.

    c. teach a family member how to assist the patient.

    d. plan extended training sessions with much repetition.

120. A 20-year-old patient has a severe exacerbation of asthma with pronounced wheezing and dyspnea. The patient is only able to give one- to two-word responses and is using accessory muscles to breathe. The nurse should expect which of the following to be the first-line treatment?

    a. short-acting B_2-Agonist (albuterol) and corticosteroid

    b. theophylline and non-specific B-adrenergic agent (epinephrine)

    c. anticholinergic (ipratropium) and heliox

    d. short-acting B_2-agonist and intravenous magnesium

121. The nurse is aware that a patient is extremely nervous about having an MRI and takes a CD by the patient's favorite singer to the imaging lab so that the patient can listen to the music during the procedure. This is an example of

    a. response to diversity.

    b. collaboration.

    c. patient advocacy.

    d. caring practices.

122. A patient asks the nurse many questions about her medical treatment; but, when the physician is present, the patient becomes very quiet and asks no questions despite the nurse's encouragement to do so. The best solution for the nurse is to

    a. prompt the patient when the doctor is present.

    b. ask the patient why she doesn't ask the doctor questions.

    c. prepare a list of the patient's questions for the physician.

    d. tell the physician that the patient has many questions.

123. A nurse mentors peers new to the profession. Which of the Standards for Acute and Critical Care Nurses under the Standards of Professional Performance does this support?

    a. quality of care
    b. education
    c. collaboration
    d. collegiality

124. A patient who is critically ill has been "talking" with her husband, who has actually been dead for many years, and describing a beautiful place. The nurse recognizes these as signs of

    a. delirium.
    b. dementia.
    c. impending death.
    d. opioid toxicity.

125. A nurse on the unit states she has no interest in the politics of work and just wants to work with the patients and not worry about other departments and institutional problems. This represents

    a. dedication to the nursing profession.
    b. incompetent practice of nursing.
    c. old-fashioned attitude toward the nursing profession.
    d. barrier to systems thinking.

126. A staff nurse repeatedly makes mistakes with electronic charting, insisting that the system is too difficult and inefficient, that the institution made a big mistake in forcing staff to use the computer system, and that most staff agree with this assessment. This is an example of

    a. having an autocratic view.
    b. arriving at weak consensus.
    c. displaying displaced anger.
    d. failing to adapt.

127. Which of the following is the most common cause of hypoxemia?

    a. alveolar hypoventilation.
    b. physiologic shunting.
    c. ventilation/perfusion (V/Q) mismatch.
    d. intrapulmonary shunting.

128. A patient is admitted with partial obstruction of the airway after aspiration of a metal screw 24 hours earlier. The patient is able to speak with difficulty but is dyspneic and having severe bouts of coughing and complains of chest pain. Which treatment option should the nurse anticipate?

    a. bronchodilator and postural drainage
    b. flexible bronchoscopy
    c. rigid bronchoscopy
    d. bronchotomy

129. A patient with progressive pulmonary arterial hypertension must be monitored for signs of

    a. left ventricular heart failure.
    b. right ventricular heart failure.
    c. ventricular fibrillation.
    d. cardiomyopathy.

130. What is the minimum time period that heliox should be administered to gain full effects?

    a. 20 minutes
    b. 40 minutes
    c. 60 minutes
    d. 90 minutes

131. Some hospital units are overstaffed, according to patient census, while others are understaffed, requiring nurses to work overtime and resulting in increased costs. While most understaffed units are requesting additional full-time nurses, one-unit leader suggests that the hospital switch to acuity-based staffing and increase the number of float nurses from current staff and train them in more than one discipline in order to cut overall costs and meet the needs of multiple units. This suggestion is an example of

    a. divergent thinking.
    b. parallel thinking.
    c. systems thinking.
    d. convergent thinking.

132. When considering the validity of written material, the most important thing to consider is the

    a. source.
    b. author.
    c. date.
    d. statistical evidence.

133. Adhesive atelectasis, caused by surfactant deficiency, is most often associated with

    a. necrotizing pneumonia.
    b. space-occupying lesions.
    c. asbestos exposure.
    d. acute respiratory distress syndrome (ARDS).

134. A patient who underwent a thoracic laminectomy developed increasing dyspnea and hypoxemia with cough, hemoptysis, substernal pain, and subcutaneous emphysema of neck and chest within 4 hours of extubation. The most likely cause is

    a. tracheal perforation.
    b. surgical trauma to chest.
    c. esophageal perforation.
    d. pneumothorax.

135. A patient has undergone bilateral lung volume reduction per video-assisted thoracoscopic surgery (VATS) for severe emphysema. What postoperative complication is most common?

   a. pneumonia
   b. air leaks
   c. aspiration of gastric contents
   d. respiratory failure

136. A patient has suffered blunt chest trauma in an accident with bilateral lung contusions. During what time period should the nurse anticipate possible onset of symptoms of acute respiratory distress syndrome?

   a. 1 to 2 hours
   b. 4 to 12 hours
   c. 12 to 24 hours
   d. 24 to 48 hours

137. A 68-year-old patient with severe asthma is lethargic and somnolent and arouses with difficulty. His PaO_2 has fallen to 58 mmHg on low-flow oxygen and $PaCO_2$ has increased to 56 mmHg while the pH is 7.28. Which of the following is the most likely cause of these symptoms?

   a. acute respiratory failure
   b. pulmonary embolism
   c. sepsis
   d. pneumonia

138. A 20-year-old man who had been practicing football in extreme heat is admitted with heat stroke. Which of the following symptoms is typically found with exertional heat stroke as opposed to non-exertional?

   a. anhidrosis
   b. temperature above 41 °C (106 °F)
   c. high risk for rhabdomyolysis
   d. low risk for renal failure

139. An 18-year–old woman comes to the hospital 18 hours after she took "a bottle" of extra-strength acetaminophen. She feels slight nausea but has no other symptoms. At what beginning serum acetaminophen level should N-acetylcysteine (NAC) be administered?

   a. 10 mcg/mL
   b. 50 mcg/mL
   c. 160 mcg/mL
   d. 200 mcg/mL

140. A patient with a history of severe allergic reaction to bananas and kiwis is at risk for allergy to

   a. plastics.
   b. penicillins.
   c. vitamin supplements.
   d. latex.

141. With intrarenal causes of acute renal failure, the expected level of urine sodium is

a. less than 20 mEq/L.
b. greater than 20 mEq/L
c. greater than 30 mEq/L.
d. greater than 40 mEq/L.

142. Which of the following is the most important factor in delegation?

a. determining if the task is appropriate based on the person's skills and available time
b. providing clear instructions, including expected objectives and timeline
c. monitoring progress and ensuring that tasks were performed correctly
d. reviewing the final results when the task is completed and recording outcomes

143. A patient who is supposed to be on a low carbohydrate diet has gained weight and reports eating frequent convenience foods that are high in carbohydrates. When questioned, the patient is knowledgeable about the diet, but states that poor vision and arthritis in her hands make food preparation difficult. The most appropriate referral for the patient is

a. nutritionist.
b. occupational therapist.
c. social worker.
d. home health agency.

144. The nurse must inform the family of a patient that the patient is dying. Which of the following is an effective strategy?

a. provide the information quickly
b. tell the family and then leave and allow them to grieve
c. ask the family if they have questions
d. advise the family to ask the physician about the patient's condition

145. The nurse is coaching a new graduate nurse in carrying out a procedure, utilizing a mannequin; however, the graduate nurse makes many errors and appears anxious. What is the best strategy for helping the graduate nurse master the procedure?

a. point out errors as the nurse makes them
b. provide positive feedback, stressing the nurse's correct actions
c. suggest the graduate nurse research the procedure and memorize the steps
d. remind the graduate nurse that her lack of knowledge could endanger patients

146. A patient who is dependent on peritoneal dialysis is admitted to the critical care unit with cardiac dysrhythmias. Which renal replacement therapy does the nurse anticipate will be used during hospitalization?

a. intermittent hemodialysis
b. continuous venovenous hemofiltration
c. peritoneal dialysis
d. continuous arteriovenous hemofiltration

147. A patient is to undergo a left renal biopsy. What is the correct position to place the patient in for the procedure?

a. prone
b. upright leaning over bedside table
c. right side-lying
d. knee-chest position

148. A patient who is undergoing deep sedation while mechanically ventilated is monitored with the bispectral index system (BIS). Which of the following values indicates that the patient is unconscious with low likelihood of recall?

a. 50-60
b. 90-100
c. 40-50
d. Less than 20

149. Which of the following drugs used for sedation provides the most prolonged sedation?

a. diazepam
b. lorazepam
c. propofol
d. midazolam

150. A patient is unconscious with severe generalized tonic-clonic status epilepticus leading to periods of apnea with cause unknown. The patient is administered lorazepam (Ativan) initially and again in 5 minutes when there is no response, but seizures continue. What should the nurse anticipate will be the next step?

a. administration of another dose of lorazepam
b. rapid sequence intubation
c. addition of fosphenytoin
d. addition of phenobarbital

Answer Key and Explanations

1. C: The optimal temperature range for therapeutic hypothermia is 32-36 °C (89.6-96.8 °F) according to the American Heart Association. Patients may be placed between two cooling blankets, or ice packs may be used to lower temperature. If using ice packs, they should be applied to the femoral area, axillae, and sides of the neck as well as the sides (but not the top) of the chest. Patients must be carefully monitored for oxygen saturation and dysrhythmias. The MAP should be maintained at greater than 80 mmHg for neuroprotection. The head of bed should be elevated to 30°.

2. D: The electrolyte imbalance that is the most life threatening for patients with renal failure is hyperkalemia (greater than 5.5 mEq/L). Hyperkalemia may cause cardiac abnormalities and ECG changes (peaked or tented T-waves) as well as changes in general condition. Treatment for hyperkalemia includes sodium polystyrene sulfonate (Kayexalate), which can be administered orally or as a retention enema. Kayexalate exchanges sodium ions for potassium ions in the intestines. Unstable patients may receive IV dextrose 50% with insulin and calcium to shift potassium from the blood into the cells. Nebulized albuterol may also lower potassium levels.

3. A: The best method to improve a patient's motivation is to provide positive feedback about tasks the patient is able to complete at the time he is doing the tasks because that helps the patient focus on concrete improvements. Focusing on long-term or even short-term goals may seem overwhelming in the initial stages of rehabilitation, especially if the patient is depressed. Comparing present abilities and initial abilities focuses on the past more than the present and future, and the nurse should never make overgeneralizations that include "everyone" because each person is individual.

4. C: These symptoms are consistent with sepsis and part of the continuum leading to septic shock. The diagnostic criteria for sepsis include many variables. General signs of infection and impending shock are usually present (fever, tachycardia, hypotension, fever) as well as edema and flushing resulting from massive arterial and venous vasodilation in early stages. WBC may be elevated (greater than 12,000) or decreased (less than 4000). Hyperglycemia and coagulopathies are common, and urine output falls because of decreased intravascular volume.

5. C: Clinical pathways should be developed by interdisciplinary teams that include physicians as well as nurses and other healthcare providers who may participate in patient care, such as respiratory and occupational therapists and nutritionists. The team must select the patient group, diagnosis, and procedures based on analysis of evidence through observation, literature review, and interviews. The group should discuss issues and reach consensus and should clearly outline levels of care and days covered by the pathway. Pilot testing and staff education should precede utilization.

6. A: A well-written learning objective should clearly outline expectations of the learning process and usually contains 4 elements: the condition or testing situation ("after attending a workshop about hypertension"); the identity of the learner, not the instructor ("the patient"); the expected behavior ("will be able to state"); and the measurable criterion ("4 causes for high blood pressure").

7. D: Because carbon dioxide acts as a vasodilator, dilating cerebral blood vessels and causing cerebral edema and increased ICP, the optimal $PaCO_2$ level is 27 to 32, which is lower than the normal $PaCO_2$ level of 35 to 45. Ventilation, usually per tracheal intubation, is provided to provide oxygenation and control CO_2 levels although hyperventilation, which constricts cerebral blood vessels, should be avoided (especially during the first 5 post-operative days) or used only for short periods since it may induce ischemia.

8. B: While state laws may vary somewhat, nurses are mandated reporters for both child abuse and elder abuse, so the nurse should report the observations to adult protective services. Bruises on the parts of the body covered by clothes are characteristic of those inflicted by an abuser who wants to hide evidence of abuse. Arm bruises are often defensive. The nurse should not confront the suspected abuser, as this may put both the nurse and the patient at risk.

9. C: While at one time tidal volume for ARDS was set at 12 mL/kg predicted body weight (PBW), current studies indicate that 6 to 8 mL/kg PBW (low tidal volume ventilation) has a more protective effect on the lungs and reduces mortality rates. PEEP may need to be set higher than usual to prevent atelectasis. Initial settings: tidal volume of 8 mL/kg PBW; respiratory rate of 35/min; PEEP of 5 cmH$_2$O or higher; FiO$_2$ less than 70% when possible but high enough to maintain oxygen saturation of 88 to 95%; and tidal volume reduced to 7 mL/kg PBW and then 6 mL/kg PBW over 4 hours or less.

10. A: The two treatments used for GBS are IV Ig or plasmapheresis (plasma exchange). IV Ig may reduce recovery time by 50% by neutralizing myelin antibodies and promoting remyelination although it poses a risk of thromboembolic events, so low doses of heparin may be given. Plasmapheresis may also be used to remove autoantibodies, cytotoxic constituents and immune complexes from serum. There is no advantage to providing both IV Ig and plasmapheresis. Corticosteroids do not improve GBS. Immunoadsorption is still in the trial stage but shows promise.

11. C: This patient is exhibiting typical indications of acute heart failure with dyspnea, orthopnea, basilar rales, lateral displacement of the apical beat (from enlarged left ventricle), peripheral edema, tachycardia, elevated blood pressure, and hypoxia. CPAP or BiPAP should be administered since this may increase oxygenation and reduce the need for endotracheal intubation with mechanical ventilation. Nitrates may also be administered to decrease pre-load. While a loop diuretic, such as furosemide, may be indicated, diuretics are no longer considered first-line treatments as they may result in hypotension.

12. B: While many of these symptoms can be found with all of these conditions, two are specific to pneumopericardium: the mill wheel murmur and the shifting tympany. Hamman's sign—a popping or crunching sound heard over the mediastinum—may or may not be present but is more commonly associated with pneumomediastinum. Pneumopericardium can be confirmed CT. Treatment includes needle aspiration and insertion of drainage tube or thoracotomy as well as oxygen therapy. Asymptomatic pneumopericardium may be treated conservatively.

13. D: This pattern of pain—severe epigastric pain radiating to the back—that is exacerbated by lying flat or walking is consistent with pancreatitis. Generally, the upper abdomen is tender but without rigidity or guarding, which may be present with other disorders. Abdominal distention and jaundice may occur in some patients. Fever to 39 °C is common as is tachycardia and pallor. Serum amylase and serum lipase may be elevated up to 3 times normal values within 24 hours, and leukocytosis (10,000 to 30,000) may be evident.

14. A: One of the barriers to adequate pain management is nurses' preconceptions about physiological and emotional responses to pain and what a patient in pain should look like. Some patients moan and cry while others show little outward sign of pain, but pain is what the patient says it is, and if a patient requests pain medication for severe pain, then the nurse should give the opioid. A patient may try to not to show pain to family members or friends even when the patient is very uncomfortable.

15. C: It's very important that an impermeable covering be placed over the insertion site until the chest tube can be reinserted to prevent air from sucking into the pleural cavity. If no plastic or petroleum gauze dressing is available, the nurse can cover the insertion site with a clean gloved hand while calling for assistance. The physician must be notified as soon as the insertion site is secured. The patient's arterial blood gases should be assessed as soon as possible.

16. C: The CT-PA is most diagnostic for PE. D-dimer is almost always elevated with PE as endogenous fibrinolysis results in decreased levels of fibrinogen and increased D-dimer as the body attempts to digest the clot. A normal D-dimer generally can rule out PE, but an abnormal D-dimer is common in hospitalized patients and not diagnostic alone. Usually both the D-dimer and CT-PA are used. While hypoxemia and hypocapnia are common with PE, arterial blood gas values may alter for other reasons and remain within normal range even with pulmonary emboli. Pulmonary angiogram is rarely used, and chest radiograph is not diagnostic.

17. A: A potassium level of 3.2 mEq/L indicates hypokalemia, which increases the risk of digoxin toxicity. Immediate treatment includes withholding digoxin (the number of doses or the need for reduction in dosage depends on the severity of the reaction as well as the cause). With hypokalemia, potassium supplement should be administered as well as supportive therapy, such as acetaminophen for headache and an antidiarrheal. The digoxin antidote, digoxin immune Fab, is not routinely given but may be administered if indicated, usually because of severe toxicity with hyperkalemia, severe cardiac dysrhythmias, or digoxin overdose.

18. D: Pain and local swelling, erythema, and itching are common after bee sting and may extend to an entire limb or extended area, but urticaria, edema, and itching occurring in areas distant from the sting site suggest a systemic reaction leading to anaphylaxis. Patients may feel lightheaded and nauseated and may have tightness in the chest, dyspnea, and lingual edema as well as generalized hives because of vasodilation and edema. Hypotension, bronchospasm, laryngospasm, and loss of consciousness may lead to respiratory and cardiac arrest.

19. C: Cocaine: euphoria, restlessness, hyperactivity, tachycardia, hypertension, dilated pupils, and rhinitis (from sniffing cocaine). Patients may show damage to the nasal septum and may develop severe cardiac problems, including myocardial infarction. Peak effect occurs in 2 to 30 minutes and persists 30 to 60 minutes. Barbiturate (such as Valium): relaxed state, lack of inhibition, inability to concentrate, drowsiness, slurred speech, and sleepiness. Heroin: euphoria, lethargy, constricted/pinpoint pupils, drowsiness, and lack of motivation. Amphetamines: hyperactivity, agitation, euphoria, inability to sleep, and loss of appetite.

20. B: The patient receiving adenosine should be carefully monitored for transient asystole since the drug slows AV node conduction, sometimes resulting in heart block and development of new dysrhythmias, including atrial fibrillation. Facial flushing is a common side effect and is short-lived (usually only lasting one to two minutes) as the drug is very fast acting with a half-life of less than 10 seconds. Other adverse effects can include dizziness, numbness and tingling in the arms, headache, nausea, and dyspnea.

21. A: Because potassium-sparing diuretics markedly increase the risk of hyperkalemia in patients with chronic kidney disease, they are usually used only with patients who have persistent hypokalemia or hypertension. Risk is highest in patients whose glomerular filtration rate is less than 30 mL/min/1.73 m² and are also receiving ACEI or ARBs. Dosages should begin low and be increased slowly. Electrolyte levels must be monitored frequently. Hyporeninemic hypoaldosteronism is a contraindication for the use of potassium-sparing diuretics.

22. D: Wellens syndrome can occur in patients with unstable angina, indicating marked stenosis of the left anterior descending coronary artery and impending acute anterior wall myocardial infarction. Cardiac enzymes are usually within normal range or show only slight elevation. This is an emergency situation that requires immediate cardiac catheterization for angioplasty or stent placement before complete occlusion occurs. The R waves remain intact because the myocardial infarction has not yet taken place. ST segments (V1 and V3) may be normal or show slight elevation, and terminal T-wave inversion occurs (V2-V3) during pain-free periods.

23. B: This pattern is consistent with atrial fibrillation. Atrial fibrillation results in ineffective beats that do not adequately empty the atria so that blood begins to pool, increasing the risk of thrombus formation and emboli. While stroke volume decreases, the ventricular rate increases to compensate but the decreased cardiac output can result in myocardial ischemia. Treatment may include cardioversion (per electrical cardioversion or pharmaceutical), ventricular pacing, and anticoagulant therapy if the atrial fibrillation lasts more than 24 hours.

24. C: If bubbling occurs in the water seal container, this indicates that there is an air leak somewhere in the system. The first step is to check the chest tube by clamping the drainage tube just below the chest tube. If this stops the bubbling, then the leak is superior to the clamp from the chest tube or the patient's chest. If bubbling continues after clamping, then the leak is in the system below the clamp, so the drainage system should be changed.

25. A: Myasthenic crisis (usually due to too little medication) and cholinergic crisis (due to too much medication) both present with similar symptoms—profound weakness, respiratory distress, anxiety—and the Tensilon test (also used to diagnose myasthenia gravis) is used to differentiate the two. The Tensilon (edrophonium) test consists of administration of small doses (up to a total of 10 mg) of edrophonium. A positive response (improvement in muscle strength) indicates myasthenic crisis and a negative response (no improvement) indicates a cholinergic crisis.

26. C: With transcutaneous pacing, the rate is usually set at 60 to 70 bpm with the current increased slowly until capture, after which the current is slowly lowered if possible. Electrodes (gel-covered paddles/pads) are usually placed on the left chest and left back so that the heart is between them. Leads connect to a computerized ECG and defibrillator, which is synchronized so the electrical current is delivered during QRS (ventricular depolarization). It's important that the current be delivered at the correct time or ventricular tachycardia or ventricular fibrillation may occur.

27. A: While all of these are risk factors for hospital-associated pneumonia (HAP), 80% of HAP is the result of ventilator-associated pneumonia (VAP), a subgrouping of HAP that may occur 48 or more hours after initiation of ventilation per endotracheal tube or tracheostomy. When patients are receiving mechanical ventilation, they have depressed epiglottal and cough reflexes, increased secretions, and decreased cilia activity, all increasing the risk of aspiration and colonization of bacteria in the lungs. Two common pathogens associated with HAP are *Pseudomonas aeruginosa* and *Staphylococcus aureus*.

28. B: Mannitol tends to form crystals at low temperatures, so it should always be administered through a filter. Crystals are more likely to form with concentrations of over 15%. Mannitol solutions may be kept in a warming device to prevent crystal formation but should be cooled to body temperature prior to administration. Test doses are indicated for patients with renal impairment. Mannitol is usually administered over a 30- to 60-minute period while the patient is carefully monitored for changes in ICP and cerebral perfusion.

29. C: With status asthmaticus, indications for intubation and mechanical ventilation include peak expiratory flow rate less than 40% of predicted as well as FEV1 less than 20% of predicted. On initial presentation, hyperventilation usually results in ABGs showing hypocapnia and respiratory alkalosis, but if the patient's condition worsens, hypoxemia and hypercapnia develop, resulting in respiratory and metabolic acidosis. Patients may exhibit decreased level of consciousness, diminished or absent breath sounds, inability to breathe in supine position, and pulsus paradoxus greater than 25 mmHg.

30. D: The pacing mode that is most commonly used with temporary transvenous pacing is VVI. The electrode is placed in the ventricle and paces the ventricle first, senses ventricular activity, and inhibits ventricular output when it senses intrinsic ventricular depolarization. This is the fastest type of pacing to use in emergency situations because it is more difficult to position and maintain a temporary atrial lead. VVI is also the pacing mode often used with epicardial leads after cardiac surgery, especially in the presence of third-degree AV block.

31. C: These symptoms are consistent with disseminated intravascular coagulation, so a DIC panel is indicated to determine if factors necessary for clotting are decreased and if clotting times are prolonged (if so, these findings may confirm DIC). DIC occurs as secondary to another disorder, such as bacteremia or sepsis, trauma, necrotizing enterocolitis, cancer, malaria, and placenta abruptio. With DIC, both excess clotting and hemorrhage may occur at the same time. Identifying and treating the underlying cause is critical to treatment.

32. A: The two most commonly used drugs to treat delirium are lorazepam and haloperidol. Anticholinergics, such as benztropine, may trigger delirium, especially in older adults. Delirium has similar symptoms as dementia; but with delirium the symptoms tend to fluctuate, so patients may have both periods of lucidity and profound confusion. Delirium may be triggered by many conditions, such as trauma, depression, surgery, untreated pain, and electrolyte imbalance. A patient's attention deficit may be noted if the patient is unable to count backward from 1 to 20 or spell his first name backward.

33. B: Patients who develop West Nile virus flaccid paralysis are at high risk for respiratory failure, which may require mechanical ventilation and is the primary cause of mortality. WNV flaccid paralysis is similar to poliomyelitis with damage to anterior horn cells. It may involve paralysis of one limb or all four limbs. A similar manifestation is WVN-associated Guillain-Barré syndrome. Patients may also develop WNV meningitis and/or encephalitis. Treatment is supportive and depends on symptoms, as no specific medication is available for WNV.

34. D: Inflation must be timed exactly to the beginning of diastole at the dicrotic notch. Inflation and deflation must be coordinated with the patient's cardiac cycle to achieve hemodynamic stability. If inflation occurs too early, it may force the aortic valve to close prematurely, impairing ejection. If inflation occurs too late, the assistive function is shortened (although this does not directly cause harm to the patient). The balloon should deflate at the end of diastole just prior to the aortic upstroke.

35. C: To increase reading ease for patients, the maximum word length for a sentence should be 20 words, keeping in mind that a word count of 13 to 20 is approximately equivalent to a seventh-grade reading level, 7 to 12 equivalent to sixth-grade reading level, and 3 to 6 equivalent to a fifth-grade reading level. Complex sentence structures should be avoided and materials presented in active voice and second person (you). Language should be simple and conversational, avoiding technical terms.

36. A: Sodium nitroprusside is often given initially to treat hypertensive crisis related to cardiac ischemia because it provides very fast-acting vasodilation. Treatment must be given immediately to lower blood pressure and prevent damage to vital organs because a diastolic BP greater than 120 mmHg is considered a hypertensive emergency. The goal is usually not to lower BP to normal levels, and a decrease in 10% to 15% may reduce symptoms. With hypertensive urgency, when organs are not in immediate danger, the goal is one-third reduction in six hours, one third in the next 24 hours, and one-third over 2-4 days.

37. B: Cimetidine carries a high risk of drug interactions, especially in older adults, because it binds hepatic enzymes that metabolize many different drugs. Cimetidine inhibits oxidation of the drugs and may raise blood concentrations. It is especially a concern with drugs, such as warfarin and theophylline, which have a narrow therapeutic index. Cimetidine, like all H_2 antagonists, may inhibit absorption of drugs that require an acidic gastric environment. Cimetidine is the oldest H_2 antagonist, and newer drugs, such as famotidine, have far fewer drug interactions.

38 A: When the Passy-Muir valve is placed on a tracheostomy tube, the cuff must be completely deflated. If mechanical ventilation is used, the tidal volume should also be increased. The Passy-Muir valve is a one-way valve that opens on inhalation so that air can enter the lungs and closes on exhalation, forcing the air over the vocal cords and out the mouth instead of out the tracheostomy tube. The valve may be used to help the patient regain normal breathing patterns, improve swallowing, and decrease the risk of aspiration.

39. B: The primary concern with combining these drugs is that hydrochlorothiazide can interfere with the action of antidiabetic agents, decreasing hypoglycemic effects; so, patients may develop hyperglycemia and should be advised to careful monitor their blood glucose levels when beginning treatment since the dosage for the antidiabetic agent may need to be increased. Patients should also be advised to avoid licorice, which may cause increased potassium loss, and alcohol, which may cause orthostatic hypotension.

40. D: Because the lungs are especially sensitive to the inflammatory changes that occur with SIRS, the pulmonary system is often the first to fail and the subsequent lack of oxygen causes other systems to fail as well. While there is much variation in the manner in which systems fail, some sequentially and others failing at the same time, the most common progression is from the lungs to the liver, the GI system, the kidneys, and the heart. MODS may be primary from direct injury or secondary, such as from SIRS.

41. D: Prone positioning is used with ALI to improve oxygenation to the less damaged parts of the lungs and to improve ventilation/perfusion matching and decrease intrapulmonary shunting. Prone positioning should improve PaO_2 by more than 10 mmHg within 30 minutes, although no minimum or maximum time period for prone positioning has been established, and the treatment is usually reserved for those with life-threatening conditions because of the difficulty in positioning patients and preventing pressure. Special frames, such as the Vollman Prone Positioner, or pillows must be used so that the abdomen hangs free so the diaphragm descent is not impaired.

42. C: When oxygen is delivered via a mask with a reservoir bag, the estimated FiO_2 is 10 times the setting: 6 is equal to 60% estimated FiO_2. The flow rate should be set from 6 to 10. With a nasal cannula or catheter, the base setting of a flow rate of 1 is FiO_2 of 24 and each increase in the flow rate increases the FiO_2 by 4 percentage points: 1—24%, 2—28%, 3—32%, 4—36%, 5—40%, 6—

44%. With an oxygen mask, each increase in flow rate increases the FiO_2 by 10%: 5-6 is 40%, 6-7 is 50%, and 7-8 is 60%.

43. D: Syndrome of inappropriate secretion of antidiuretic hormone (SIADH) can be triggered by many different disease processes and many medications, but a common cause is bronchogenic small (oat) cell carcinoma because these abnormal cells synthesize and release ADH. The initial symptoms (lethargy, anorexia, nausea, and vomiting) result from dilutional hyponatremia; however, as the sodium level falls to critical levels (below 120 mEq/L), neurological symptoms become more evident as the patient becomes increasingly confused and unable to concentrate. Without treatment, the patient will progress to seizures, coma, and death. The first-line treatment is fluid restriction.

44. D: These findings are consistent with tension pneumothorax, which will require insertion of a chest tube on the left side. Tension pneumothorax can occur in COPD patients with rupture of lung bullae and also may occur in patients on mechanical ventilation. Patients are usually in severe respiratory distress with tachycardia and tachypnea. Classic signs include tracheal shift, decreased lung expansion, increased percussion notes, decreased breath sounds, and distended jugular veins, although many patients do not exhibit all of these signs.

45. A: The three characteristics most often associated with cardiogenic shock include increased preload, increased afterload, and decreased contractility. These characteristics combine to cause decreased cardiac output and increased systemic vascular resistance as a compensatory measure to protect internal organs. Tissue perfusion and coronary artery perfusion decrease as cardiac output falls. Because the left ventricle cannot adequately pump the blood, the fluid backs up, causing pulmonary edema and right ventricular failure. Patients exhibit hypotension, tachycardia, decreased heart sounds, chest pain, basilar rales, tachypnea, pallor, and cool clammy skin.

46. B: The ejection click, a brief high-pitched sound that occurs immediately after S1, is associated with aortic valve stenosis. Gallop rhythms include S3, which occurs after S2 and may indicate left ventricular failure in older adults, although it may be a normal finding in children and young adults; and S4, which occurs before S1 and may indicate ventricular hypertrophy, coronary artery disease, or aortic valve stenosis. The opening snap, an unusual high-pitched sound that occurs immediately after S2, is associated with mitral valve stenosis. The friction rub, which is a harsh grating sound during systole and diastole, is associated with pericarditis.

47. C: At one time, patients were routinely shielded from bad news, but the pendulum has swung in the opposite direction and now it is generally believed that patients should always be told the truth. This is a cultural belief more common in the West than the East. In some cultures, people are often not told that they are dying or have cancer, especially if no cure is possible. In this case, the nurse should respect the family's wishes.

48. D: While balloon tamponade can be maintained for up to 24 hours, it should be left in place for the shortest period possible because of the risk of serious complications, such as airway obstruction, esophageal injury, and aspiration (especially if the gastric balloon ruptures and the tube migrates upward or if the patient is confused and pulls on the tube). When removing the tube, the esophageal tube is deflated first and the patient observed for bleeding for a few hours prior to deflation of the gastric balloon.

49. C: Atrial fibrillation is often treated with cardioversion, a timed electrical shock to the heart to convert a tachydysrhythmia to a sinus rhythm. An anticoagulant, such as warfarin, is usually prescribed 3 weeks prior to the procedure in order to reduce the risk of emboli. Patients on digoxin must discontinue the drug at least two days prior to the procedure. In some cases, antiarrhythmics, such as diltiazem hydrochloride (Cardizem) or amiodarone hydrochloride (Cordarone) may be prescribed prior to the cardioversion to slow the heart rate.

50. C: Azotemia: dehydration, increased BUN, and increased urinary specific gravity. Management includes decreasing amino acids in PN formula or changing to NephrAmine. Hypoglycemia: decreased serum glucose, diaphoresis, pallor, lethargy, confusion, and weakness. Management includes stopping insulin and increasing concentration of dextrose as well as slowing infusion rate and evaluating for sepsis. Hyperammonemia: lethargy, change in mental status, asterixis. Management includes decreasing protein concentration in PN formula and evaluating for hepatic insufficiency. EFA deficiency: dry skin, thrombocytopenia. Management includes increasing lipid intake (at least 2 times weekly), oral fats (if possible), and topical fats.

51. D: Amylase levels are often elevated after CPB, but only 3% or fewer patients develop pancreatitis; however, levels over 1000 UI/L indicate increased risk, so patients must be monitored carefully. The increased amylase level may develop because of decreased renal excretion. Patients may exhibit nausea, anorexia, and ileus. Treatment is primarily supportive. If pancreatitis develops, it typically results from necrosis associated with lengthy CPB and prolonged decreased cardiac output. Patients with a history of alcoholism are at increased risk.

52. D: These nonspecific signs and symptoms of decline are characteristic of failure to thrive, which is commonly associated with depression in older adults, so the Geriatric Depression Scale should be administered. GDS is a simple 15-question questionnaire that requires only "yes" or "no" answers with a score of greater than 5 "yes" answers indicating depression. Failure to thrive may result from medications (anticonvulsants, antidepressants, opioids, SSRIs, neuroleptics, diuretics, beta-blockers, anticholinergics, alpha-antagonists, and benzodiazepines), chronic illness, socioeconomic factors, and abuse or neglect.

53. B: The normal height of the jugular vein pulsation above the sternal angle is 4 cm or less. If the measurement is greater than 4 cm, this can indicate increased pressure in the right atrium and right heart failure. However, pericarditis and tricuspid stenosis may also increase pressure as well as laughing or cough (which can trigger the Valsalva response). The jugular venous pressure is a non-invasive method of estimating central venous pressure although the procedure is usually not accurate with heart rate of over 100/min.

54. C: Red clover is contraindicated with clopidogrel because it increases the risk of bleeding. NSAIDs and salicylates also increase risk of bleeding and should be avoided or monitored carefully. Clopidogrel is an antiplatelet inhibitor (adenosine diphosphate inhibitor). It inhibits platelet aggregation and forming of a clot by changing the membrane so that it can no longer receive the signal to aggregate. Adverse effects include bleeding, chest pain, hypertension, edema, flu-like symptoms, abdominal pain, indigestion, diarrhea, epistaxis, rash, pruritus, bradycardia, dizziness, edema, leg and pelvic pain, and chills.

55 A: The balloon for a pulmonary artery catheter is usually inflated when the catheter tip reaches the right atrium, allowing it to float through the right ventricle and into the right pulmonary artery. The balloon should be inflated to a maximum of 1.5 mL of air. The waveforms and pressures should be recorded as the catheter passes from the right atrium into the pulmonary artery where it occludes the vessel in position for recording of pulmonary artery wedge pressure (PAWP). Once the PAWP is obtained, the balloon is deflated and the catheter secured.

56. D: Patients with delirium tremens (onset usually greater than 48 hours after drinking cessation) frequently exhibit global confusion, hallucinations, delusions, fever, tachycardia, and hypertension. Patients may become very aggressive and violent as they respond to feelings of paranoia and fear. Many patients feel as though something is crawling on their skin and may believe they are dying. DTs occur in about 5% of patients undergoing alcohol withdrawal and can be fatal without prompt treatment. Patients may progress from alcohol intoxication to alcohol withdrawal, to DTs.

57. A: Spontaneous wedging can occur if the catheter becomes displaced, often from the patient moving about or from migration of the catheter. The first action should be to try to dislodge the catheter by turning the patient onto the opposite side of the catheter placement. Other interventions include asking the patient to raise or straighten the arm or turn the head and gently cough. If this does not resolve the problem, then the catheter may need to be repositioned.

58. B: Celiac disease results in malabsorption of folate and iron, so patients are often anemic. Additionally, damage to the lining of the small intestines from gluten sensitivity interferes with absorption of fats and calcium, so patients may exhibit osteomalacia and bone pain and steatorrhea. Celiac disease is an autoimmune disorder in which antibodies to gluten in the diet cause inflammation and damage to intestinal villi. Patients must be maintained on a strict gluten-free diet. Gluten is found in some grains, such as wheat.

59. D: An intra-abdominal pressure of more than 25 mmHg indicates the need for immediate surgical decompression to prevent cardiovascular and renal damage. Normal intra-abdominal pressures range from 0 to 5 mmHg, but perfusion of internal organs may be impaired with pressures above 13 mmHg. Below 25 mmHg, treatment usually includes hypervolemic therapy to expand volume and improve perfusion. If decompression is indicated, crystalloids are usually administered first to prevent too rapid reperfusion, which can cause acidosis and cardiac arrest.

60. B: CPAP is titrated at bedtime after the patient has participated in a demonstration of the equipment and usually begins with the pressure set at low at about 5 cm H_2O until the patient falls asleep after which the pressure is slowly increased by 1 cm H_2O every 15 minutes with the patient carefully observed until relief of symptoms occurs. During titration, the patient is usually placed in supine position. The pressure may be adjusted up and down until optimal pressure is achieved.

61. C: In order to calculate the stroke volume, the patient's cardiac output and heart rate must be known. If the cardiac output is 5.6 L/min, this equals 5600 mL. If the heart rate is 80, then the calculation is: CO/HR = SV, 5600/80 = 70 mL. Normal cardiac output ranges from 4 to 6 L per minute. Normal SV is 60 to 70 mL per heartbeat.

62. A: Oxygen should help relieve hypoxemia. Inotropes, such as dobutamine, improve contractility of the heart, increasing the CO (normal 4-6 L/min) and SV (normal 60-70 mL/beat). Vasodilators, such as nitroprusside, should decrease the SVR and PAWP. Combined action should decrease the heart rate and improve the blood pressure, which should in turn increase the MAP, which is barely within normal range (70 to 110 mmHg). MAP of at least 60 mmHg is required for adequate perfusion.

63. C: Characteristics of a Q-wave myocardial infarction include peak CK levels at 27 hours (compared to 12 to 13 hours for non-Q-wave MI). Infarction of the coronary artery is usually prolonged with coronary occlusion complete in 80 to 90%. Most but not all Q-wave MIs are transmural. As the tissue damage approaches the full-thickness of the heart muscle, Q waves (wide and deep) begin to appear on the ECG, especially early in the morning because of adrenergic activity. The mortality rate for Q-wave MI is about 10%.

64. B: Fluid intelligence is the ability to see relationships, reason, and think abstractly—all qualities needed to facilitate learning. Older adults tend to have altered time perception so that time seems to pass more quickly than when they were younger, so they may focus more on the here and now rather than on future needs. Other changes include increased test anxiety, decreased short-term (rather than long-term) memory, increased processing and reaction time, and persistence of stimuli (confusing older learning with newer).

65. A: The femoral nerve may become damaged during the fem-pop bypass procedure, resulting in numbness and tingling in the anterior and medial aspects of the thigh. The femoral nerve activates muscles used to extend the leg and move the hips, so damage may impair mobility (depending upon the degree). The damage may occur as direct injury or from compression related to edema and inflammation. The symptoms may recede over time, although some patients will need physical therapy to strengthen muscles.

66. D: The two types of drugs most commonly implicated in acute hypoglycemia are insulins and sulfonylureas, including glipizide (Glucotrol), which stimulates beta cells in the pancreas to produce more insulin. The hypoglycemic effect of sulfonylureas may be potentiated by other medications that compete for binding sites on albumin. Patients with sulfonylurea-induced hypoglycemia and altered mental status require hospitalization, IV glucose, and careful monitoring, since oral ingestion of carbohydrates alone may not prevent relapses, which may occur for days.

67. B: Because bronchiolitis obliterans is a progression of allograft rejection, the usual treatment approach is to increase immunosuppression, often initially with methylprednisolone, although there is little evidence this actually improves the condition, and it may further increase risk of infection. Bronchiolitis obliterans results in inflammation of the small airways and fibrosis with development of intraluminal polyps and hyperplasia that obstructs the bronchioles and may extend into the alveolar ducts and distal alveoli. Prognosis is poor.

68. B: Because warfarin decreases the clotting time, warfarin should be discontinued two to three days prior to the procedure and the INR should be under 2. Vitamin K or fresh frozen plasma may be administered to reverse the effects of warfarin if necessary. Aspirin and other antiplatelet medications are usually given before cardiac catheterization. Heparin therapy can be continued during cardiac catheterization but discontinued for removal of the sheath.

69. C: These signs and symptoms are characteristic of complete small bowel obstruction (especially not passing flatus for more than 12 hours), the dilated loops of small bowel, and the lack of air in the colon and rectum; so, the initial intervention is likely to be exploratory surgery since the risk for ischemia is high. If the blockage is in the proximal part of the small bowel, abdominal distention may not be evident. Laboratory studies, such as the complete blood count and electrolytes, may be normal or abnormal, depending on many factors.

70. B: These signs and symptoms are consistent with acute pulmonary edema; and since the client is dyspneic and cyanotic, the nurse should immediately sit the patient upright and administer 100% oxygen per mask to relieve the patient's hypoxemia and achieve a PO_2 above 60%. Some patients may require BiPAP or endotracheal intubation and mechanical ventilation. Morphine sulfate (2 to 8 mg) may be administered subcutaneously or intravenously in severe cases. Other treatments include loop diuretics to promote venous dilation and diuresis, nitrates, bronchodilators, digoxin (if tachycardia present), and ACE inhibitors to reduce afterload.

71. D: Signs and symptoms of retroperitoneal hemorrhage may be nonspecific, especially at first, but as blood accumulates, back and flank pain may occur. Pulse rate increases and blood pressure will fall as the patient becomes increasingly hypotensive. Hemoglobin may show an abrupt decrease. A CT scan of the abdomen should show the mass. This is a medical emergency, and the patient must be transferred immediately back to the cath lab for angiography to locate the site of perforation and leakage. A vascular closure device may be used, and/or a balloon inflated over the bleeding site to control bleeding.

72. C: When undergoing pericardiocentesis, the patient should be positioned upright at 45 degrees because this allows good visualization and easy access and brings the heart closer to the chest wall. Patients often receive atropine before the procedure to prevent vasovagal reactions. A nasogastric tube may need to be inserted if the patient has abdominal distention. After the needle is inserted, the obturator is removed and a syringe attached to aspirate blood or fluid. A sterile alligator clamp is attached from the needle to a precordial lead of the ECG for monitoring to ensure that the ventricle is not punctured.

73. D: Stimulation threshold testing is conducted to determine the minimum output necessary to consistently capture the heart. Once the output for consistent capture is determined, the output should be set at 2 to 3 times this level, so if threshold testing shows consistent capture at 2 mA, the output should be set at 4 to 6 mA. The procedure for sensitivity testing is: first, verify paced rhythm, increasing rate temporarily if necessary, to override intrinsic rhythm; then watch monitor while slowly decreasing output and not when loss of capture occurs; gradually increase output until 1:1 capture resumes; and set output.

74. B: The symptoms are consistent with thoracic aortic aneurysm. Patients with Marfan syndrome are at risk for thoracic aortic aneurysms and should be monitored carefully to prevent rupture. Surgery is indicated for aneurysms of 5 cm or more. With MFS, the aneurysm usually occurs at the sinuses of Valsalva (aortic root) and in most cases is ascending with type A dissection. It the aneurysm is in the ascending aorta or arch; open surgical repair is indicated and carries a higher risk than repairs in the descending aorta. Beta-blockers may slow aneurysm dilation.

75. A: Wool, plastics, and polyurethane foam produce cyanide gas when burned, so the patient is at risk for cyanide poisoning and should receive hydroxocobalamin as the antidote of choice. It is usually administered with sodium thiosulfate, which potentiates the effects. Hydroxocobalamin combines chemically with cyanide to form vitamin B_{12}, which can be excreted through the kidneys. Sodium nitrite can also be used for cyanide poisoning but has more adverse effects and is contraindicated with severe smoke inhalation.

76. D: Flexor (decorticate) posturing indicates hemispheric damage. Brainstem damage results in flaccidity and areflexia while midbrain and upper pons damage results in extensor (decerebrate) posturing. Anoxic encephalopathy can occur within 5 minutes if the brain is without oxygenation. Absence of pupillary responses and elicited eye movements indicates severe brain damage. If there is damage to the frontal or occipital areas of the brain but the midbrain and pons are intact, horizontal movement of the eyes may be evident.

77. C: Patients are at high risk for fatal or non-fatal MI if they have unstable angina and the following findings: ECG changes including transient ST-segment changes greater than 0.05 mV, persistent VT, and BBB; troponin T elevated to greater than 0.1 ng/mL; increased ischemic symptoms in previous 48 hours; rest pain longer than 20 minutes; pulmonary edema, new or increased MR murmur, S3 or increased rales; decreased BP; bradycardia or tachycardia; and advanced age (over 75). T-wave inversion, pathologic Q waves, and slight elevation of Troponin T (<0.1 ng/mL) are moderate risk factors.

78. A: Pulmonic stenosis constricts blood flow from the right ventricle to the lungs, resulting in right ventricular hypertrophy as the pressure increases in the right ventricle. Respiratory symptoms develop as pulmonary blood flow is decreased, including dyspnea and mild cyanosis. Depending on the degree of stenosis, some patients may be asymptomatic, or symptoms may develop slowly and not be evident until adulthood. Treatment includes balloon valvuloplasty to separate valve cusps in younger children and pulmonary valvotomy for adults and older children.

79. A: Primary graft dysfunction (reperfusion injury) is a major cause of illness and death in lung recipients with symptoms and treatment similar to ARDS. Indications include frequent oxygen desaturation, general malaise, increased dyspnea and work associated with the act of breathing, and intolerance to activity. Causes may include increased capillary permeability, interrupted lymphatic drainage, edema, and mismatch in compliance and vascular resistance between donor and recipient. Treatment includes high oxygen concentrations, decreased tidal volumes, PP ventilation for those intubated, and increased oxygen supplementation and pulmonary toileting for those extubated.

80. D: The best approach is to attempt to collaborate with the patient, allowing the patient to feel more in control: "Let's talk about how we can work together to make this easier for you." There can be many reasons why patients are uncooperative and have an exaggerated response to pain. The patient may simply be frustrated, or the patient may be tired or fearful. It's possible that the pain medication isn't adequate, but the nurse needs to really listen to the patient to try to determine the best solution.

81. B: SvO_2 measures oxygen saturation in mixed venous blood via a catheter in the pulmonary artery. Normal value is 60 to 80%. SaO_2 measures oxygen saturation in arterial blood with a gas analyzer. Normal value is 96 to 100%. SpO_2 measures oxygen saturation with a pulse oximeter. Normal value is also 96 to 100%. $ScvO_2$ measures oxygen saturation in mixed venous blood from the head, neck, arms and upper thorax per a fiber-optic catheter or central venous catheter. Normal value is greater than 70% and is usually 5 to 10% higher than SvO_2 value.

82. D: Extra gastric hemorrhage most often occurs 24 to 48 hours after surgery and may present with sudden onset of hypotension, tachycardia, and diminished urinary output. Peritoneal drains may show some bloody or blood-tinged discharged while NG aspirant remains essentially clear. Symptoms may mimic myocardial infarction. CT scan is used for diagnosis. Causes of bleeding include lacerated spleen, liver injury (from retractors), pancreatic bed hemorrhage, and improperly secured vessels. If blood transfusions do not stabilize the patient, then exploratory laparotomy is indicated.

83. B: A high-fat, high-protein, and low-carbohydrate diet is recommended for patients after gastric surgery to prevent or minimize dumping syndrome. Carbohydrates are absorbed more quickly than fats or proteins, increasing dumping symptoms. Additionally, a high-carbohydrate diet may exacerbate the postprandial hypoglycemia that often occurs two to three hours after a patient eats because of the sudden bolus of high carbohydrates that enters the small intestine and triggers release of insulin. Lying down after eating helps to slow the movement of food through the GI tract, decreasing symptoms.

84. A: The patient is exhibiting signs of mild lithium toxicity. Symptoms of mild toxicity are evident with levels 1.5 to 2.5 mEq/L. The therapeutic level of lithium for maintenance therapy is 0.6 to 1.2

mEq/L and 1.0 to 1.5 mEq/L for acute episodes of mania. Lithium has a narrow therapeutic index and levels should be monitored weekly initially and then monthly with patients educated about signs of toxicity. More severe life-threatening symptoms (ECG abnormalities, seizures, coma) can occur with blood levels above 2.5 mEq/L.

85. C: Although the patient's platelet count remains above 100,000, a reduction of 30% to 50% with evidence of thrombi and vascular occlusion is indicative of heparin-induced thrombocytopenia Type II, which is an immune-mediated response to heparin. While most often associated with unfractionated heparin, it can also be caused by low-molecular-weight heparin, so the intervention is to immediately discontinue the heparin and administer lepirudin or argatroban. HIT Type II can be confirmed with the functional assays heparin-induced platelet aggregation (HIPA) and serotonin release assay (SRA). ELISA can be used to identify presence of HIT antigen.

86. B: The primary problem with basing research on qualitative data is that the data are subjective, and objective data have more validity for research. However, both may provide valuable information. Qualitative data are usually described verbally or in graphic form. Gathering qualitative data can require considerable time because it may involve interviewing numerous participants. Quantitative data, which are described statistically, may be derived from surveys, questionnaires, and other methods of obtaining numerical data.

87. A: The most critical concern after AVM repair (surgery or embolization) is reperfusion bleeding, so strict control of BP to prevent it from exceeding the maximum established (usually 140 systolic) must be maintained. As feeder arteries are occluded, blood is diverted into vessels that are maximally dilated and tissues that have often suffered from chronic ischemia, so the increased pressure from additional blood flow may cause leakage of blood from the vessels. To prevent reperfusion bleeding, AVM repair is often done in two to four stages with partial embolization or excision done at each stage.

88. D: The patient has burns covering approximately 27% of his body. The Rule of 9s is used to estimate total body surface area burned in order to calculate the need for fluid replacement and other treatments. Rule of 9s: each arm 9% (4.5% anterior and 4.5% posterior), each leg 18% (9% anterior and 9% posterior), groin area 1%, upper chest 9%, abdomen 9%, upper back 9%, lower back/buttocks 9%, head 9% (4.5% anterior and 4.5% posterior).

89. C: While idiopathic thrombocytopenia purpura is often self-limiting, because the patient is exhibiting symptoms, this puts her at risk for more serious complications (such as intracerebral hemorrhage), so the usual initial treatment is a course of oral corticosteroids, which usually results in an increase of the platelet count to normal level within 2 to 6 weeks. If symptoms are severe, then IV Ig may be used to suppress the antibody response. High-dose IV methylprednisolone may also be administered. Following IV Ig or methylprednisolone, platelet transfusions are recommended. If no response to medical treatment, splenectomy may be considered.

90. B: The patient is in uncompensated respiratory acidosis, indicating hypoventilation: PaO_2 of 88 mmHg (normal value 80 to 100) indicates the patient is not hypoxemic; pH of 7.28 (normal value 7.35 to 7.45) indicates acidosis since it is greater than 7.4; $PaCO_2$ of 48 mmHg (normal value 35 to 45) represents respiratory acidosis resulting from hypoventilation since the value if greater than 45 (less than 35 would represent respiratory alkalosis); HCO_3^- of 23 mEq/L (normal value 22 to 26) remains normal. Because both the pH and the $PaCO_2$ are abnormal, this indicates uncompensated ABGs, since the pH has not returned to normal level.

91. A: Usually for severe dehydration related to DKA, 1 to 1.5 L of 0.9% normal saline with insulin is administered at the rate of 1 L/hour, after which serum sodium levels should be determined. If the serum sodium is low, IVs and insulin are continued with 0.9% normal saline at the rate of 4 to 14 mL/kg, but if sodium is normal or high, the IV fluids are switched to 0.45% sodium chloride at the rate of 4 to 14 mL/kg until serum glucose reaches 250 mg/dL. Then IV fluid is changed to 5% dextrose with 0.45% sodium chloride (150-250 mL/hr.).

92. C: These laboratory values are consistent with diabetes insipidus. Desmopressin acetate is used to increase water resorption in the nephron. Central DI often develops secondary to neurosurgery, traumatic brain injury, meningitis, and encephalitis. Inadequate amounts of vasopressin are secreted, resulting in dilute urine with decreased osmolality and specific gravity with frequent urination while serum osmolality and serum sodium increase, resulting in increased thirst. Thiazide diuretics are used with nephrogenic DI and hypertonic saline solution and demeclocycline with severe SIADH.

93. B: The primary difference between HHNK and DKA is that HHNK does not involve breakdown of fats (into ketones) and DKA does because some insulin production remains with HHNK although it is inadequate to prevent hyperglycemia (greater than 600 mg/dL). HHNK is a disease that occurs in those with diabetes and insulin resistance, leading to persistent hyperglycemia and osmotic diuresis. As fluid shifts from intracellular to extracellular spaces, glucosuria and dehydration cause hypernatremia and increased serum osmolality (greater than 350 mOsm/L). Treatment is similar to DKA: insulin and IV fluids.

94. C: Asking a nurse on another unit about his experience with a procedure is an example of informal collaboration because the collaboration does not stem from established organization or protocol, such as teams or hierarchical structures. When members of a team help each other, this represents formal collaboration because that is the purpose of a team. Collaboration is a continuous process in nursing, occurring almost every time a healthcare provider interacts with other healthcare providers, patients, or family members. Both informal and formal collaboration may be equally valuable.

95. B: All of the laboratory values are within normal limits except for the BUN, which is elevated to 26 from a normal of 7 to 17 mg/dL (reference values may vary somewhat). While this is outside the normal range, it is usually evaluated with creatinine to determine if there is kidney damage, and the creatinine level is normal. BUN values may be elevated by dehydration and some commonly-used drugs, such as acetaminophen and ibuprofen.

96. D: The best response is the one that provides the reason for early surgery: "The risk of re-bleeding increases every day, putting you at grave risk if you delay." Approximately 4% of patients experience re-bleeding during the first 24 hours with a 1 to 2% chance of re-bleeding every day for at least a month. Re-bleeding carries a mortality rate of approximately 70%. Surgical repair, which may include clipping or embolization, is usually scheduled within 48 hours for grades I and II and for some grade III SAH.

97. C: The immediate intervention for directly observed aspiration is suction of the upper airway to prevent further aspiration by removing remaining gastric contents. Following this, oxygen should be administered as needed while the patient awaits bronchoscopy for removal of large particles. Bronchoalveolar lavage poses the risk of disseminating the aspirant throughout the lung fields, causing more damage. The most common sites for aspiration infiltration are the right middle lobe and lower lobes, but this can vary depending on the patient's position and volume of aspirant.

98. B: The first-line treatment for obstructive sleep apnea (OSA) is CPAP. OSA occurs when the pharynx collapses during sleep because of narrow or restricted airway. It is most common in those who are overweight, especially middle-aged males. It is characterized by heavy snoring with apneic periods that may last up to one minute, usually at least 30 times per night. CPAP delivers pressurized room air to a nasal or oral interface/mask and allows for adjusting of airflow and expels carbon dioxide through a vent or valve. Most machines can provide pressures ranging from 2 to 20 cmH$_2$O.

99. A: If dysrhythmias occur during apnea testing, the nurse should obtain a blood sample for ABGs and reconnect the ventilator, since the testing should not be the cause of death. Apnea testing includes disconnecting the ventilator and administering 100% oxygen at 6L/min per endotracheal tube. The patient is observed closely for respiratory movements and a blood sample obtained for ABGs after 8 minutes. Then, the patient is reconnected to the ventilator. During the test, the patient's core body temperature should be maintained at 36.5 °C or higher with a systolic BP at 90 mmHg or higher. Euvolemia and eucapnia (PaCO$_2$ about 40 mmHg) should be established.

100. B: The most important factor in having a patient sign a consent form is the patient's ability to give informed consent. This means that the patient must have the legal right by age or emancipation and must be able to comprehend. If a patient is cognitively impaired because of dementia, sedation, or condition, this can pose a problem because patients cannot legally give consent if they are unable to understand. If patients don't speak English, a translator should be provided.

101. D: Controlled mandatory ventilation (CMV): This mode provides a specified volume of air and rate with no triggering required of the patient and respiratory response decreased through medication. Synchronized intermittent mandatory ventilation (SIMV): This mode provides a specified tidal volume that is synchronized with the patient's breathing. Assist control ventilation (ACV): This mode is triggered by the patient's own breathing, but if apneic periods occur, the machine will initiate respirations at a specified tidal volume. Pressure support ventilation (PSV): This mode requires the patient to initiate all breaths, which are supplemented by positive pressure.

102. D: While bilateral periorbital ecchymosis (Raccoon's eyes) may indicate eye trauma (as well as multiple myeloma and disseminated neuroblastoma), it is likely that the patient has a basilar skull fracture because of the previous car accident. Raccoon's eyes may not be evident for two to three days after an injury, but the "salty" taste in the patient's mouth suggests leakage of cerebrospinal fluid. In some cases, Battle's sign—ecchymosis in the mastoid area behind the ear—may be present as well.

103. B: While it's very unlikely that a miracle cure will occur as a result of positive thinking, patients often need to hold onto hope to cope with dying, and thinking positively may help them to find some peace, so the nurse should be supportive without making false claims, dismissing the idea, or trying to dissuade the person with reason. Additionally, positive thinking may increase the release of endorphins, which may help to alleviate some discomfort.

104. B: For ventilator management, the fraction of inspired oxygen (FiO$_2$) should be maintained below 40% (0.4) to avoid oxygen toxicity although the patient may initially need a higher concentration of oxygen. Normal room air provides 21% (0.2). The flow rate will vary depending on the type of oxygen delivery system used. For example, with a nasal cannula at flow rate of 5 L/min, FiO$_2$ is 40%. With a Venturi mask and flow rate of 8 L/min, FiO$_2$ is 35 to 40%.

105. D: The best and only legal action is to ignore the parents, as they have no standing. Rights go with the individual patient, not the one for paying for insurance. Because the patient is 18 years old and legally an adult, he has the right to decide who visits or not, and the parents should have been advised of this. The nurse cannot legally contact the parents about the patient without his permission. He should be advised of the parents' action so that he can deal with the issue.

106. A: Because the patient sustained a head injury and is at risk for increased intracranial pressure, the patient should have a CT of the brain prior to the procedure so it can be reviewed for signs of a brain shift that may indicate ICP. With increased ICP, when pressure is suddenly relieved by withdrawing of cerebral spinal fluid, the brain structures may herniate through the foramen magnum, compressing the brainstem, which is critical for regulation of cardiac and respiratory function.

107. A: Trauma patients should be provided 1 to 1.5 g/kg/day of protein. Higher amounts show no benefit. Trauma results in increased breakdown of protein because of catabolism in addition to protein losses that may have occurred with blood loss. Patients may lose as much as 10% of lean body mass within 10 days. When 25% or more of lean body mass is lost, protein malnutrition is severe and can result in increased mortality. Protein is more critical than total calories and the increased catabolic rate resists protein supplementation although synthesis of protein increases with infusions of amino acids.

108. C: About 25% of those with subarachnoid hemorrhage develop hydrocephalus as a late complication because blood that has been absorbed by arachnoid villi may result in villi obstruction and decreased absorption of cerebrospinal fluid. In about half of these cases, the condition is self-limiting and resolves without intervention, so if patients remain awake and responsive and do not have severe symptoms, observation for 24 hours is the usual initial intervention. If the patient's condition worsens, then in some cases serial lumbar punctures are done to drain fluid, but the most common treatment is ventriculostomy or ventriculoperitoneal shunt.

109. B: Patients often establish close relationships with nurses caring for them and begin to develop dependency, so the best solution is for the nurse to make the transfer as easy as possible is by accompanying the patient to her new room and introducing her to staff, ensuring that the patient is settled into her new unit without difficulty. The nurse should not make unrealistic promises (such as daily visits) that she may not be able to keep.

110. C: Phenytoin may cause gingival hyperplasia, so patients should be advised to carefully maintain dental care and to see dentists regularly. Patients may have monthly blood tests initially but once stabilized blood tests are usually done every six months. Patients should be advised to avoid alcohol entirely when taking any anticonvulsant drug. Stopping anticonvulsant drugs abruptly may trigger rebound seizures, so if adverse effects occur, the patient should be advised to immediately contact the physician for guidance in withdrawing the drug if necessary.

111. C: Intracranial hypertension occurs with intracranial pressure greater than 20 mmHg. Normal intracranial pressure ranges from 7 to 15 mmHg. Because of the constraints of the skull, the volume in the brain is fixed and has 3 components: blood, tissue, and cerebrospinal fluid. According to the Kelli-Moore hypothesis, an increase in one component requires a compensating decrease in another component. The brain may accommodate some increase in volume with little increase in ICP, but when the brain's volume limit is reached, even a small increase in volume may result in a significant increase in ICP.

112. A: When patients receiving CCRT exhibit increased heart rate, decreased blood pressure and ECG abnormalities, the nurse should suspect electrolyte imbalance. Electrolyte levels must be carefully monitored and output values checked at least every hour. Hypotension may also decrease the ultrafiltration rate as blood flow through lines decreases. Fluid volume must also be monitored since too much or too little fluid may result in changes in mentation and increased or decreased CVP or PAOP.

113. B: While in most cases it is inappropriate to use family members—especially children—to interpret, the granddaughter can be asked to assist because the directions for the test are relatively simple ("How old are you? What is the date today?"). In all cases, the nurse may use some type of pantomime to assist the patient, such as demonstrating how to show the teeth when scoring facial palsy. The patient's first response should be recorded. The granddaughter should be asked not to coach the patient in any way or give hints.

114. A: The usual contraindications to recombinant tPA apply to people who have had strokes and appear for treatment within the 3-hour window after the stroke, but additional exclusions apply to those who appear in the 3- to 4.5-hour window. This patient is excluded from treatment because he is over 80 years old. Other exclusions include a history of both stroke and diabetes, score on the NIH stroke scale of more than 25, and any current use of oral anticoagulants.

115. D: Metabolic acidosis is associated with acute renal failure because the impaired kidneys are unable to excrete increased levels of acids due to decreased excretion of phosphates and other organic acids and because the tubules are unable to excrete ammonia or reabsorb sodium bicarbonate. Characteristics of metabolic acidosis include low (acidic) pH level and decreased bicarbonate. Symptoms may vary, but with chronic renal failure, the patient may remain asymptomatic until the bicarbonate level falls to 15 mEq/L or less.

116. B: With fractures of ribs 8 and above on the right side, the primary concern is injury to the spleen. Fractured ribs are usually the results of severe blunt trauma, so underlying injuries are common. With fractures of ribs 8 and above on the left side, the primary concern is injury to the liver. Fractures of the upper two ribs (either one side or both) pose a risk of injury to the trachea, bronchi, and great vessels. If three or more adjacent ribs are fractured both anteriorly and posteriorly, a flail chest results.

117. C: Studies show that most adults experience a period of low energy in the afternoon (the reason for afternoon naps). About 55% of adults are most alert and work and study best in the early morning while about 28% do best in the evening, so group education is probably best planned for morning while individual education should be more flexible according to the patient's preference whenever possible. Most people are aware whether they are "morning" or "evening" people.

118. D: Displacement: The patient directs anger at other individuals (the wife in this case) rather than directing it at the person (physician), who is the actual source of bad news (threat). Projection: The patient believes that others are exhibiting the patient's own unacceptable characteristics (seeing in others what the person cannot recognize in himself/herself). Reaction formation: The patient behaves or expresses the opposite of how the patient actually feels. Sublimation: The patient converts repressed feelings into actions that are socially acceptable.

119. B: Patients who are legally blind often have developed the ability to compensate for lack of vision with increased acuity in other senses, including the sense of touch, smell, hearing, and taste. Patients who are blind should be encouraged to handle and manipulate equipment while the nurse explains, using as much verbal description as possible. Patients may have developed improved memory skills that allow them to learn quickly from spoken words. Family members may want to learn about the equipment as well, but the focus should be on teaching the patient to use it independently.

120. A: The first-line treatment for acute exacerbations of asthma is short-acting B$_2$-agonsit, such as nebulized albuterol and a corticosteroid, such as oral prednisone or IV methylprednisolone. While corticosteroids will not have immediate effect, it is important to administer the drug early to maintain control. Nonspecific B-adrenergic agents, such as epinephrine, are usually reserved for treatment before intubation for patients unresponsive to other treatments. Anticholinergic medications, such as ipratropium bromide, may be added to albuterol. Theophylline has many side effects so is often avoided. IV magnesium and heliox are usually given only if patients do not respond to other treatments.

121. D: The nurse provided the CD for the patient to help relieve the patient's anxiety and to show caring. This is an example of caring practice in which the nurse carries out acts of kindness and provides a supportive caring relationship for the patient. Caring practices require the nurse to take a creative approach to care and to look at the needs of the whole person. The nurse makes a choice to take action for the benefit of the patient, often beyond that which is required.

122. C: Many patients are afraid of their doctors or don't want to bother them, so prompting the patient or telling the physician that the patient has questions may still not elicit them. The best method is to prepare a list of the patient's questions for the physician and to explain the patient's reluctance to ask the physician the questions directly. The patient may not be able or willing to articulate the reasons for not asking questions directly.

123. D: Collegiality: interacting with others and contributing to professional development of peers and other healthcare providers. Quality of care: evaluating the quality of care in a systematic manner. Education: acquiring and maintaining both current knowledge and competencies necessary to provide care to the critically ill. Collaboration: working together with patients, families, and health care providers to provide excellence in patient care. Ethics: making decisions and acting in an ethical manner. Individual practice evaluation: reflecting knowledge of professional and legal standards, laws, and regulations. Research: using clinical inquiry. Resource utilization: considering safety, effectiveness, and cost.

124. C: Talking to people who aren't there and who have died is often a sign of impending death. Patients nearing death may also say they must prepare for a trip and may describe a place they appear to be able to see. Some patients express awareness that they are dying. The role of the nurse is to remain supportive to the patient and the family and provide as much comfort care as possible. When treatments are no longer necessary or effective because the patient is dying, the nurse should request discontinuation of the treatments.

125. D: There are three barriers to systems thinking here. Identifying with professional role instead of purpose: looking only at one's own role and needs and not considering the roles of others and the institution as a whole. Feeling victimized: blaming others (institution, administration, other healthcare professional) for own shortcomings and believing nothing can be done to improve situations. This feeling may become institutionalized, making changes difficult. Relying on past experience: persisting in trying to apply old solutions to new problems.

126. D: There are four barriers to systems thinking here. Failing to adapt: feeling very threatened by changes, such as the switch to electronic charting. Some may feel they cannot learn new procedures and may react angrily or withdraw. Having an autocratic attitude: believing that only their perceptions or practices are the correct one and focusing on narrow views and short-term outcomes. Arriving at weak consensus: superficially solving problems without really delving into all issues. Displaying displaced anger: directing anger at someone or something other than the cause of the problem.

127. C: V/Q mismatch, which occurs when well-ventilated alveoli lack adequate perfusion while poorly-ventilated alveoli have adequate perfusion, is the most common cause of hypoxemia. This is true because many common respiratory disorders can result in V/Q mismatch, including asthma, COPD, pulmonary embolus, pneumonia, and pulmonary hypertension. With V/Q mismatch, administration of 100% oxygen should increase oxygen saturation because oxygen improves uptake of oxygen in areas with poor ventilation. Dead space occurs when there is ventilation but no perfusion (such as in the trachea), and a shunt occurs where there is perfusion but no ventilation.

128. C: Rigid bronchoscopy is the treatment option of choice for removal of foreign bodies from the respiratory tract because the larger diameter makes retrieval less difficult. In some cases, flexible bronchoscopy may be used first to isolate the location of the foreign body, but the diameter is generally too small to withdraw foreign objects and attempting to grasp the object at the end of the scope and remove it in that manner may result in significant tissue damage. Bronchotomy is indicated if removal per bronchoscopy is unsuccessful. Bronchodilators and postural drainage is useful in only a small number of asymptomatic cases.

129. B: A patient with progressive pulmonary arterial hypertension must be monitored for signs of right ventricular heart failure, a common complication. With PAH, the pulmonary vascular bed becomes obstructed or damaged so that it cannot dilate adequately for increased blood flow, so this blood then increases pulmonary artery pressure, which in turn increases pulmonary vascular resistance. This requires increased workload for the right ventricle, leading to hypertrophy and failure. The patient may begin to have peripheral edema, ascites, liver engorgement, crackles, distended jugular veins, and heart murmur.

130. A: Heliox should be administered for at least 20 minutes in order for the patient to gain the full effects. Heliox is usually administered in mixtures of 80% He/20% O_2 or 70% He/30% O_2. The 70/30 mixture is indicated for patients with hypoxemia, so this mixture is more commonly used. Heliox is used to reduce airway resistance in order to increase oxygenation. Recent studies indicate that evidence is insufficient to recommend use of heliox for acute asthma or COPD exacerbations, although it is frequently ordered.

131. C: The nurse who suggested the switch to acuity-based staffing is exercising systems thinking by looking at the organization as a whole and determining what best serves the organization and the patients rather than looking at only the needs of the unit. Systems thinking requires an understanding of interrelationships and structures as well as the ability to anticipate outcomes and understand how different actions affect outcomes. The nurse has applied a practical solution to a systems problem.

132. A: While all of these are important considerations when evaluating the validity of written material, the source of the material is the primary concern followed by the author's credentials. Articles printed in the popular press must meet different standards than articles printed in juried journals (such as *The New England Journal of Medicine*). The Internet has few rules, so much that is found on websites may look authentic but have no validity whatsoever. Wikipedia, while often helpful, cannot ever be used for evidence.

133. D: Adhesive atelectasis, caused by surfactant deficiency is most often associated with acute respiratory distress syndrome because surfactant production, which is critical to maintaining alveolar surface tension, is reduced, so alveoli collapse. With ARDS, alveolar collapse occurs widely throughout both lungs rather than in isolated areas, such as may occur with other causes of atelectasis. PEEP must be adequate to prevent further alveolar collapse in order to improve oxygenation.

134. A: Increasing dyspnea and hypoxemia with cough, hemoptysis, substernal pain, and subcutaneous emphysema of neck and chest are consistent with perforation of the trachea, which is a complication of endotracheal intubation. Perforation, especially in the posterior trachea, can occur during intubation or extubation. With this surgery, repositioning after surgery could also increase risks. Slight perforations may heal spontaneously with artificial airway that seals the perforation, but many, especially those who have cardiovascular instability, cannot adequately ventilate the lungs, or have tears greater than 4 cm, will require thoracotomy to repair.

135. B: Air leaks are a very common complication following bilateral lung volume reduction regardless of the surgical approach (VATS or median sternotomy). Patients return from surgery with two chest tubes in each hemithorax, and these are usually placed immediately in water seal drainage. Other complications include pneumonia, cardiac dysrhythmias, and infection. A small number of patients may go into respiratory failure and require reintubation. Adequate pain control is important to allow the patient to clear secretions and to encourage movement.

136. D: While onset of symptoms varies depending on many factors, including the severity of injury, usual signs and symptoms of acute respiratory distress syndrome (the most common complication of lung contusion) usually occur within 24 to 48 hours when hypoxemia becomes more obvious. Contusion results in pulmonary edema because of torn capillaries and micro-hemorrhage. Alveoli collapse and atelectasis are common. Inflammation occurs, increasing risk of respiratory failure. Ventilation/perfusion mismatch decreases oxygen saturation. Damage from chest contusion may not be visible on chest radiograph for a number of hours. CT scans or ultrasounds are more accurate.

137. A: These symptoms (decreased PaO_2 less than 60 mmHg, increased $PaCO_2$ greater than 45 mmHg, and decreased pH) are consistent with acute respiratory failure, type II, which is usually the result of alveolar hypoventilation and hypoxemia. With chronic respiratory failure, which usually develops over a period of days, the pH is closer to normal because of compensation. Patients with hypoventilation should be positioned in semi-erect position. Treatment includes oxygen, ventilation, bronchodilators, steroids, sedatives, and analgesics, nutritional support, correction of acidosis, and monitoring for complications.

138. C: Patients with exertional heat stroke (EHS) are at high risk for rhabdomyolysis, DIC, and renal failure, while these are rare with non-exertional heat stroke (NEHS). Because patients with EHS can still sweat and exhibit diaphoresis, temperatures tend to be well below the highs (over 41 °C or 106 °F) seen with NEHS, which is associated with anhidrosis. CNS system manifestations may be similar at times. Those with EHS often suffer syncope and loss of consciousness while those with NEHS may exhibit very mild irritability to deep coma.

139. C: The 72-hour protocol for N-acetylcysteine (NAC) is provided with serum levels greater than 150 mcg/mL. Patients often show no symptoms or only slight gastrointestinal upset for the first 24 hours after ingestion of acetaminophen, but evidence of hepatic damage usually is evident by the second day. Toxic dosages are greater than 140 mg/kg in one dose or greater than 7.5 g in 24 hours. Serum levels should always be done because patients often overestimate or underestimate the number of drugs taken.

140. D: Patients who are allergic to bananas, kiwis, avocados, and chestnuts are at increased risk of allergy to latex because of cross reactivity and should be maintained in a latex-free environment. Reactions may occur with 5 types of exposure: inhalational, contact, mucous membrane, internal (surgical, invasive procedures), intravascular (IV). Other patients at higher risk include those with multiple surgeries, those with neural tube defects, those with congenital urogenital disorders, and those who work in the rubber industry, and those with allergies to anesthetics.

141. D: Sodium levels vary according to the underlying cause of acute renal failure. Prerenal causes: Urine sodium is decreased to below 20 mEq/L with urine osmolality increased to 500 mOsm. Urine specific gravity is increased. Intrarenal causes: Urine sodium is increased to more than 40 mEq/L, while urine osmolality is usually about 350 mOsm. Urine specific gravity is low normal. Postrenal causes: Urine sodium varies but is usually decreased to 20 mEq/L or less. Urine osmolality also varies but may be equal to or more than the serum level. Urine specific gravity also varies.

142. A: While all of these are important, assigning a task to someone who does not have the necessary skills or time to complete the task can result in the task not being completed correctly or even danger to the patient, so the first thing the nurse must do is determine if the task is appropriate for the person to whom it is delegated. This must be followed by clear instructions, monitoring progress, reviewing the final results, and recording outcomes as the responsibility for the task remains with the delegating nurse.

143. B: The most appropriate referral for the patient is an occupational therapist who can help the patient develop strategies and skills needed to compensate for poor vision and arthritis and provide information about adaptive equipment that the patient can use to prepare food. The occupational therapist can help the patient establish goals for independent food preparation and help the patient modify tasks. The occupational therapist may also help the patient learn how to better manage her arthritis to minimize symptoms.

144. C: Providing sensitive information to patients or family members should be done slowly rather than quickly so that they have time to digest the information. The nurse should ask if they have questions and should avoid technical jargon and consider psychosocial implications and well as cultural differences. It's important to respond to people's feelings and discuss follow-up. The nurse should exercise patience, understanding that people respond to bad news in very different ways, including both anger and silence.

145. B: The best strategy when coaching another nurse is usually to provide positive feedback, stressing the nurse's correct actions rather than focusing on errors because the latter may increase the graduate nurse's anxiety and result in more errors. The nurse may use questioning to help the graduate nurse recognized problem areas. The nurse should provide a demonstration and encourage the graduate nurse to ask questions. The primary objective should be to help the learner gain both confidence and skills.

146. C: Most patients who are maintained of peritoneal dialysis at home should continue to receive PD after admission to a critical care unit unless there are specific contraindications, which include recent abdominal surgery, significant pulmonary disease, peritonitis, and need for rapid removal of fluid. The most common complications of PD are peritonitis and infection of exit site, so the nurse must carefully monitor laboratory values and patient condition for signs of infection. Patients usually are very knowledgeable about the amount and type of dialysate to be infused and the frequency of infusion.

147. A: The patient undergoing a renal biopsy should be placed in prone position because the biopsy is done from the posterior aspect. A small pillow may be placed under the patient's abdomen. The procedure is done under a local anesthetic (1% lidocaine). After removal of the biopsy needle, pressure should be applied. After the site is bandaged, the patient should be placed in supine position for 6 to 8 hours, and the patient should be observed for at least 12 hours to ensure bleeding does not go undetected.

148. A: The bispectral index system (BIS) can be used to both monitor the degree of consciousness for those who are receiving deep sedation and response to analgesia. BIS applies an algorithm to EEG activity and displays the result as a number (0 to 100) rather than a tracing. A value of 50 to 60 is usually the goal for deep sedation in which the patient is unconscious with low likelihood of recall. With values over 70, the patient is probably aware, while a score above 95 indicates an awake state. Brain waves are suppressed with values under 20.

149. A: Diazepam: Onset is 2 to 5 minutes, but the half-life ranges from 20 to 120 hours with prolonged sedation. Lorazepam: Onset is 5 to 20 minutes, and half-life is 8 to 15 hours with prolonged sedation. Propofol: Onset is 1 to 2 minutes with a half-life of 2 to 8 minutes when used for short-term sedation. If administered continuously, the sedative effect may last for 26 to 32 hours. Midazolam: Onset of action is rapid (2 to 5 minutes) and half-life ranges from 3 to 11 hours. Sedative effect is prolonged with continuous administration.

150. B: Because of the risk that periods of apnea associated with severe seizures can lead to respiratory failure and death, if a patient with status epilepticus does not respond to the first two doses of the benzodiazepine anticonvulsant medication, the next step is usually rapid sequence intubation so the patient can be ventilated while treatment continues. Fosphenytoin and phenobarbital may be added, but this may cause apnea, so intubation is necessary prior to administration of the drugs.

How to Overcome Test Anxiety

Just the thought of taking a test is enough to make most people a little nervous. A test is an important event that can have a long-term impact on your future, so it's important to take it seriously and it's natural to feel anxious about performing well. But just because anxiety is normal, that doesn't mean that it's helpful in test taking, or that you should simply accept it as part of your life. Anxiety can have a variety of effects. These effects can be mild, like making you feel slightly nervous, or severe, like blocking your ability to focus or remember even a simple detail.

If you experience test anxiety—whether severe or mild—it's important to know how to beat it. To discover this, first you need to understand what causes test anxiety.

Causes of Test Anxiety

While we often think of anxiety as an uncontrollable emotional state, it can actually be caused by simple, practical things. One of the most common causes of test anxiety is that a person does not feel adequately prepared for their test. This feeling can be the result of many different issues such as poor study habits or lack of organization, but the most common culprit is time management. Starting to study too late, failing to organize your study time to cover all of the material, or being distracted while you study will mean that you're not well prepared for the test. This may lead to cramming the night before, which will cause you to be physically and mentally exhausted for the test. Poor time management also contributes to feelings of stress, fear, and hopelessness as you realize you are not well prepared but don't know what to do about it.

Other times, test anxiety is not related to your preparation for the test but comes from unresolved fear. This may be a past failure on a test, or poor performance on tests in general. It may come from comparing yourself to others who seem to be performing better or from the stress of living up to expectations. Anxiety may be driven by fears of the future—how failure on this test would affect your educational and career goals. These fears are often completely irrational, but they can still negatively impact your test performance.

> **Review Video: 3 Reasons You Have Test Anxiety**
> Visit mometrix.com/academy and enter code: 428468

285

Elements of Test Anxiety

As mentioned earlier, test anxiety is considered to be an emotional state, but it has physical and mental components as well. Sometimes you may not even realize that you are suffering from test anxiety until you notice the physical symptoms. These can include trembling hands, rapid heartbeat, sweating, nausea, and tense muscles. Extreme anxiety may lead to fainting or vomiting. Obviously, any of these symptoms can have a negative impact on testing. It is important to recognize them as soon as they begin to occur so that you can address the problem before it damages your performance.

> **Review Video: 3 Ways to Tell You Have Test Anxiety**
> Visit mometrix.com/academy and enter code: 927847

The mental components of test anxiety include trouble focusing and inability to remember learned information. During a test, your mind is on high alert, which can help you recall information and stay focused for an extended period of time. However, anxiety interferes with your mind's natural processes, causing you to blank out, even on the questions you know well. The strain of testing during anxiety makes it difficult to stay focused, especially on a test that may take several hours. Extreme anxiety can take a huge mental toll, making it difficult not only to recall test information but even to understand the test questions or pull your thoughts together.

> **Review Video: How Test Anxiety Affects Memory**
> Visit mometrix.com/academy and enter code: 609003

Effects of Test Anxiety

Test anxiety is like a disease—if left untreated, it will get progressively worse. Anxiety leads to poor performance, and this reinforces the feelings of fear and failure, which in turn lead to poor performances on subsequent tests. It can grow from a mild nervousness to a crippling condition. If allowed to progress, test anxiety can have a big impact on your schooling, and consequently on your future.

Test anxiety can spread to other parts of your life. Anxiety on tests can become anxiety in any stressful situation, and blanking on a test can turn into panicking in a job situation. But fortunately, you don't have to let anxiety rule your testing and determine your grades. There are a number of relatively simple steps you can take to move past anxiety and function normally on a test and in the rest of life.

> **Review Video: How Test Anxiety Impacts Your Grades**
> Visit mometrix.com/academy and enter code: 939819

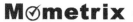

Physical Steps for Beating Test Anxiety

While test anxiety is a serious problem, the good news is that it can be overcome. It doesn't have to control your ability to think and remember information. While it may take time, you can begin taking steps today to beat anxiety.

Just as your first hint that you may be struggling with anxiety comes from the physical symptoms, the first step to treating it is also physical. Rest is crucial for having a clear, strong mind. If you are tired, it is much easier to give in to anxiety. But if you establish good sleep habits, your body and mind will be ready to perform optimally, without the strain of exhaustion. Additionally, sleeping well helps you to retain information better, so you're more likely to recall the answers when you see the test questions.

Getting good sleep means more than going to bed on time. It's important to allow your brain time to relax. Take study breaks from time to time so it doesn't get overworked, and don't study right before bed. Take time to rest your mind before trying to rest your body, or you may find it difficult to fall asleep.

Review Video: The Importance of Sleep for Your Brain
Visit mometrix.com/academy and enter code: 319338

Along with sleep, other aspects of physical health are important in preparing for a test. Good nutrition is vital for good brain function. Sugary foods and drinks may give a burst of energy but this burst is followed by a crash, both physically and emotionally. Instead, fuel your body with protein and vitamin-rich foods.

Also, drink plenty of water. Dehydration can lead to headaches and exhaustion, especially if your brain is already under stress from the rigors of the test. Particularly if your test is a long one, drink water during the breaks. And if possible, take an energy-boosting snack to eat between sections.

Review Video: How Diet Can Affect your Mood
Visit mometrix.com/academy and enter code: 624317

Along with sleep and diet, a third important part of physical health is exercise. Maintaining a steady workout schedule is helpful, but even taking 5-minute study breaks to walk can help get your blood pumping faster and clear your head. Exercise also releases endorphins, which contribute to a positive feeling and can help combat test anxiety.

When you nurture your physical health, you are also contributing to your mental health. If your body is healthy, your mind is much more likely to be healthy as well. So take time to rest, nourish your body with healthy food and water, and get moving as much as possible. Taking these physical steps will make you stronger and more able to take the mental steps necessary to overcome test anxiety.

Review Video: How to Stay Healthy and Prevent Test Anxiety
Visit mometrix.com/academy and enter code: 877894

Mental Steps for Beating Test Anxiety

Working on the mental side of test anxiety can be more challenging, but as with the physical side, there are clear steps you can take to overcome it. As mentioned earlier, test anxiety often stems from lack of preparation, so the obvious solution is to prepare for the test. Effective studying may be the most important weapon you have for beating test anxiety, but you can and should employ several other mental tools to combat fear.

First, boost your confidence by reminding yourself of past success—tests or projects that you aced. If you're putting as much effort into preparing for this test as you did for those, there's no reason you should expect to fail here. Work hard to prepare; then trust your preparation.

Second, surround yourself with encouraging people. It can be helpful to find a study group, but be sure that the people you're around will encourage a positive attitude. If you spend time with others who are anxious or cynical, this will only contribute to your own anxiety. Look for others who are motivated to study hard from a desire to succeed, not from a fear of failure.

Third, reward yourself. A test is physically and mentally tiring, even without anxiety, and it can be helpful to have something to look forward to. Plan an activity following the test, regardless of the outcome, such as going to a movie or getting ice cream.

When you are taking the test, if you find yourself beginning to feel anxious, remind yourself that you know the material. Visualize successfully completing the test. Then take a few deep, relaxing breaths and return to it. Work through the questions carefully but with confidence, knowing that you are capable of succeeding.

Developing a healthy mental approach to test taking will also aid in other areas of life. Test anxiety affects more than just the actual test—it can be damaging to your mental health and even contribute to depression. It's important to beat test anxiety before it becomes a problem for more than testing.

Review Video: Test Anxiety and Depression
Visit mometrix.com/academy and enter code: 904704

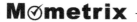

Study Strategy

Being prepared for the test is necessary to combat anxiety, but what does being prepared look like? You may study for hours on end and still not feel prepared. What you need is a strategy for test prep. The next few pages outline our recommended steps to help you plan out and conquer the challenge of preparation.

STEP 1: SCOPE OUT THE TEST

Learn everything you can about the format (multiple choice, essay, etc.) and what will be on the test. Gather any study materials, course outlines, or sample exams that may be available. Not only will this help you to prepare, but knowing what to expect can help to alleviate test anxiety.

STEP 2: MAP OUT THE MATERIAL

Look through the textbook or study guide and make note of how many chapters or sections it has. Then divide these over the time you have. For example, if a book has 15 chapters and you have five days to study, you need to cover three chapters each day. Even better, if you have the time, leave an extra day at the end for overall review after you have gone through the material in depth.

If time is limited, you may need to prioritize the material. Look through it and make note of which sections you think you already have a good grasp on, and which need review. While you are studying, skim quickly through the familiar sections and take more time on the challenging parts. Write out your plan so you don't get lost as you go. Having a written plan also helps you feel more in control of the study, so anxiety is less likely to arise from feeling overwhelmed at the amount to cover.

STEP 3: GATHER YOUR TOOLS

Decide what study method works best for you. Do you prefer to highlight in the book as you study and then go back over the highlighted portions? Or do you type out notes of the important information? Or is it helpful to make flashcards that you can carry with you? Assemble the pens, index cards, highlighters, post-it notes, and any other materials you may need so you won't be distracted by getting up to find things while you study.

If you're having a hard time retaining the information or organizing your notes, experiment with different methods. For example, try color-coding by subject with colored pens, highlighters, or post-it notes. If you learn better by hearing, try recording yourself reading your notes so you can listen while in the car, working out, or simply sitting at your desk. Ask a friend to quiz you from your flashcards, or try teaching someone the material to solidify it in your mind.

STEP 4: CREATE YOUR ENVIRONMENT

It's important to avoid distractions while you study. This includes both the obvious distractions like visitors and the subtle distractions like an uncomfortable chair (or a too-comfortable couch that makes you want to fall asleep). Set up the best study environment possible: good lighting and a comfortable work area. If background music helps you focus, you may want to turn it on, but otherwise keep the room quiet. If you are using a computer to take notes, be sure you don't have any other windows open, especially applications like social media, games, or anything else that could distract you. Silence your phone and turn off notifications. Be sure to keep water close by so you stay hydrated while you study (but avoid unhealthy drinks and snacks).

Also, take into account the best time of day to study. Are you freshest first thing in the morning? Try to set aside some time then to work through the material. Is your mind clearer in the afternoon or evening? Schedule your study session then. Another method is to study at the same time of day that you will take the test, so that your brain gets used to working on the material at that time and will be ready to focus at test time.

STEP 5: STUDY!

Once you have done all the study preparation, it's time to settle into the actual studying. Sit down, take a few moments to settle your mind so you can focus, and begin to follow your study plan. Don't give in to distractions or let yourself procrastinate. This is your time to prepare so you'll be ready to fearlessly approach the test. Make the most of the time and stay focused.

Of course, you don't want to burn out. If you study too long you may find that you're not retaining the information very well. Take regular study breaks. For example, taking five minutes out of every hour to walk briskly, breathing deeply and swinging your arms, can help your mind stay fresh.

As you get to the end of each chapter or section, it's a good idea to do a quick review. Remind yourself of what you learned and work on any difficult parts. When you feel that you've mastered the material, move on to the next part. At the end of your study session, briefly skim through your notes again.

But while review is helpful, cramming last minute is NOT. If at all possible, work ahead so that you won't need to fit all your study into the last day. Cramming overloads your brain with more information than it can process and retain, and your tired mind may struggle to recall even previously learned information when it is overwhelmed with last-minute study. Also, the urgent nature of cramming and the stress placed on your brain contribute to anxiety. You'll be more likely to go to the test feeling unprepared and having trouble thinking clearly.

So don't cram, and don't stay up late before the test, even just to review your notes at a leisurely pace. Your brain needs rest more than it needs to go over the information again. In fact, plan to finish your studies by noon or early afternoon the day before the test. Give your brain the rest of the day to relax or focus on other things, and get a good night's sleep. Then you will be fresh for the test and better able to recall what you've studied.

STEP 6: TAKE A PRACTICE TEST

Many courses offer sample tests, either online or in the study materials. This is an excellent resource to check whether you have mastered the material, as well as to prepare for the test format and environment.

Check the test format ahead of time: the number of questions, the type (multiple choice, free response, etc.), and the time limit. Then create a plan for working through them. For example, if you have 30 minutes to take a 60-question test, your limit is 30 seconds per question. Spend less time on the questions you know well so that you can take more time on the difficult ones.

If you have time to take several practice tests, take the first one open book, with no time limit. Work through the questions at your own pace and make sure you fully understand them. Gradually work up to taking a test under test conditions: sit at a desk with all study materials put away and set a timer. Pace yourself to make sure you finish the test with time to spare and go back to check your answers if you have time.

After each test, check your answers. On the questions you missed, be sure you understand why you missed them. Did you misread the question (tests can use tricky wording)? Did you forget the information? Or was it something you hadn't learned? Go back and study any shaky areas that the practice tests reveal.

Taking these tests not only helps with your grade, but also aids in combating test anxiety. If you're already used to the test conditions, you're less likely to worry about it, and working through tests until you're scoring well gives you a confidence boost. Go through the practice tests until you feel comfortable, and then you can go into the test knowing that you're ready for it.

Test Tips

On test day, you should be confident, knowing that you've prepared well and are ready to answer the questions. But aside from preparation, there are several test day strategies you can employ to maximize your performance.

First, as stated before, get a good night's sleep the night before the test (and for several nights before that, if possible). Go into the test with a fresh, alert mind rather than staying up late to study.

Try not to change too much about your normal routine on the day of the test. It's important to eat a nutritious breakfast, but if you normally don't eat breakfast at all, consider eating just a protein bar. If you're a coffee drinker, go ahead and have your normal coffee. Just make sure you time it so that the caffeine doesn't wear off right in the middle of your test. Avoid sugary beverages, and drink enough water to stay hydrated but not so much that you need a restroom break 10 minutes into the test. If your test isn't first thing in the morning, consider going for a walk or doing a light workout before the test to get your blood flowing.

Allow yourself enough time to get ready, and leave for the test with plenty of time to spare so you won't have the anxiety of scrambling to arrive in time. Another reason to be early is to select a good seat. It's helpful to sit away from doors and windows, which can be distracting. Find a good seat, get out your supplies, and settle your mind before the test begins.

When the test begins, start by going over the instructions carefully, even if you already know what to expect. Make sure you avoid any careless mistakes by following the directions.

Then begin working through the questions, pacing yourself as you've practiced. If you're not sure on an answer, don't spend too much time on it, and don't let it shake your confidence. Either skip it and come back later, or eliminate as many wrong answers as possible and guess among the remaining ones. Don't dwell on these questions as you continue—put them out of your mind and focus on what lies ahead.

Be sure to read all of the answer choices, even if you're sure the first one is the right answer. Sometimes you'll find a better one if you keep reading. But don't second-guess yourself if you do immediately know the answer. Your gut instinct is usually right. Don't let test anxiety rob you of the information you know.

If you have time at the end of the test (and if the test format allows), go back and review your answers. Be cautious about changing any, since your first instinct tends to be correct, but make sure you didn't misread any of the questions or accidentally mark the wrong answer choice. Look over any you skipped and make an educated guess.

At the end, leave the test feeling confident. You've done your best, so don't waste time worrying about your performance or wishing you could change anything. Instead, celebrate the successful

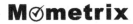

completion of this test. And finally, use this test to learn how to deal with anxiety even better next time.

Important Qualification

Not all anxiety is created equal. If your test anxiety is causing major issues in your life beyond the classroom or testing center, or if you are experiencing troubling physical symptoms related to your anxiety, it may be a sign of a serious physiological or psychological condition. If this sounds like your situation, we strongly encourage you to seek professional help.

Thank You

We at Mometrix would like to extend our heartfelt thanks to you, our friend and patron, for allowing us to play a part in your journey. It is a privilege to serve people from all walks of life who are unified in their commitment to building the best future they can for themselves.

The preparation you devote to these important testing milestones may be the most valuable educational opportunity you have for making a real difference in your life. We encourage you to put your heart into it—that feeling of succeeding, overcoming, and yes, conquering will be well worth the hours you've invested.

We want to hear your story, your struggles and your successes, and if you see any opportunities for us to improve our materials so we can help others even more effectively in the future, please share that with us as well. **The team at Mometrix would be absolutely thrilled to hear from you!** So please, send us an email (support@mometrix.com) and let's stay in touch.

> **If you'd like some additional help, check out these other resources we offer for your exam:**
> **http://mometrixflashcards.com/CCRN**

Additional Bonus Material

Due to our efforts to try to keep this book to a manageable length, we've created a link that will give you access to all of your additional bonus material.

Please visit http://www.mometrix.com/bonus948/ccrnadult to access the information.

Made in the USA
Las Vegas, NV
21 August 2022